Asian Septorhinoplasty

Eun Sang Dhong

Asian Septorhinoplasty

Septal L-Strut Extension Graft

Springer

Eun Sang Dhong
Department of Plastic Surgery
Korea University Guro Hospital
Seoul, Korea (Republic of)

ISBN 978-981-96-6126-8 ISBN 978-981-96-6127-5 (eBook)
https://doi.org/10.1007/978-981-96-6127-5

This Springer imprint is published by the registered company Springer Nature Singapore Pte Ltd.
The registered company address is: 152 Beach Road, #21-01/04 Gateway East, Singapore 189721, Singapore

Preface

It has been 3 years since I authored *Asian Septorhinoplasty: Conundrums and Solutions*. The completion of "Septal L-Strut Extension Graft" is particularly significant, as it was a subject I had long wished to explore and write about. Achieving success in Asian rhinoplasty necessitates an approach and strategy that diverges entirely from Western techniques.

To alleviate the profound suffering endured by patients through numerous surgeries, I have penned this book with an unwavering commitment to safety, rather than merely striving for superficial aesthetics. This book serves not only as a manual for attaining the highest standards of surgical excellence but also as a testament to our deep-seated responsibility.

Hence, this book is not merely a conclusion; it is a pledge. In an era marked by rapid changes and societal expectations, we remain resolute. We sculpt not just faces but futures, and shape not just bodies but better tomorrows. With scalpel in hand and heart aligned, we endeavor to create not just outcomes, but enduring legacies in the field of plastic surgery.

In the art of healing, what matters is not the swift and easy path but the sincere pursuit of excellence.

– I dedicate this book to my beloved Minwha, Hyunseung, and my dear parents.

Seoul, Republic of Korea
June, 2024

Eun Sang Dhong

Contents

Part I

Analysis

Soft Tissue Cephalometric Analysis (STCA) for an Easy Start of Primary Septorhinoplasty

1

Pearls

- Standardized 2D photographs serve as crucial data for surgical quality control. Adjusting the roll in frontal views and the pitch in lateral views is essential for surgical planning.
- Measuring the nasion can be challenging, particularly when positioned too low to mark in the lateral view.
  It is advisable to employ a modified lateral view that captures the beginning of the opposite eyebrow to address this issue.
- Standardizing magnification, roll, and pitch is relatively straightforward; however, correcting for yaw is not feasible with 2D photographs. Therefore, ensuring that a single, accustomed photographer takes photographs is crucial to maintain consistency and accuracy.
- Determining the ideal positions for the sellion (Si) and subnasale (Subi) marks the commencement and culmination of the analytical process.
- For Asian individuals, the ideal height of the sellion (Si) is preferably positioned between the lowest point of the upper eyelid and a horizontal line extending through the mid-pupil, or at most 2 mm above this line. The depth of Si should ideally fall within 2–4 mm behind the most anterior point of the glabella.
- Ideally, the Subi should be positioned 0–2 mm below the point two-thirds along the distance from the Si to the stomion.
- The determination of Ti automatically follows the identification of Si and Subi. Both the columellar-lobular angle and the double break to the lobular tip angle are essential considerations.
- Once the tip has been strategically planned, it is crucial to assess the alar crease junction (ACJ) and pogonion. Patients often overlook these aspects.

1.1 Perspectives in Consultation

Prolonged pre-surgical analysis and goal-setting can detract from the primary focus of surgery preparation. Drawing upon the experience from prior cases, where the author effectively established case-specific objectives using PowerPoint, the author was able to streamline this process through the adept use of photo editing and copy-paste techniques. The attention primarily centers on key surgical landmarks, notably the sellion and subnasale, whose identification is crucial. Pinpointing these critical points simplifies the process of defining the remaining ideal landmarks.

This chapter delves into the methods of crafting and applying standardized STCA points in surgical planning, utilizing photo editing software. This approach, requiring merely 1–5 min, presents a time-efficient method for envisaging the expected surgical results. It seamlessly merges the patient's aspirations with viable surgi-

E. S. Dhong, *Asian Septorhinoplasty*, https://doi.org/10.1007/978-981-96-6127-5_1

cal options, optimally preparing for the forthcoming procedure.

Take photos in advance, and perform a simple analysis the day before or on the day of the surgery. If photos need to be taken on the day of the surgery, it will require more time, but if pre-taken images are used, the analysis can be completed in the time it takes to drink a cup of coffee.

1.1.1 Natural Head Position (NHP)

The Frankfort horizontal and sella-nasion planes serve as established reference points in cephalometry. Since the 1950s, the concept of the natural head position (NHP) has attracted significant attention and research within dentistry. Criticisms of analyses that rely on 2D photographs frequently concern the authenticity of the NHP as representative of the patient's typical posture and the accuracy of the true vertical line [1].

Improving the reproducibility of NHP can be achieved by allowing patients to view themselves in a mirror [2]. It is crucial for a rhinoplasty surgeon to conduct patient analysis in a convenient and reproducible manner. Although the approach outlined here may slightly differ from the patient's comfortable head position, it offers a quick analysis method that closely mimics the patient's natural posture. The surgeon must operate according to subjective standards. It is necessary to manipulate the minor angles of photos to establish reference points using standardized images. This means adjusting the angle of the entire photo, not changing its proportions.

Removing any tension from the shoulders is advisable for photographing, particularly in seated patients. The patient should be instructed to sit and stand from the stool multiple times, directing their gaze at a mirror or a distant object, thereby adopting a natural stance for the photograph. Ensuring that these images are taken at a consistent eye level and with the Frankfurt Horizontal (FH) line aligned with the photographer's perspective enhances the accuracy and standardization of the images.

Comparing the patient's relaxed posture with the photograph adjusted for roll in the anteroposterior (AP) view helps understand their NHP for the analysis. Individuals with a short nasal structure, significant nasal deviation, and facial asymmetry might display an atypical NHP.

Rotating the patient's entire body while taking photographs is crucial to mitigate the minor discrepancies introduced by yawing. Simply rotating the head, including the neck, often makes obtaining standardized images difficult, primarily due to the varying degrees of neck muscle relaxation. It is also imperative to capture an extensive series of photographs to mitigate the subtle variations introduced by yawing, rolling, and pitching movements.

Review the images with the patient to assess discomfort and discuss their preferred midline. Compare the patient's relaxed posture with the photograph adjusted for roll in the anteroposterior (AP) view to understand their NHP.

The surgeon's view on the midline and the patient's usual perception of their facial midline should not be established on the day of the surgery plan but through several in-depth consultations to ensure compliance.

1.1.2 Overcoming the Difference Between Real and Imaginary

The author's primary reason for refraining from using virtual surgical imagery for patient counseling is the potential for creating unrealistic expectations. Patients often become accustomed to the altered images, leading to feelings of suspicion and discomfort toward the actual postoperative outcomes.

When assessing facial symmetry, drawing a line from the lateral canthus to the cheilion in the frontal view can be insightful, especially when comparing the size discrepancy of the left and right sides of the face. Additionally, observing the horizontal line connecting the mid-pupils and noting variations in the occlusal plane while the patient bites a tongue depressor can reveal inherent asymmetries. It is often found that these lines do not remain parallel when one side of the face is more prominent than the other. Research has demonstrated that duplicating only one side of the face to create a full facial image can result in distinctly different appearances [3].

Presenting patients with a mirrored image of their photograph can be an effective strategy to help them adjust to the post-surgical changes and overcome the initial unfamiliarity with their new appearance. This approach is particularly beneficial for patients with deviated noses. Showing them mirrored images of their preoperative state can better prepare them for the changes they will experience post-surgery.

1.1.3 Primary Rhinoplasty Vs. Secondary Rhinoplasty

The approach to planning primary rhinoplasty significantly differs from that of secondary rhinoplasty. The preoperative strategies and photographs discussed below can be effectively utilized for primary rhinoplasty. However, these methods often prove inadequate in the context of secondary rhinoplasty for various reasons, which will be explored in greater detail in Chap. 2.

- Predicting how much the soft tissue envelope can be stretched becomes challenging without direct dissection.
- The previous application of alloplastic implants may not always align with expectations.

1.2 Soft Tissue Cephalometric Analysis (STCA) Using 2D Photo

In jaw surgery, lateral cephalometry is a standard tool; similarly, employing a lateral photographic view is advantageous for surgical planning in rhinoplasty. Particularly in Asian patients, the nasion tends to be positioned lower, which can result in its concealment by the leading edge of the pupil in an accurate lateral view. Consequently, adopting a modified lateral view that captures the medial portion of the contralateral brow is beneficial, facilitating a more informed surgical strategy (Fig. 1.1).

The concept of natural head position is subject to considerable debate. It is commonly observed that patients tend to elevate their chins by an average of 4°. Surgeons rely on photographs for planning, inherently presenting a perspective contrary to what patients observe in the mirror. Consequently, the midline perceived by the patient may diverge from the surgeon's observation. This discrepancy can result in the patient feeling awkward post-surgery, akin to the disorientation experienced when one's reflection is observed between mirrors positioned in front and behind.

Soft tissue cephalometric analysis (STCA) employs photographs from frontal and modified lateral views and is instrumental in surgical preparation. The surgeon adjusts the orientation of the frontal photographs and anglings the lateral views to ensure precise planning and execution.

The author refrains from providing patients with virtual predictions and using 3D-manufactured dorsal implants. This approach is not due to insensitivity; instead, it is based on the understanding that 3D scanning, while helpful in observing outcomes before and after surgery, may not accurately predict intraoperative needs due to the dynamic nature of intraoperative septal procedures and variability.

Due to the many unpredictable aspects of the changes in the framework during surgery, it is tough to accurately predict the outcome of an Asian rhinoplasty that involves altering the elongation or projection of the nose.

Outcomes also can significantly vary based on factors such as the volume of local anesthetics administered during surgery and the extent of flap dissection. In my practice, combining hyaluronidase with local anesthetics occasionally led to temporary thinning of the dorsal skin envelope, necessitating an unneeded larger dorsal graft than initially planned. This is an example of a case where intraoperative changes prevent accurate 3D prediction. It is crucial to understand that showing patients virtual surgical outcomes and setting such expectations can lead to postoperative dissatisfaction. While 3D simulations can be valuable research tools, their application in patient counseling should be cautiously approached due to potential negative repercussions.

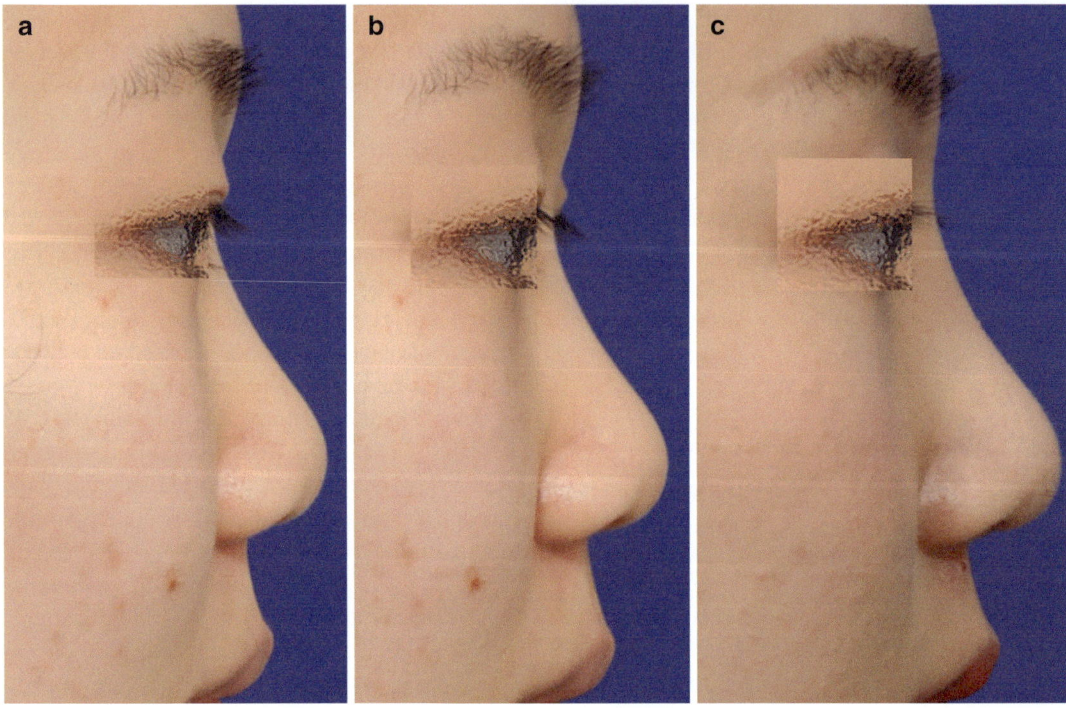

Fig. 1.1 How to capture a modified lateral view. (**a**) True lateral view. (**b**) Modified lateral view: Capture a lateral view with a slight yawing to reveal the upper left eyelash or the beginning of the brow. (**c**) Postoperative modified lateral view of the same patient: The visibility of the left eyelash is reduced due to the elevation of the nasion relative to the preoperative state in (**b**). However, the starting point of the brow remains visible

1.3 Standardization of 2D Photo

The following method does not involve manipulating the photos; instead, it refers to incrementally standardizing the angles of the already-taken photos. The diagonal proportions of the photos must not be altered, but the overall size can be adjusted.

There are four factors to consider to maintain standardization for 2D photos.

- Magnification
- Pitch
- Roll
- Yaw

Magnification, pitch, and roll variables can be standardized by adjusting the 2D images that have already been captured. However, controlling for yaw poses a challenge. Suppose the degree of yaw differs too much in the preexisting photographs. In that case, these images may be unreliable for comparison before and after surgery or for assessing the patient's natural head position. Although magnification, pitch, and roll can be corrected by rotating the overall angle of the photo using software, yaw cannot be corrected. Although the techniques described in this chapter are straightforward and replicable, their effectiveness is contingent upon high-quality photography. Hence, it is crucial to engage a skilled photographer to ensure consistency in the images taken before and after surgery.

The software employed should be user-friendly to facilitate the surgeon's tasks. I utilize Microsoft Picture Manager® (Microsoft Corp., Redmond, WA, USA), which is not part of the standard software package and requires separate downloading, possibly from Microsoft SharePoint. Other software may also be used.

1.3.1 Standardizing the Magnification

Drawing a line from the mid-pupil to the cheilion and using this line as a baseline for standardization proves beneficial for standardizing multiple photographs, particularly for pre-and postoperative comparisons (Fig. 1.2). In certain instances, a line can also be drawn from the lateral canthus to the cheilion. One can ascertain consistent magnification across photographs by resizing images to ensure these lines are of identical length. Furthermore, maintaining uniformity in the direction of these lines ensures that the pitching is also appropriately adjusted.

1.3.2 Control Pitching

The software enables the pitching adjustment for the entire photograph in the lateral and modified lateral views. In photography, establishing the Frankfort horizontal line is not feasible, leading to discrepancies regarding the true vertical line. Nonetheless, the operator has the flexibility to modify the pitching of the photograph as needed. In Microsoft Picture Manager®, you can use the "rotate and flip" function to adjust in 1-degree increments (Fig. 1.3). In situations involving significant jaw thrusting or retraction, it is crucial to adjust the pitching to achieve a vertical line that facilitates comfortable operation for the practitioner. If the reference line used for magnification adjustments maintains consistent length and direction, aligning the pitching accordingly becomes straightforward.

The authors superimposed the adjusted photographs within Microsoft PowerPoint software (Microsoft Corp., Redmond, WA, USA) to facilitate the comparison of preoperative and postoperative images alongside reference lines. Adobe's software is more detailed and complicated, so the author stopped using it.

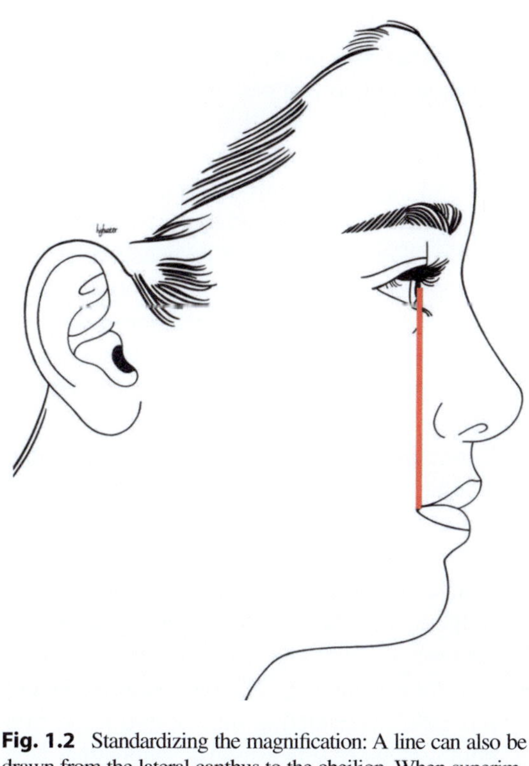

Fig. 1.2 Standardizing the magnification: A line can also be drawn from the lateral canthus to the cheilion. When superimposing photographs using the image program, make these lines equal in length to standardize the scale of the photographs

1.3.3 Control Rolling

Rolling adjustments can be made in the anteroposterior (AP) view, allowing surgical preparation to align with the desired vertical line using photo management software. It also utilizes the "rotate and flip" function as above.

This vertical line is defined by connecting the mid-pupil of each eye to the horizontal line. Suppose the patient exhibits minimal rolling in their most natural posture. In that case, it is advantageous for the surgeon to use the horizontal plane, drawn through the left and right mid-pupils, as the basis for planning. This view is crucial for assessing the need to correct the axial deviation or perform alar reduction (Fig. 1.4).

However, strictly adhering to this vertical line may result in lower facial disharmony and severe deviations. Therefore, a compromise is necessary.

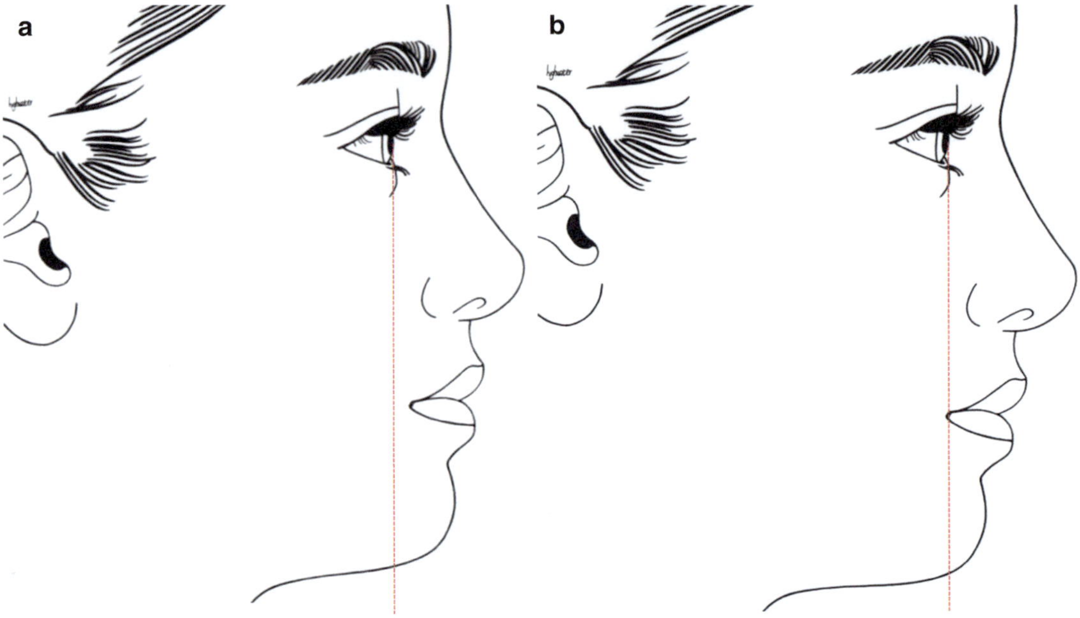

Fig. 1.3 Control pitching. (left) Before rotating the lateral schematic. (right) Use the "rotate and flip" function to rotate it clockwise. In this illustration, the line extending from the pupil to the chelion became vertical

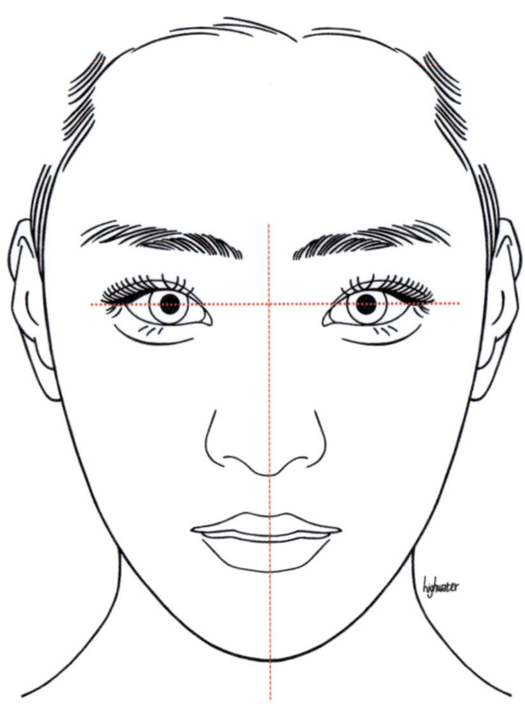

Fig. 1.4 Control rolling: Rotate the photo clockwise or counterclockwise using the "rotate by degree" function to ensure the horizontal line connecting the mid-pupils on both sides. Then, measure the angle between this line and the bony or cartilaginous axis to target deviation correction

1.3.4 Control Yawing

Standardizing yaw in the modified lateral view involves using two complex reference lines. It is feasible to capture multiple photographs and select the one where the distances from the tragus to the mid-pupil and from the tragus to the cheilion remain constant, serving as the basis for measurement (Fig. 1.5). However, since adjusting these distances within a single 2-D photograph is not possible, the photo with the slightest discrepancy between these two distances can serve as a basis for pre- and postoperative comparison and standardization.

Correcting yaw in a 2D photo is impossible once it has been taken. This allows for the selection of images with the most similar views.

- Adjust the roll in the frontal view and the pitch in the lateral view to analyze and prepare for surgery.
- Controlling yaw in 2D photography is not possible, necessitating the capture of several photographs in advance. The photo that best aligns before and after surgery should be used for comparative analysis.

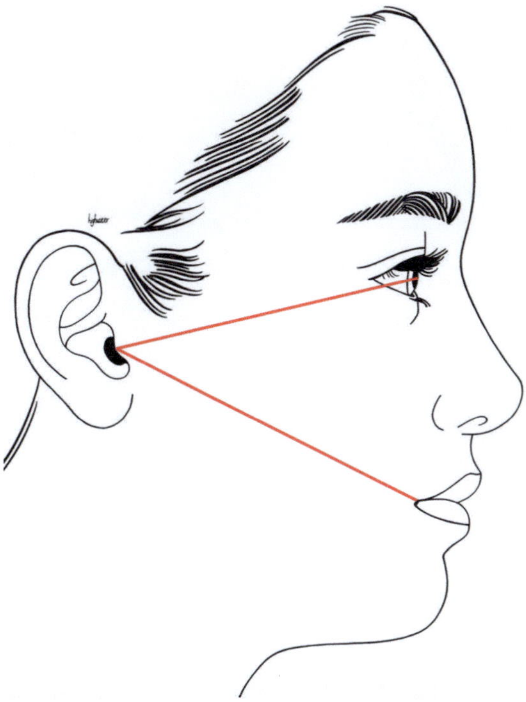

Fig. 1.5 Control yawing: Standardizing yaw in the modified lateral view involves using two complex reference lines, ensuring that the distances from the tragus to the mid-pupil and from the tragus to the cheilion remain constant

1.4 Soft Tissue Cephalometric Analysis (STCA) in 3D Software

With the advent of 3D measurement technology, 3D scanning has become an invaluable tool for postoperative evaluation, complementing traditional 2D analysis. For preoperative planning, the author relies on 2D photographs, while for postoperative assessment, I utilize 3D data in conjunction with standardized photographs as previously described. Various scanners are available to capture 3D images; I use Morpheus 3D (Morpheus Co. Ltd., Seoul, Korea) to build a database. Ultimately, the choice of technology depends on the surgeon's preference and comfort with the equipment.

Measuring volume before and after surgery is crucial, and for surgeons aiming to specialize in rhinoplasty, having such measurement equipment is no longer optional but necessary. Each device has unique features, so selecting one that accurately captures the details of the nostrils is advisable. Additionally, choosing a device that offers continuous updates is beneficial. While the current Morpheus 3-D model may not fully delineate concave structures like the nostrils, future scanners are expected to provide more comprehensive and valuable data.

1.5 STCA for Primary Rhinoplasty (Author's Method)

Microsoft Picture Manager® (Microsoft Corp., Redmond, WA, USA) was used to rotate the photographs. Micro Office SharePoint enabled the program to run in Microsoft Office® or Office 365 according to the manufacturer's guide. This program is now outdated and no longer receives updates. I hope you will consider trying other software.

Once you've obtained frontal and modified lateral photos using the method mentioned in Sect. 1.2 above, here is a simple analysis example.

1.5.1 Analyze Frontal Photos

Observing the patient's natural frontal facial posture during the consultation is essential for accurately predicting the degree of head rotation in a frontal photograph. Pay particular attention to habitual head tilting, which can influence the assessment.

The initial step involves measuring the nose's length. This is achieved by comparing the midfacial height (MFH) to the lower facial height (LFH) in a frontal photograph. It is crucial to consider the relationship between MFH and LFH in these images. Notably, a preference for a smaller LFH is often observed in younger individuals.

1. Begin by establishing the patient's head position: draw a line connecting the midpoints of the pupils across both eyes. Compare this line

to the absolute horizontal line of the screen. Draw a vertical line from above. This step aids in identifying habitual head tilting (rolling).

2. To determine the nasal midline, envisage a line extending from what is presumed to be the midline of the rhinion to the center of the cupid's bow. The midpoint from the sellion to the rhinion constitutes the bony axis, while the portion from the rhinion's midpoint to the nasal tip's midpoint is regarded as the cartilaginous axis.
3. The distance from the soft tissue glabella (G) to the alar base plane (ABP) is referred to as the midfacial height (MFH), and the span from the ABP to the soft tissue menton (Me) is termed the lower facial height (LFH) (Fig. 1.6).
4. In the frontal view, draw a vertical line downward from the bilateral medial canthus to evaluate its alignment with the bilateral alar crease junction. Alar flaring is identified if the lateral alar margin extends beyond this line by more than 2 mm. An alar reduction is unnecessary if the lateral alar margin falls within 0–2 mm of this vertical line (Fig. 1.7).

Ricketts' golden proportion may be contemplated; however, its application involves intricate aesthetic evaluations, rendering it less practical for preoperative analysis. The authors devise and execute surgical procedures grounded on the aforementioned streamlined measurements. Despite the simplification, outcomes may only sometimes align with initial expectations.

In the frontal examination, attention is directed toward the nasal proportions relative to the entire face, assessing the integrity of the bony and cartilaginous axes and the extent of alar flaring.

1.5.2 Analyze Modified Lateral Photos

Analyzing the Asian true lateral view presents challenges, often due to the low position of the radix area, which results in the eyeball obscuring the nasion in a true lateral perspective.

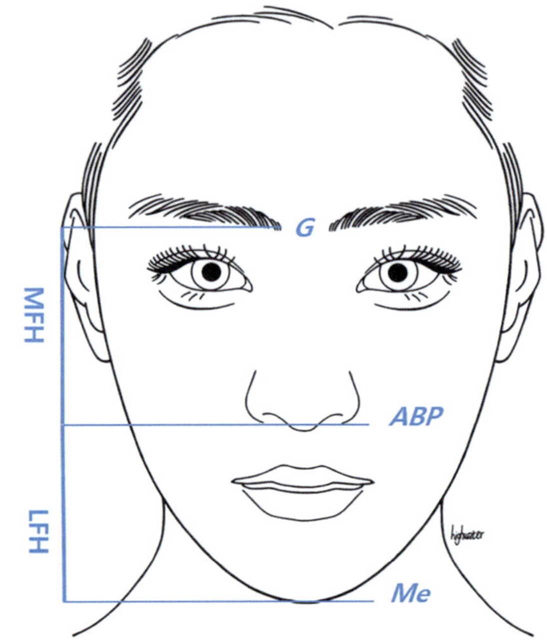

Fig. 1.6 Two facial heights: Midfacial height (MFH) and lower facial height (LFH)

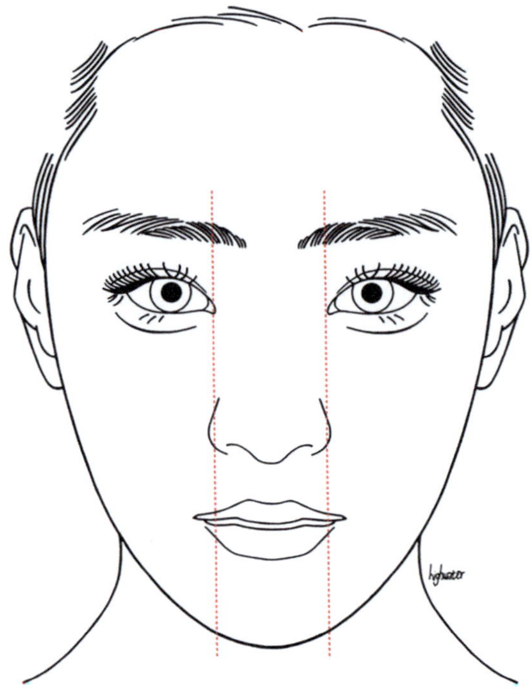

Fig. 1.7 Determination of alar width: Draw a vertical line from the bilateral medial canthus downward to the bilateral alar crease junction

As mentioned, a modified lateral view is recommended to circumvent this. Capturing images with a slight yaw, such that the contralateral brow or eyelash is faintly visible, facilitates an effective comparison of pre- and postoperative states.

It is difficult to adjust the amount of yaw precisely, and some patients may not want excessive augmentation of the nasion, so a sufficient yaw that reveals the nasion may be necessary (Fig. 1.8).

1.5.3 Steps of Achieving Ideal Sellion and Subnasale

The initial phase of direct surgical planning involves measuring the nose's length in the lateral view. Using the five key landmarks below, a straightforward strategy can be formulated and illustrated (Fig. 1.9). It's important to note that the subnasale is not depicted in the figure but is discussed subsequently.

Surgeons can modify each of these five landmarks using surgical techniques. However, the position of the ideal tip is inherently dictated by the optimal angle. Since the surgeon can adjust and finalize the position of each landmark, the term "ideal" (i) is appended to signify this adjustability.

1.5.3.1 Determination of the Length of the Nose in Primary Cases

The length of the nose is measured from the ideal sellion (Si) to the ideal tip (Ti). As previously mentioned, determining the ideal tip can be challenging because its position is naturally dictated. Therefore, the first step involves establishing the height and depth of the ideal sellion (Si). The subsequent step is to determine the position of the ideal subnasale (Subi).

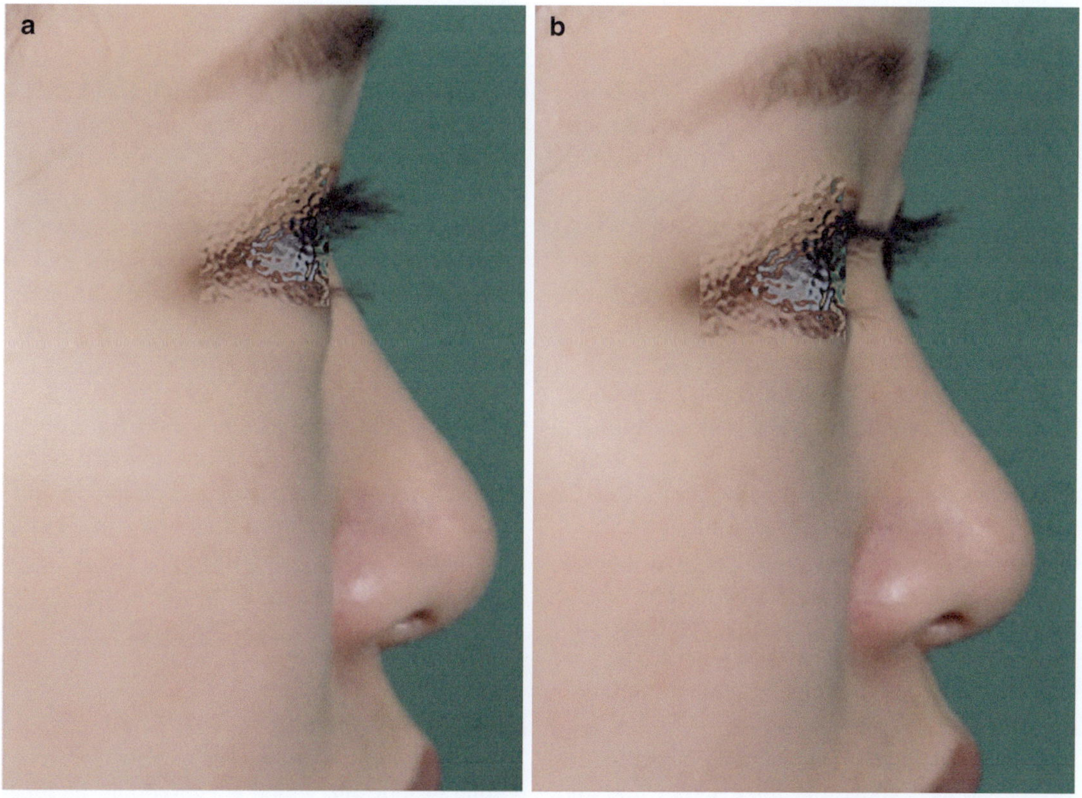

Fig. 1.8 Modified lateral view: It should be a commitment to the amount of yaw, pitch, and roll from when the photo is taken. It is difficult to adjust the amount of yaw precisely (**a**) True lateral view. (**b**) Modified lateral view

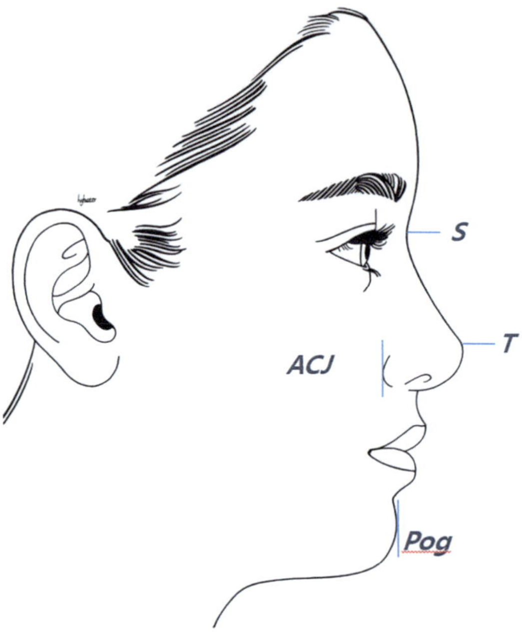

Fig. 1.9 Four anthropometric points: S (sellion), T (tip), ACJ (alar crease junction), Pog (pogonion). The remaining one point is Subi (subnasale)

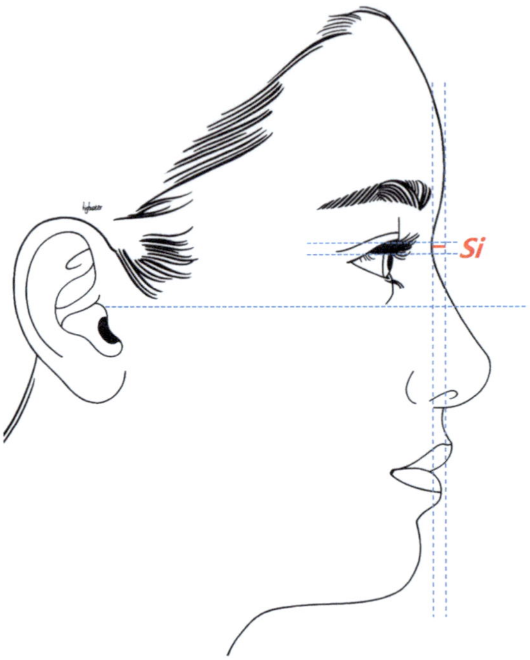

Fig. 1.10 Deciding the ideal sellion (Si): The first ideal point

Ideal Sellion (Si)

Photo analysis cannot rely on the bony nasion; instead, it must be based on the soft tissue equivalent, the sellion (Si). In the lateral view, it is crucial to ascertain Si′s depth and height, which vary between males and females. This determination involves analyzing the patient's radix shape, considering the forehead's most anterior point, and accounting for frontal bossing.

The positioning of Si significantly influences the perceived length of the nose: a more cephalically placed Si gives the impression of a longer nose, whereas a more caudally positioned Si makes the nose appear shorter. Although numerous studies exist, Western data may not directly apply to Asian surgical practices. For height assessment, the intercanthal horizontal line is utilized, and for depth, the anterior point of the glabella is considered, with a typical variation ranging from 6 to 13 mm [4, 5].

In Western populations, the sellion should ideally be situated above the intercanthal line and behind the most anterior point of the glabella. However, various authors propose different ideal locations due to the preferred angles and depths influenced by the ideal nasofrontal angle. This angle is typically 130° for Western men and 134° for Western women. Applying these standards to Asian individuals can be challenging, as anatomical and aesthetic preferences may differ significantly [6, 7]. Fewer angles should be considered in Asians. The author sets goals based on the following criteria:

- For Asian individuals, the ideal height of the sellion (Si) is preferably positioned between the lowest point of the upper eyelid and a horizontal line extending through the mid-pupil, or at most 2 mm above this line. The depth of Si should ideally fall within 2–4 mm behind the most anterior point of the glabella (Fig. 1.10).

Ideal Subnasale (Subi)

To determine the subnasale, apply Ricketts' golden proportion, which suggests that the ideal position for the subnasale is at two-thirds of the distance from the sellion (Si) to the stomion. This means that a third of this length from Si toward the stomion is considered the optimal location for the rhinion [8, 9].

The LFH should be slightly smaller than the MFH for patients who prefer to look younger.

- The ideal subnasale position in Asians is typically 0–2 mm below the point that marks two-thirds of the distance from the sellion (Si) to the stomion.
- Additionally, it is optimally positioned 2–4 mm behind the superior labrale of the lateral lip. While this positioning is influenced by maxillary protrusion and incisor inclination, it is presented in simplified terms to facilitate establishing an ideal nasal relationship (Fig. 1.11).

In primary rhinoplasty, modifying the subnasale's (Subi) position, either raising or lowering it, is generally straightforward. In contrast, during secondary rhinoplasty, the final position of the Subi is determined intraoperatively because the soft tissue exhibits less elasticity, complicating adherence to the initial surgical plan. Extending a shortened nose under these circumstances can be incredibly challenging.

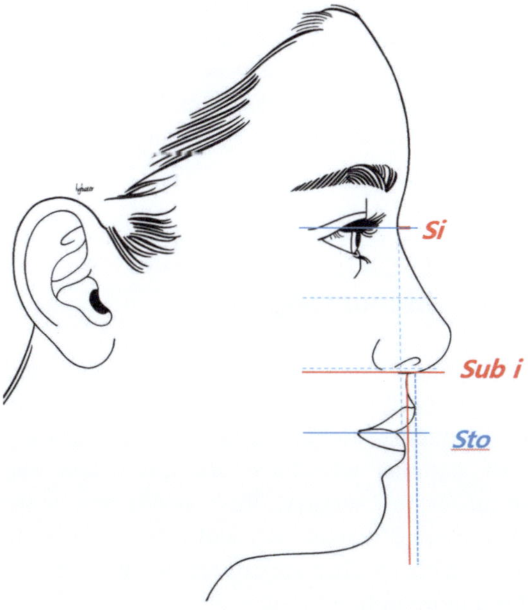

Fig. 1.11 Deciding the ideal subnasale (Subi): The second ideal point

Ideal Tip (Ti)

It is incorrect to consider the ideal tip position (Ti) in isolation when determining it. Multiple factors influence the determination of Ti and naturally follow the establishment of the sellion (Si) and subnasale (Subi) positions. This means that Ti is automatically determined, not that you set Ti and then choose the rest.

Ti is derived from the preferred nasofacial angle, which originates from the sellion, and the preferred columellar-labial angle, which begins at the subnasale. These angles collectively contribute to the natural determination of the Ti.

- The authors typically adopt around 30° as a guideline for the nasofacial angle and seldom exceed this angle for patients desiring a higher tip position (Ti). Regarding the columellar-labial angle, a recommendation of 90° is made for men, with an allowance of up to 105 degrees for women.
- Once the sellion (Si) and subnasale (Subi) are established, the determination of the tip position (Ti) becomes relatively automatic. It is essential also to consider a double break, factoring in the columellar-lobular angle, to achieve a harmonious and natural-looking nasal tip (Fig. 1.12).

In Asian rhinoplasty, achieving the desired projection level often raises the question of what materials to use. Much of the projection can be attained through additional grafting beyond the lower lateral cartilage (LLC). Therefore, even with a well-developed LLC, substantial grafting is required, and it's fair to say that the tip position (Ti) can be sculpted through this method. If the LLC is not robust, more extensive efforts will be necessary to achieve the desired outcome.

Ideal Alar Crease Junction (ACJi)

In the lateral view, the ideal alar crease junction (ACJi) should be anterior to the vertical line extending from the lateral canthus. An anterior positioning of more than 2 mm is considered aesthetically pleasing. This region is relatively safe for alloplastic implants in Asian rhinoplasty, as it

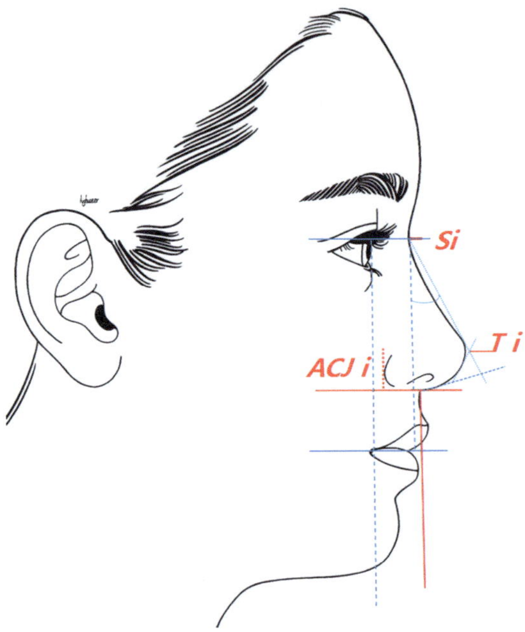

Fig. 1.12 Automatically determined Ideal Tip (Ti): The ideal point is determined thirdly; it can be adjusted higher or lower depending on the patient's specific needs

is enveloped by thick and soft cheek tissue, providing a protective cushion [10] (Fig. 1.12).

Ideal Pogonion (Pog i)

Specifically, a common guideline suggests that when a line is drawn from the pogonion to the ideal tip, the upper lip should be positioned approximately 2 mm behind this line, with the lower lip slightly anterior to it, enhancing facial harmony and balance. This alignment ensures that the chin and the nose complement each other, contributing to the overall aesthetic appeal of the face. Adjustments to the pogonion, such as through sliding genioplasty or the placement of a chin implant, can enhance facial harmony by creating a more favorable relationship between the chin and the nasal tip.

1.5.3.2 Deciding the Nasal Width

In frontal photographs, it is essential to determine the width and length of the nose. Ideally, the width of the bilateral ACJ should be within 0–2 mm of the bilateral medical canthus by drawing a vertical line from either side of the bilateral ACJ. Consider alar cinching or alar base reduction if it is wider than this (Fig. 1.7).

1.5.3.3 Order of Establishing Preoperative Ideal Points for Primary Case

1. Determination of nasal length
2. Determination of Si (sellion)
3. Determination of Subi (subnasale)
4. Determination of Ti (tip position)
5. Determination of alar width

1.6 Copy and Paste the Ideal Points to a New Analysis

The ideal STCA points mentioned above can generally be applied to both male and female patients, except in cases where a higher tip is desired. For patients whose analysis has been completed, copying only the ideal points from the patient's PPT and pasting them into a new PPT is possible. Of course, first, a photo with the adjusted angle must be saved in the picture manager, and this photo should be loaded into the new PPT as a background before overlaying each ideal point on it. Even in this case, by simply adjusting the proportions, it is possible to quickly draw the goals for a new patient using the ideal points from a previous patient. Only the ideal sellion and ideal subnasale need to be redefined. If this method seems too insincere, you can perform the abovementioned tasks from **1.2** to **1.5** in a new PPT. But the copy-and-paste method is more convenient, so it is recommended to try it.

1.7 STCA for Secondary Rhinoplasty

The general rules of the methods mentioned above significantly rarely govern the planning of secondary surgery. Since we are dealing with patients who have had more than one unsuccessful surgery, their needs are more specific and demanding, and they often come to us with specific requirements and a desire for a more defined look.

Chapter 2 will discuss the surgery's planning in detail, but for various reasons, the author does not show patients what they will look like after virtual surgery. This is not because he is not confident in doing so but because the surgeon cannot predict 100% of the exceptions that may occur during secondary surgery. The more complex the previous surgical method, the more destructive the remaining tissue, and the surgery may have to be terminated without achieving its purpose.

Preparing for surgery or taking various measures is more than twice as complex as a secondary operation, so it requires more thorough planning, 180° different from Western rhinoplasty, which will be discussed in more detail in Chaps. 2 and 4. In Asian surgery, the presence of alloplastic implants is an entirely different consideration, as there are many grafts from previous surgeries, and there is a need to be prepared for the possibility of running out of grafts to use.

The core focus of this book is on reconstructing the nasal framework, mainly through the use of septal L-strut extension grafts. Similar to primary cases, the surgery adheres to the same five ideal points.

However, it is crucial to emphasize that the outcome of the surgery is significantly influenced by the condition of the mucosal layer enveloping the framework, the extent of elongation, and the degree to which the skin and soft tissue envelope are released. This is because the success of the graft implantation depends not only on the precision of the framework construction but also on its adequate coverage by the surrounding tissues.

References

1. Madsen DP, Sampson WJ, Townsend GC. Craniofacial reference plane variation and natural head position. Eur J Orthod. 2008;30:532–40.
2. Cooke MS, Wei SH. The reproducibility of natural head posture: a methodological study. Am J Orthod Dentofacial Orthop. 1988;93:280–8.
3. Rhodes G, Proffitt F, Grady JM, Sumich A. Facial symmetry and the perception of beauty. Psychon Bull Rev. 1998;5:659–69.
4. Mowlavi A, Meldrum DG, Wilhelmi BJ. Implications for nasal recontouring: nasion position preferences as determined by a survey of white north Americans. Aesthetic Plast Surg. 2003;27:438–45.
5. Byrd HS, Hobar PC. Rhinoplasty: a practical guide for surgical planning. Plast Reconstr Surg. 1993;91:642–54; discussion 655–6.
6. Daniel RK. The radix. In: Daniel RK, editor. Rhinoplasty: an atlas of surgical techniques. New York: Springer New York; 2002. p. 1–21.
7. Hwang NH, Han SK, Dhong ES. Adaptive planning and overcoming pitfalls in Asian rhinoplasty. Arch Aesthetic Plast Surg. 2014;20:8–14.
8. Guyuron B. Precision rhinoplasty. Part I: the role of life-size photographs and soft-tissue cephalometric analysis. Plast Reconstr Surg. 1988;81:489–99.
9. Ricketts RM. Divine proportion in facial esthetics. Clin Plast Surg. 1982;9:401–22.
10. Lee T-Y, Chung H-Y, Dhong E-S, Jeong S-H, Han S-K. Paranasal augmentation using multi-folded expanded polytetrafluorethylene (ePTFE) in the east Asian nose. Aesthet Surg J. 2019;39:1319–28.

2 Analytical Difference of Secondary Asian Rhinoplasty

Pearls

- It is not recommended to rely solely on the patient's memory for medical procedures due to potential unrecalled alloplastic implants in situ. A patient may have a history of silicone, Gore-Tex, and Medpor use that they don't remember.
- The damage to the nasal structure post-removal of such materials is often unpredictable.
- Challenges arise, especially after removing dorsal implants, where the implant and capsule might maintain the nasal structure, necessitating different surgical approaches based on the status of the underlying framework.
- Assessing the mucosal integrity of the septum is critical, especially for patients with Medpor, as mucosal coverage may be compromised upon removal.
- Complications such as severe inflammation can occur from surgical site infections after using PCL mesh, posing significant challenges in nasal reconstruction.
- The presence and condition of the membranous septum are also crucial, mainly when using septal extension grafts, as they affect nasal tip mobility.
- There is a significant difference between the conventional implant-made sellion and the bony nasion below the implant.
- The presence or absence of the caudal septal cartilage is essential in determining the difficulty of reconstruction.
- The degree of cellulitis is an index that determines whether a secondary operation is possible, as in the surgical site infection.

Supplementary Information The online version contains supplementary material available at https://doi.org/10.1007/978-981-96-6127-5_2.

2.1 Unique Considerations in Asian Secondary Surgery

The preoperative analysis methods outlined in Chap. 1 seldom apply intraoperatively in secondary surgery planning. Given that these patients have undergone multiple unsuccessful surgeries, their clinical needs are particularly complex and demanding. They often seek a more definitive outcome and have precise expectations, which, in practice, can be challenging to fulfill. The true extent of the necessary corrections frequently remains unclear until surgical dissection is performed. A thorough understanding of the following key aspects is crucial for effective surgical planning.

2.1.1 Various Alloplastic Materials: Need to Know, but It's Hard to Know

The identification of alloplastic materials used in dorsal augmentation can be challenging. While CT scans can reveal variances in shadows, distin-

E. S. Dhong, *Asian Septorhinoplasty*, https://doi.org/10.1007/978-981-96-6127-5_2

guishing between materials such as silicone, Gore-Tex, and Medpor is often speculative and may not always be accurate. This uncertainty is compounded in patients with extensive surgical histories, where the complete procedural background can be unclear or difficult to ascertain.

In such cases, it is crucial to carefully analyze the imaging shadows and make informed predictions about the types of implants that might be present within the residual capsule and scar tissue. This assessment is essential for planning subsequent dissection and anticipating potential complications from interactions with the existing alloplastic materials.

- The challenge arises when there is a history of using multiple alloplastic materials, such as silicone, Gore-Tex, and Medpor, concurrently in a single patient. In such cases, distinguishing between these materials preoperatively becomes particularly difficult. Identifying the types of implants used and their locations is impossible without the surgical procedure. This complexity underscores the importance of thorough surgical planning and preparedness for various scenarios encountered during the operation.

2.1.2 Silicone and Gore-Tex

Silicone and Gore-Tex are two common materials that show a hyperlucent shadow on CT scans (Figs. 2.1 and 2.2).

However, the difference in the density between the two is not different at the bone and mediastinum settings. Even in physical examination, it's hard to tell the difference between the two.

Very soft silicone has a similar hardness to Gore-Tex, but Gore-Tex tends to shrinkage into a harder texture over time. When considering the removal of such an implant, the integrity of the underlying nasal framework becomes a key consideration. This framework consists of bone and cartilage, and its condition can vary significantly from one individual to another due to factors like previous surgeries and anatomical differences. If the underlying framework remains solid and intact after removing the dorsal implant, simple options for reconstructive strategies are presented. In such cases, the surgeon may choose to use additional grafts or implants to achieve the desired aesthetic outcome without compromising the structural integrity of the nose. These grafts can be sourced from autografts, depending on the specific needs and goals of the surgery.

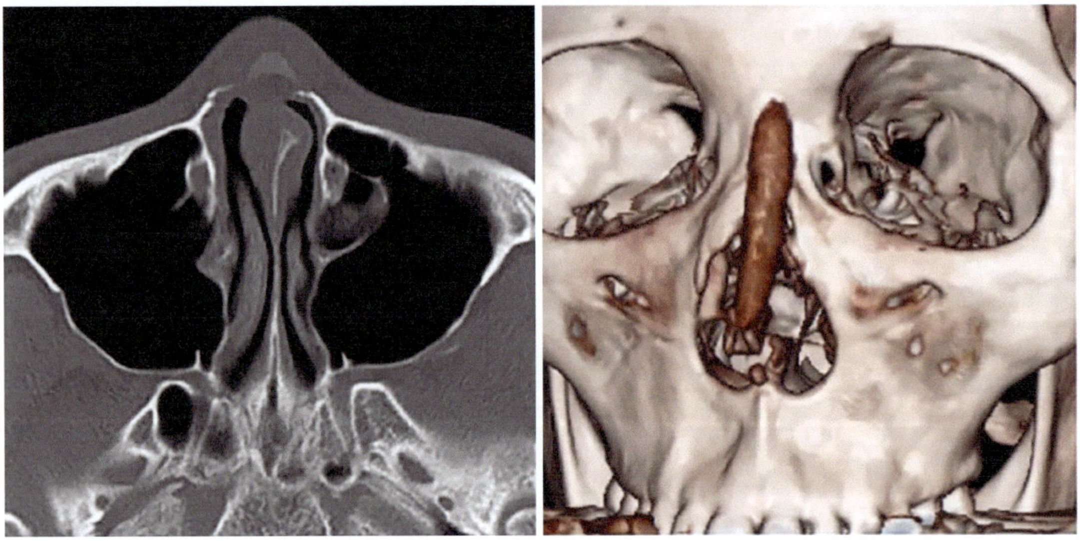

Fig. 2.1 CT findings of silicone. (Left) Axial view in bone setting. (Right) 3D view

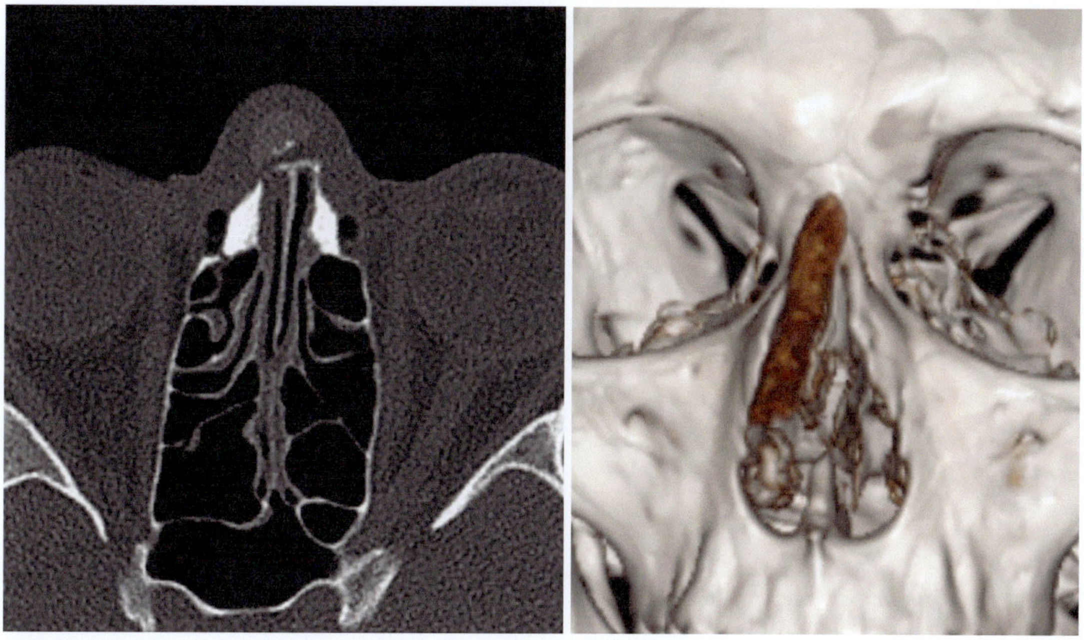

Fig. 2.2 CT findings of Gore-Tex. (Left) Axial view in bone setting. (Right) 3D view

- It is crucial to acknowledge that the contour of the nose is preserved, whether by structural support or by the longitudinal implant.
- The integrity of the underlying framework is a critical determinant in selecting the surgical approach upon removing the implant.
- If the foundational structure remains robust following dorsal implant extraction, reconstruction using an alternative graft or implant is often feasible. Conversely, if broken platforms are discovered after implant removal, they are often impossible to camouflage without a framework rebuilding.

2.1.3 Medpor

Medpor is typically hypolucent on CT imaging and is often located in the anterior or caudal segments of the septum, necessitating adjustments in contrast for optimal visualization (Fig. 2.3). Hypolucency, when observed, does not correlate with palpability upon gentle nasal manipulation. Patients frequently report mild nasal dorsum or tip discomfort, particularly upon tip elevation. This discomfort is especially notable in cases with a septal extension graft or when the Medpor is positioned within the caudal septum, often prompting patients to seek pain management.

For surgical planning, it is advisable to assess the mobility of the caudal septum transnasally to evaluate the integrity of the septal mucosa. Given that Medpor is infrequently utilized for dorsal onlay grafting, it is often predominantly encountered within the intraseptal region. Consequently, removing Medpor will likely reveal a deficiency in the septal framework.

- The presence or absence of a membranous septum serves as an indicator for determining whether a prior septal extension procedure has been performed.
- It is challenging to detect a small piece of Medpor in the columella preoperatively. Persistent, unexplained nasal tip pain may raise suspicion of an undetected Medpor in the mobile tip area.
- It is critical to understand that the extraction of Medpor might lead to a compromise in septal support. Removing Medpor is expected to result in a significant defect within the anterocaudal segment of the septum.

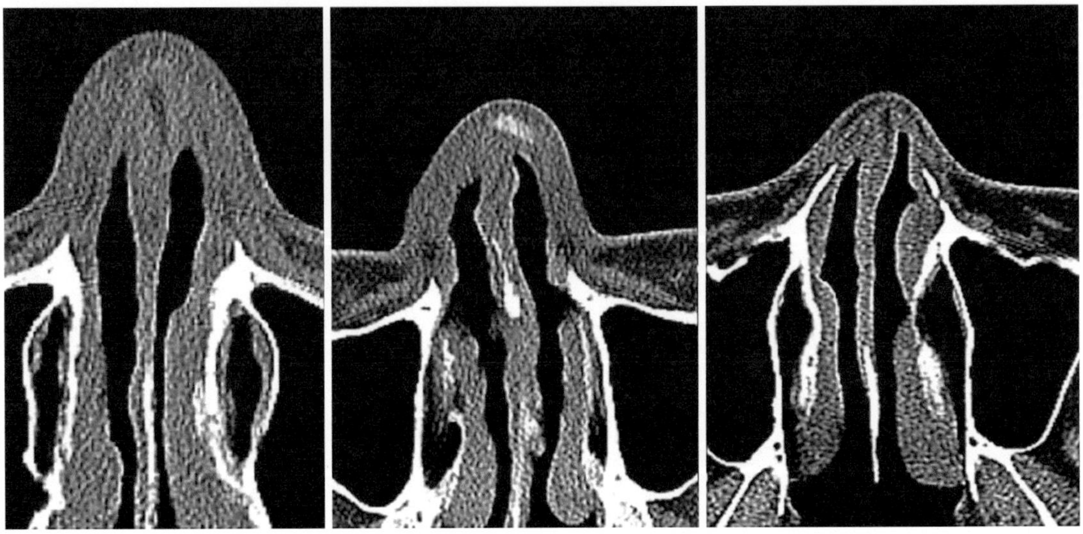

Fig. 2.3 CT findings of Medpor in three patients. (Left) High septal Medpor with a thin silicone implant. (Middle) Fractured Medpor with dorsal silicone implant. (Right) Intraseptal Medpor has the same shadow as the dorsal subcutaneous fatty shadow

2.1.4 Absorbable Mesh Plate

Absorbable mesh plates, mainly made from polylactic acid (PLA) and polycaprolactone (PCL), appear hyperlucent/hypolucent on CT imaging according to the retention period (Fig. 2.4). Yet, they can achieve a certain level of visibility based on their density relative to surrounding tissues. Hydroxyapatite can present with varying degrees of opacity, especially when combined with absorbable mesh plates.

Since the early 2010s, polydioxanone (PDS) foil has been extensively utilized for reinforcing fragmented or deformed autologous cartilage. In contrast, current PCL mesh products have been associated with chronic inflammation and significant septal cartilage defects, including surgical site infections. This is because the PCL mesh is used not in conjunction with cartilage but as a standalone framework. Despite the literature indicating promising outcomes, the experience of reoperations in clinical practice presents a considerable challenge, often resulting in outcomes far removed from typical surgical infections or delayed inflammatory reactions [1–3].

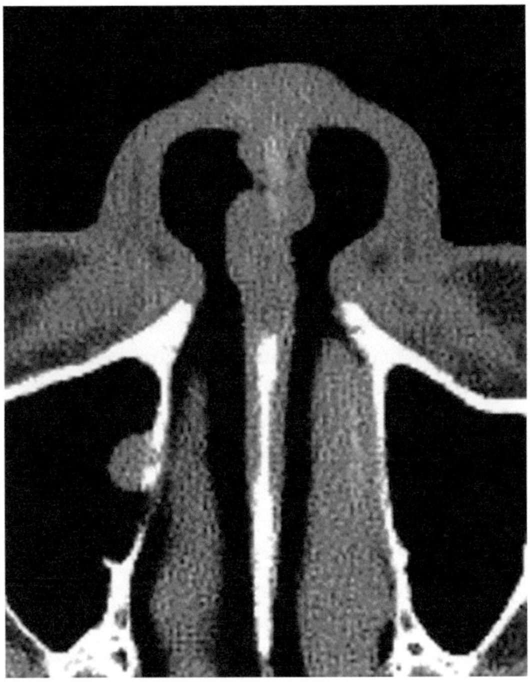

Fig. 2.4 CT finding of absorbable mesh: The shadow varies by product, but the PCL of this patient is hyperlucent

In commonly found cases of PCL mesh inflammation, central mucosal contracture presents the most significant challenge to effective reconstruction.

2.1.5 Dermofat Graft and Allodermis

In computed tomography (CT) imaging, areas that appear hypolucent often correspond to fatty compartments within the dermofat layer, occasionally containing fillers. The alloderm, in practical terms, does not exhibit clear differentiation and frequently presents similarly to scar tissue within the surgical field. When alloderm is applied in multiple folded layers, it can mimic the appearance of a scar mass. During surgical procedures, these areas may demonstrate an absence of bleeding and present as highly dense tissue, offering significant resistance to removal even with a scalpel.

2.1.6 Paraffinoma and Filler Granuloma

Prolonged exposure to paraffin can lead to the formation of granulomas. In such cases, magnetic resonance imaging (MRI) proves beneficial for diagnosis. On T1-weighted images, these granulomas appear as mixed shadows than the surrounding fatty tissue, while on T2-weighted images, they exhibit blood-sensitive sequences, reflecting the complex, heterogeneous nature typical of granulomas (Fig. 2.5). A significant concern arises when paraffin, used as a filler, infiltrates the superficial subcutaneous layer, potentially leading the skin flap to a critically compromised state. The decision to undertake complete excision, which may alter the skin's circulatory physiology, requires careful deliberation. Sometimes, opting for an aesthetically sub-optimal removal might be more prudent than resorting to a midline forehead flap despite the associated risk of paraffinoma recurrence.

2.1.7 Volume Replacement

Accurately estimating the required volume is crucial when planning volume replacement in areas requiring the removal of a capsule or alloderm. It is essential to assess the quantity of alloplastic material or scar tissue currently present (Fig. 2.6).

Removing a filler granuloma or mucoid tissue within a compromised capsule often necessitates

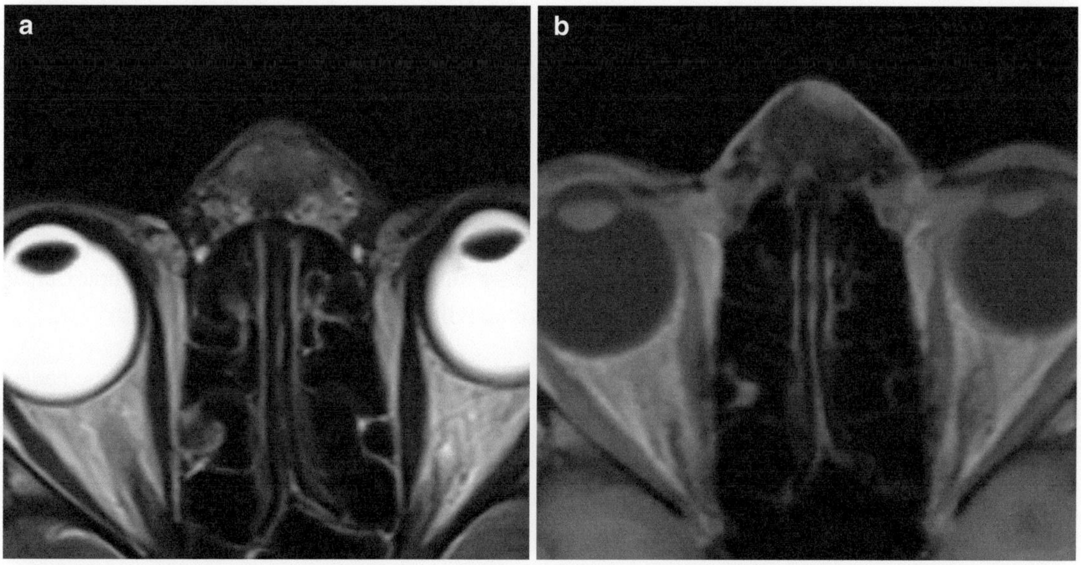

Fig. 2.5 MRI findings of paraffinoma. (**a**) T1 weighted image. (**b**) T2 weighted image

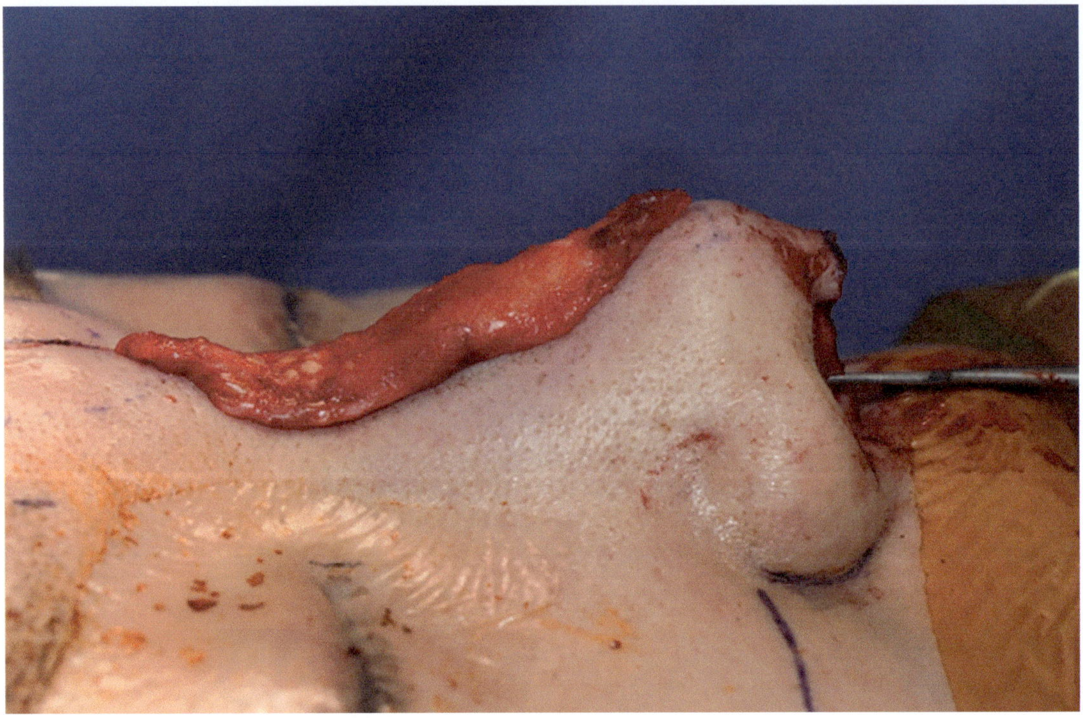

Fig. 2.6 Massive volume depletion after granuloma excision

significant volume replacement. Consequently, an ample supply of autograft material exceeding the volume to be excised is necessary.

In instances where an autograft has been previously placed, retaining a portion within the tissue might be advisable if only a moderate reduction is sought. Specifically, in cases where a considerable volume of dermofat has been previously grafted, strategizing the operation to retain some of the grafted material, rather than removing it entirely, should be considered.

This principle also extends to managing scars in lower lateral cartilages (LLCs). Attempting to excise all scar tissue and realign misaligned cartilage may prove futile if excessive cartilage graft is required.

Extensive scar tissue removal is a common challenge in secondary tip plasty. However, it is essential to recognize that completely removing the scar tissue may compromise the LLC's structural integrity.

Occasionally, preserving a portion of the scar tissue to maintain strength and proceeding with tip surgery is advisable, mainly when the actual cartilage cannot be adequately visualized and repaired (Fig. 2.7).

2.1.8 Previous Septal Surgery

Using septal cartilage for nasal extension has become prevalent in Asian procedures [4]. The nature of the secondary surgery is contingent upon the necessity for reconstructing the nasal framework. However, the septal cartilage, often required for these procedures, is typically utilized during the primary surgery. Consequently, patients who underwent submucous resection during their prior surgery will likely face more complex challenges during their secondary procedures.

- While observing the septum, touch the center with a cotton tip or freer elevator from the opposite side to see if the septum flutters. Fluttering indicates that the septum has already been harvested.
- The CT scan shows thinning of the septal mucosa.

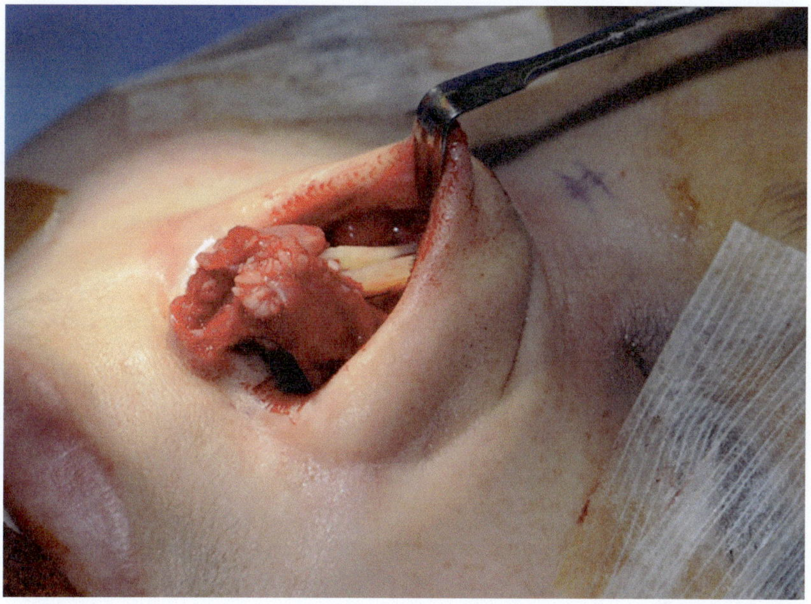

Fig. 2.7 Use of scar tissue for tip position: Completely excising the scar tissue of the destroyed LLC requires a large amount of anatomical cartilage graft

- Check the local injection of the septum in the surgical field of view.
- A poorly infiltrated septal mucosa indicates damage to the mucoperichondrium of the center (Video 2.1).
- It is essential to verify the presence of the caudal septum margin.
- The distinct caudal septal margin indicates the easy start of the framework reconstruction.

2.1.9 What Autogenous Sources Are Left?

As the frequency of revision surgeries increases, the availability of autologous tissue often becomes limited. Beyond the septal cartilage, it is not unusual to find that the cavum and cymba conchae of the auricular cartilage have been exhausted. Similarly, costal cartilage is frequently harvested to both the seventh and sixth ribs. Additionally, the sacral dermis may be harvested multiple times, underscoring the importance of an initial assessment to identify available tissues. This evaluation is crucial for determining the necessary volume for successful outcomes.

2.1.10 Previous Operative Technique

Understanding the approach taken during the initial surgery is highly beneficial if feasible. However, acquiring this information is not always possible. Given that many patients may have undergone multiple surgical procedures, it becomes crucial to ascertain the precise techniques employed. For instance, patients who received silicone implants during their fifth procedure should be informed about five distinct capsular formations. Although the significance of identifying the exact method diminishes with an increasing number of surgeries, it is advantageous for the surgeon to consult the record of the previous surgery whenever possible.

2.2 What Is Different in the Analysis of Secondary Surgery?: STCA Tracing with Simple X-Ray

Chapter 1 explored conducting soft tissue cephalometric analysis (STCA) using a patient's photo. However, this approach may not always be feasible or relevant in secondary surgery, primarily due to space-occupying alloplastic implants in the dorsum. These implants complicate the ability to predict volume augmentation and deficiency accurately. Combining simple X-rays in the lateral view and CT imaging becomes indispensable for secondary surgery analysis. These modalities can provide critical information about volumetric changes and key anatomical landmarks such as the position of the nasion, the keystone area, and the anterior nasal spine (ANS).

The STCA tracing with simple lateral X-ray highlights the nuanced understanding of the implant, alterations in sellion, implant height, or bone remodeling that may not be evident on other images.

2.2.1 Sellion Vs. Nasion

In patients undergoing secondary surgery with an alloplastic implant in place, the accurate anatomy of the nasion's undersurface remains obscured. A simple X-ray, often more intuitive than a complex CT scan, can provide valuable insights. A lateral view, complemented by a nasal bone examination, can reveal the thickness and length of the dorsum implant. It is crucial to distinguish between the actual nasion location and the sellion's position as observed in lateral X-ray.

It is advisable to carefully examine the contour of the nasion and the overlaying implant, utilizing techniques such as cephalometric tracing, and to consult CT imaging findings when available to ensure a comprehensive understanding of the surgical site's anatomy.

- In patients of short nose deformity, the sellion made by silicone may appear lower than the actual nasion, giving a descended appearance.
- In long nose deformity, the sellion often appears higher than the true nasion, typically due to a long dorsal implant (Fig. 2.8).
- Accurate measurement of the actual nasion, as it will be revealed post-implant removal, is crucial for precise surgical planning. It means that you can't know for sure without actually performing the surgery yourself.
- Enhancing the nasion's projection through grafting carries the risk of inadvertently elevating the sellion, potentially resulting in a nose that appears longer and more aged postoperatively.

2.2.2 Subnasale Vs. ANS

In secondary rhinoplasty, the subnasale often demonstrates a significant destruction in the ANS position, frequently attributed to a caudal septal extension. Contracture is common in secondary rhinoplasty, requiring a careful assessment of the condition of ANS.

A simple lateral X-ray view may not provide sufficient detail for this purpose. On the other hand, CT imaging can be more informative, especially since alloplastic materials other than silicone might not be visible. While CT scans can sometimes distinctly visualize the ANS, the clarity may be lacking in different cases.

Adequate preparation is essential to address defects or residual substances after removing an alloplastic implant. For the lengthening subnasale, a physical examination is crucial. The columella should be pulled downward sufficiently to evaluate its potential for stretching. A lack of stretchability, accompanied by rigidity, indicates the presence of contracture, which requires further assessment. A key feature of a contracted nose with a membranous nasal septum is the inability to forcefully pull the nose tip downward without causing significant pain to the patient.

- The condition of the membranous septum is a critical determinant of the extent to which the nose can be elongated in secondary surgeries.
- Considering the limited stretchability of the mucoperichondrium covering the quadrangular cartilage, perforation poses a significant challenge to releasing the membranous septum or the entire tip complex.

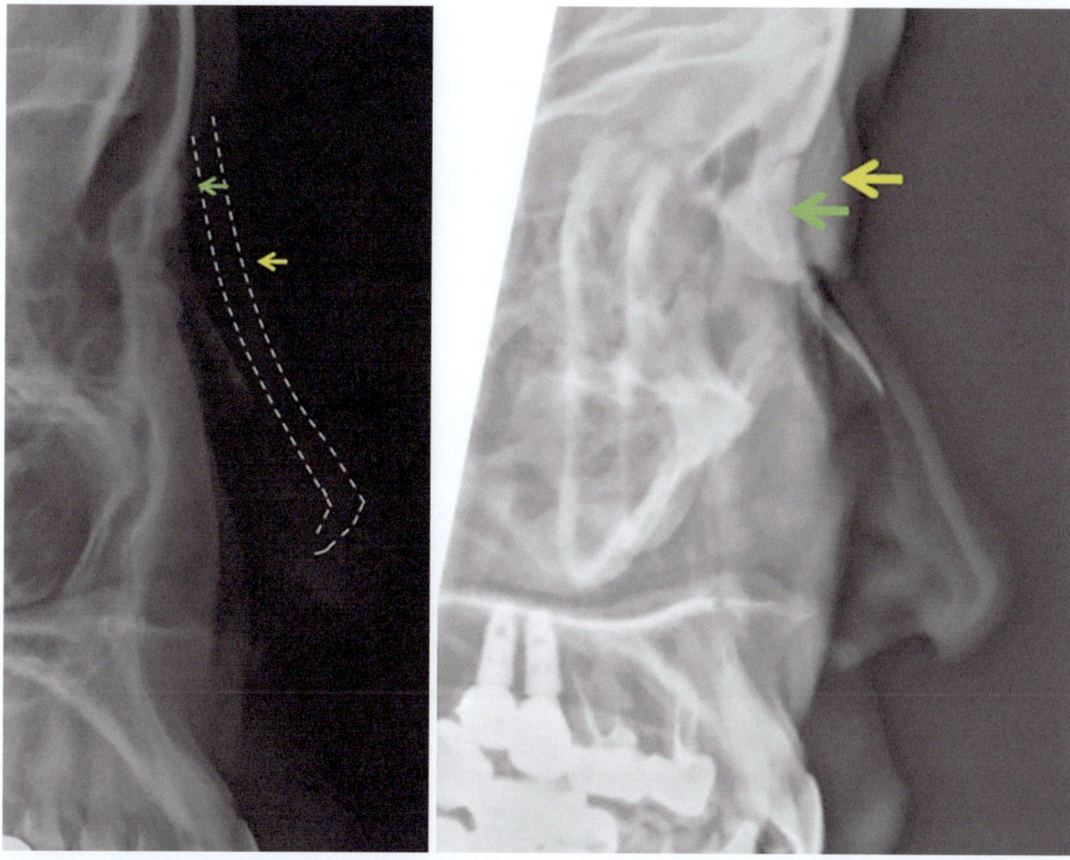

Fig. 2.8 Difference between nasion and sellion as seen on X-ray. (Right) Sellion is higher than nasion and is found in long nose deformity. (Left) Nasion higher than sellion, found in short nose deformity

2.3 Intuitive Observation and Planning: CT Scan

2.3.1 Open Roof Deformity in Asian Secondary Rhinoplasty

The phenomenon of open roof deformity beneath the implant remains undocumented in Western medical literature. This complication is uniquely associated with "reduction-augmentation rhinoplasty" practices in Asian rhinoplasty techniques. Specifically, this involves the utilization of an alloplastic implant for dorsal augmentation following the reduction of a nasal hump (Fig. 2.9).

Various factors can result in an unstable bony framework within the nasal structure. A significant contributor is the introduction of a dorsal implant after medial and lateral osteotomies. The persistent pressure from the alloplastic implant, gravitational forces, and the tension exerted by the surrounding soft tissue may jeopardize the integrity of the nasal skeletal framework over time.

In such scenarios, precise CT imaging becomes pivotal for formulating a practical surgical approach. For individuals necessitating revision surgery, the operative plan might include septal reconstruction or employing a cantilever graft to augment the nasal dorsum without an intact septum aesthetically. Implementing an extended spreader graft is crucial during septal reconstruction to provide adequate support to the anterior septum where foundational support is deficient. Furthermore, strategically placing a transcutaneous transosseous cerclage (TTC) suture is imperative to maintain structural integrity, particularly in surgeries of a broken rhinion or severe open roof deformity [5].

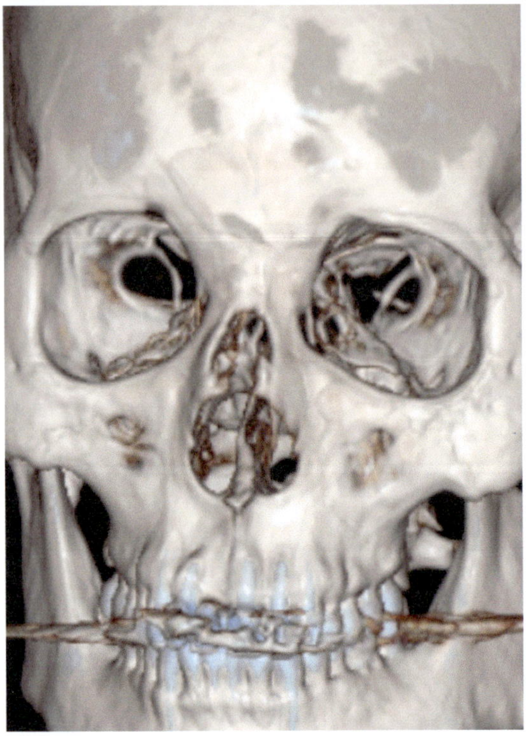

Fig. 2.9 Open roof deformity: The patient showed severe open roof deformity after silicone removal

2.3.1.1 Dorsal Aesthetic Line Vs. Implant

The lack of visible irregularities in the dorsal aesthetic lines from frontal and lateral perspectives should not be mistakenly interpreted as evidence of a uniform underlying nasal structure encompassing both the nasal bone and cartilaginous dorsum. This is especially pertinent in cases of patients who have previously undergone procedures such as hump resection or lateral nasal osteotomy. In my experience, it is not uncommon to encounter patients presenting with a collapsed framework beneath the implant despite the absence of apparent issues in the aesthetic line. This phenomenon arises when a well-defined capsule forms around the implant, concealing any irregularities in the tissue beneath. For example, regarding the dorsal line, a nose might appear to have a smooth contour despite a misaligned implant if the bony pyramid has collapsed so that it conforms to the implant's shape. This creates an optical illusion of a continuous, uninterrupted dorsal line, effectively concealing any underlying structural irregularities (Fig. 2.10).

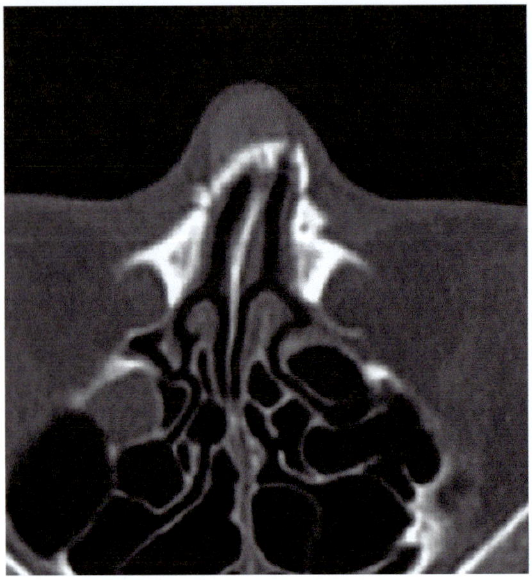

Fig. 2.10 Illusion of dorsal aesthetic line: The nasal bony pyramid under the silicone is damaged

2.3.1.2 Shape of the Implant

It is advantageous to grasp the precise shape of the implant and the degree of calcification. Depending on vague memories, patients might sometimes mix up the use of L-shaped and boat-shaped implants.

2.3.1.3 Shape of Septum and Turbinate

CT imaging is recommended during reoperation to visualize septal deviation and turbinate hypertrophy easily. Since the septum and inferior turbinate operate as an integrated unit, performing functional rhinoplasty without CT imaging is rare. This is mainly because procedures aimed at correcting the inferior turbinate frequently occur alongside submucous resection (SMR) as part of a comprehensive approach to turbinate correction.

2.3.1.4 Internal Nasal Valve (INV)

Nasal obstruction is increasingly cited as a reason for reoperation in Asian rhinoplasty. While a detailed discussion on functional issues, it's worth noting that juxtaposing acoustic rhinometry findings with CT scans are exceptionally useful in identifying problems with the internal nasal valve (INV) [6]. CT imaging plays a vital role in foreseeing necessary adjustments for nasal constriction and midline thickening that may be needed after septal reconstruction.

2.4 Physical Examination Is the Key to the Planning

2.4.1 Lower Lateral Cartilage in Secondary Tip Surgery

The appearance of a scarred nasal tip can be deceptive; it might look undamaged, but the underlying lower lateral cartilages (LLC) could be impaired due to previous dissections. It's crucial to manually evaluate the nose's elasticity by gently moving the tip upwards and downwards to assess its firmness. In significant soft tissue contraction, a technique that involves massaging the nose downwards combined with the administration of Zafirlukast may aid in softening the tissue (Fig. 2.11).

- Just as the septum beneath an implant can become indented and fractured, the lower lateral cartilage may also undergo resorption after multiple surgical interventions. In such cases, the appearance of the nasal tip might be influenced more by a huge onlay graft used during the initial surgery than by the intrinsic shape of the LLCs.

Careful examination of the incisions from previous surgeries is essential. For instance, a rim

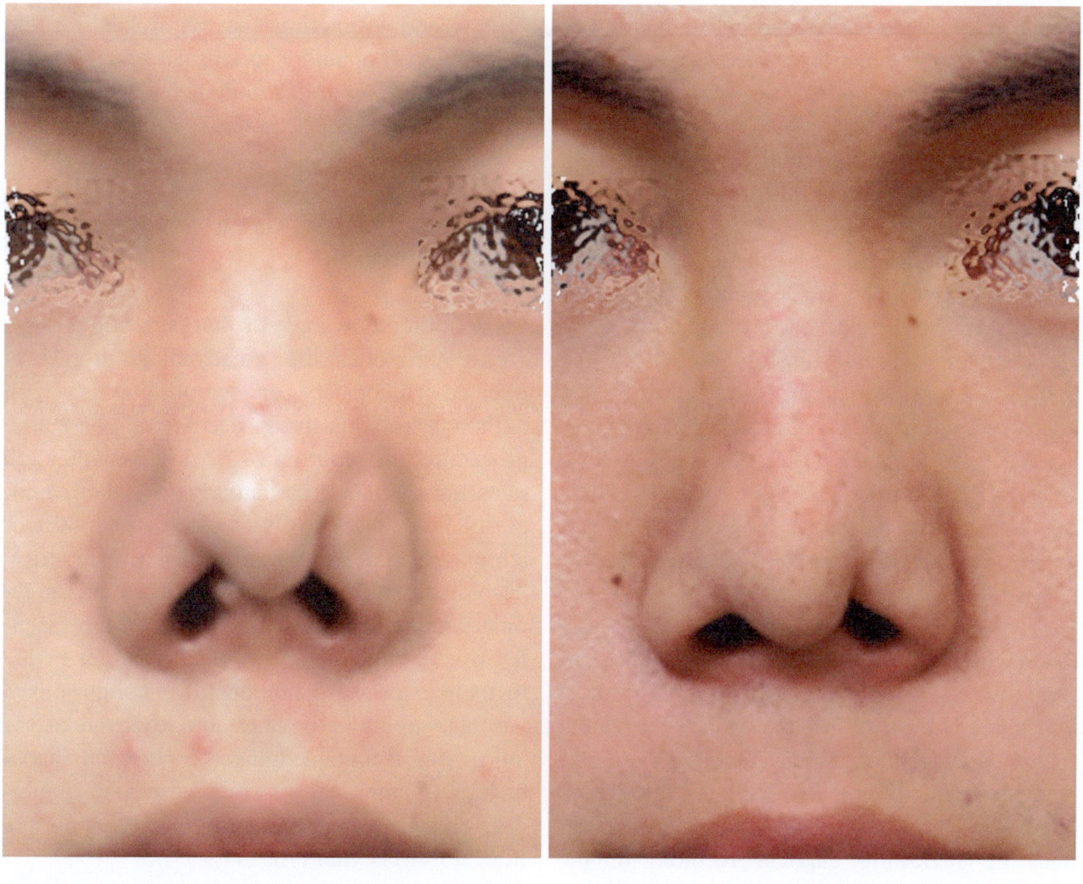

Fig. 2.11 Zafirlukast was prescribed, and the patient was instructed to massage down the nose. (Left) Before medication. (Right) One month after the medication and massage

incision might suggest an inadequate nostril flap for a soft triangle. Additionally, if tip projection was previously achieved with a columellar strut, the potential distortion of the medial and middle crura must be considered.

Alar retraction can often occur if previous incisions were made too close to the alar rim; moreover, when the nasal tip has been augmented with multiple layers of alloderm, accurately predicting the tip's original configuration before surgical exploration can be challenging.

Alloplastic materials are becoming more common for nasal augmentation. However, to reconstruct the tip, retaining a portion of the graft from the initial surgery might be necessary to preserve its projection instead of removing the entire graft. A scar healed without inflammation from the first operation can be repurposed as a soft tissue covering, whereas an inflamed or otherwise compromised scar should not be reused.

When there is a depression or a defect in the tissue due to inflammation or damage to the internal structure, restoring the skin envelope to its original condition may not be possible. If the preoperative length of the nasal tip was adequate before secondary surgery, restoring its shape and height might be possible with a significantly increased augmentation. Hence, ensuring a proper supply of soft tissue grafts is essential. The best material is the thick sacral dermis [7]. However, the superficial mastoid fascia is an area in the same surgical field that can be useful when unplanned soft tissue is suddenly needed [8].

2.4.2 Caudal Septum: Septal Extension Graft Vs. Columellar Strut

In the widespread application of the septal extension graft (SEG) technique in rhinoplasty, it is imperative to identify instances where the caudal septum is attached to the nasal tip and the membranous septum is notably small. An initial step involves verifying any previous surgical interventions by reviewing surgical records. In the absence of such records, the precise identification of the caudal septum's position during the preoperative evaluation and the confirmation of an existing SEG becomes essential.

However, similar to grafts positioned on the nasal tip, the definitive identification of grafts placed on the membranous septum or columella is contingent upon the actual surgical exposure of the graft.

2.5 When Is the Optimal Timing for the Secondary Surgery?

The author's approach to simultaneously performing septal reconstruction and autografting to the dorsum in patients experiencing pus drainage raises a critical question regarding the timing of the surgery. Determining the optimal timing is essential to ensure that the infection is adequately managed and the patient is in a suitable condition for the procedure, minimizing the risk of complications and promoting successful healing and outcomes. The author performs septal reconstruction and autograft simultaneously only when the cellulitis is under control.

2.5.1 Antibiotics Use in Secondary Rhinoplasty

Western literature suggests that peri- and postoperative antibiotics offer no advantage in uncomplicated rhinoplasty or septorhinoplasty [9]. Although rhinoplasty is deemed a non-sterile procedure, the reported 1–2% or lower infection rates are disputed, particularly in Asian rhinoplasty. Procedures involving extensive grafting or alloplastic materials, even in primary surgeries, necessitate antibiotics. There is a general agreement among rhinoplasty surgeons on the essential role of antibiotics in secondary surgeries due to their extended operation time, compromised vascular supply to the flaps, and extensive use of autografts. Acknowledging the potential inadequacies of empirical systemic intravenous antibiotics in addressing potentially infectious normal flora (PINF) is vital [10, 11].

For patients with a history of surgical site infections or those undergoing significant structural reconstruction with rib cartilage who may experience compromised flap circulation, relying on first- or second-generation cephalosporins might leave 20–30% of PINF uncovered. Therefore, selecting antibiotics based on susceptibility testing of nasal swab culture is imperative. Prescribing antibiotics based on prior experiences alone can lead to unnecessary antibiotic resistance. The authors recommend a preoperative nasal swab to identify the nasal flora and formulate an effective antibiotic ointment. A follow-up nasal swab on the day of the surgery is advised to detect any changes in the nasal flora. Systemic antibiotics, chosen based on these results, should be administered for 3–5 days postoperatively to ensure comprehensive coverage.

The role of preoperative bacteriological testing with nasal swabs and targeted antibiotics in reducing MRSA bacteremia remains debatable. Despite differing opinions, the authors acknowledge the significant benefits of preoperatively preparing the direct incision site for rhinoplasty [10].

Recent in-depth studies support the effectiveness of postoperative topical antibiotic application. Dr. Toriumi's research corroborates this, showing a decrease in postoperative infection rates to 0.62%, with proper antibiotic soaking [12].

The author endorses using a solution containing antibiotics and betadine for irrigation exclusively during surgical procedures. Utilizing this solution for irrigation inside intranasal packing or intra-dissection pockets during surgery is deemed more effective than administering 100 g of antibiotics, serving as a preventive measure for surgeries classified as clean-contaminated. While the guidelines for antibiotic use are consistent with those for surgical site infections, the preparatory steps for secondary surgeries require extra caution.

2.5.2 Late-Onset Inflammation

The authors proposed a disease category called late-onset inflammation in Asian rhinoplasty [13]. Four to five clinical stages have been subdivided clinically.

It is more accurate to say that each patient is found in one of these stages rather than the stages occurring sequentially.

More recently, the authors have been categorizing patients by pathological stage. This is introduced in Chap. 15 of the book.

1. Recurrent swelling of the nose.
2. The granulation tissue with skin lesions forms a thick scar around the implant.
3. The skin punctures with the opening of a "mucocele-like cyst."
4. Full infection with cellulitis.

Determining the ideal timing for reoperation poses a significant challenge in my practice. While some colleagues recommend waiting 6 months to a year, evaluating the patient's current position within the framework is imperative. As ridiculous as it sounds, the myth that you must wait at least 6 months for a secondary rhinoplasty did not originate from the consensus of rhinoplasty surgeons in Korea. In Korea's legal system, a judge's ruling after consulting with one doctor set a precedent and created the 6-month standard. It all started when a judge ruled against a secondary surgery performed within 6 months. Although wound stabilization, collagen production, and resorption stabilize within 6 months, it is unscientific to wait 6 months for all surgery.

It is not uncommon for patients at stage 1 to postpone surgery due to financial reasons, only to return later, perhaps after more than a year, with their condition having advanced to stage 4. At this stage, nasal contracture is considerably more severe. Interestingly, there are similarities in the pathology of capsular contracture seen with breast implants and the contracture associated with nasal silicone implants, highlighting a commonality in their physiological response.

If contracture is identified but immediate surgery is not deemed necessary, using a leukotriene receptor antagonist (LTRA) may be advantageous. Administer leukotriene receptor antagonists (LTRAs) such as zafirlukast (Accolate®, AstraZeneca) or montelukast (Singulair®, MSD) and follow-up with the patient at one-month intervals leading up to the surgery to prepare for the procedure. In cases where therapeutic options are limited, one must acknowledge that antibiotics are not applicable and corticosteroid injections prove ineffective. This scenario underscores the importance of continued follow-up and mental support, which are not negated by the absence of pharmacological interventions. Additionally, nasal massage may serve as a complementary approach to alleviate symptoms. While no conclusive evidence suggests that leukotriene receptor antagonists (LTRAs) can delay the development of nasal contracture, the absence of definitive evidence calls for further research in this area [13–15].

Choosing the right moment for surgery presents a significant dilemma. Surgeons often grapple with the uncertainty of when contracture will cease, whereas patients generally favor sooner interventions to address deformities. Occasionally, the need for immediate surgery arises due to unpredictable situations. Critical considerations in determining the timing for surgery include controlling nasal flora and assessing cellulitis severity within the soft tissue envelope. The level of cellulitis serves as a crucial indicator of the feasibility of a secondary operation. The discovery of severe cellulitis precludes the possibility of grafting or septal surgeries, except for the procedures aimed at removing the pathogen.

References

1. Hyun S, Woo S, Baek R-M. Polycaprolactone mesh for Asian rhinoplasty: outcomes and complications of composite septal extension graft compared to mesh-only graft. Facial Plast Surg. 2022;38:207. https://doi.org/10.1055/s-0041-1730962.
2. Ahn TH, Heo CY, Ahn KC. A compound osteocartilaginous graft with polycaprolactone (PCL) mesh in Asian rhinoplasty. J Plast Reconstr Aesthet Surg. 2020;73:e6–7.
3. Park YJ, Cha JH, Bang SI, Kim SY. Clinical application of three-dimensionally printed biomaterial polycaprolactone (PCL) in augmentation rhinoplasty. Aesthetic Plast Surg. 2019;43:437–46.
4. Byrd HS, Andochick S, Copit S, Walton KG. Septal extension grafts: a method of controlling tip projection shape. Plast Reconstr Surg. 1997;100:999–1010.
5. Haack S, Hacker S, Mann S, Gubisch W. Bony fixation of the nasal framework. Facial Plast Surg. 2019;35:23–30.
6. Dhong E-S, Na M-W. Nasal obstruction in Asian rhinoplasty. In: Dhong E-S, Na M-W, editors. Asian septorhinoplasty: conundrums and solutions. Singapore: Springer Nature Singapore; 2021. p. 51–65.
7. Dhong E-S, Na M-W. The resorption: the hurdle for autogenous-based Asian rhinoplasty. In: Dhong E-S, Na M-W, editors. Asian septorhinoplasty: conundrums and solutions. Singapore: Springer Singapore; 2021. p. 77–89.
8. Hong S-T, Kim D-W, Yoon E-S, Kim H-Y, Dhong E-S. Superficial mastoid fascia as an accessible donor for various augmentations in Asian rhinoplasty. J Plast Reconstr Aesthet Surg. 2012;65:1035–40.
9. Kullar R, Frisenda J, Nassif PS. The more the merrier? Should antibiotics be used for rhinoplasty and septorhinoplasty?—A review. Plast Reconstr Surg Glob Open. 2018;6:e1972.
10. Moon K-C, Jung J-E, Dhong E-S, Jeong S-H, Han S-K. Preoperative nasal swab culture: is it beneficial in preventing postoperative infection in complicated septorhinoplasty? Plast Reconstr Surg. 2020;146:27e–34e.
11. Dhong E-S, Na M-W. Nasal swab culture: the preparation for the safe surgery. In: Dhong E-S, Na M-W, editors. Asian septorhinoplasty: conundrums and solutions. Singapore: Springer Singapore; 2021. p. 29–38.
12. Toriumi DM, Kowalczyk DM, Cristel RT, Caniglia AJ, Curran N, Lombard R, et al. Evaluation of postoperative infection rates in 3084 rhinoplasty cases using antibiotic soaks and/or irrigations. Facial Plast Surg Aesthet Med. 2021;23:368–74.
13. Moon K-C, Lee K-I, Lee J-S, Kim A-R, Dhong E-S, Kim D-W, et al. Late-onset inflammation in Asian rhinoplasty using alloplastic implants. Aesthetic Plast Surg. 2021;45:670. https://doi.org/10.1007/s00266-020-01648-8.
14. Wang Y, Tian J, Liu J. Suppressive effect of leukotriene antagonists on capsular contracture in patients who underwent breast surgery with prosthesis: a meta-analysis. Plast Reconstr Surg. 2020;145:901–11.
15. Lee J-S, Tae S-S, Kim D-Y, Han S-K, Kim W-K, Dhong E-S. Do IL-3/GM-CSF effect on the myofibroblastic differentiation of human adipose derived stromal cells? Exp Cell Res. 2017;355:67–82.

3 Adaptive Planning for Primary Septorhinoplasty Using Soft Tissue Cephalometric Analysis (STCA)

3.1 The Interview Conducting Just Before the Surgery

Analyzing convenient methods before surgery is vital for streamlining the surgical process and optimizing efficiency. These methods may include imaging technologies or computer-assisted planning tools, which enable rapid and accurate assessments of nasal anatomy and surgical requirements. By integrating such efficient techniques into preoperative protocols, surgeons can minimize surgical time, reduce the risk of complications, and enhance overall patient satisfaction and outcomes.

Patients often change their minds multiple times, even after scheduling their surgery. Furthermore, the opinions of various guardians can also significantly influence the patient's decision-making process in Asia. Therefore, the interview conducted on the day of surgery holds heightened importance. It is imperative that the corresponding STCA (soft tissue cephalometric analysis) can be performed swiftly and readily available. This is because the patient's desires may have evolved considerably from those expressed during consultations months or even a year ago.

3.2 The STCA Analysis Just Before Surgery

The author invests less than the duration of enjoying a coffee before surgical preparation to conduct a 2D photograph analysis utilizing the soft tissue cephalometric analysis (STCA) mentioned in the preceding chapters. Previously, life-sized photographs were printed and displayed in the operating room for reference during surgery; however, presently, multiple photos are printed on A4 paper at an appropriate size for easier handling. Although surgery can also be performed while viewing photographs on a computer screen, the preference lies in directly printing them on paper due to the necessity of referencing CT scans and frequent logging-out issues. This task is preferably completed just before surgery to ensure clarity and organization.

3.3 Planning for a Primary Septorhinoplasty

3.3.1 What Aspects Should Be Considered for the Preoperative Plan?

A significant number of primary patients fall into the reduction-augmentation category. The concept of reduction-augmentation is relatively uncommon in Western rhinoplasty. When dealing with localized hump noses, reduction of either the bony hump or cartilaginous hump is necessary. In Asian patients, the majority often desire projection of the tip component or the lower two-third part of the dorsum below the hump in profile.

E. S. Dhong, *Asian Septorhinoplasty*, https://doi.org/10.1007/978-981-96-6127-5_3

While the diagnosis may pose challenges and subjective judgments vary, distinguishing between mild saddle nose and mild hump nose can differ depending on the patient or the surgeon. In such cases, some patients may also desire to lower the height near the keystone area but enhance the tip projection or cartilaginous dorsum. These patients typically require both reduction of the bony dorsum and augmentation of the cartilaginous dorsum simultaneously.

The central theme of this book revolves around the septal L-strut extension graft. Consequently, discussions on primary rhinoplasty that solely relies on augmentation through an implant are beyond the scope of this text.

Therefore, planning a primary septorhinoplasty naturally involves first determining whether or not it will be accompanied by septum surgery and making arrangements for the availability of adequate donor cartilage.

A practical hands-on example below involves preparing a 2D photograph based on the four essential elements of magnification, pitch, roll, and yaw. This process serves as an example for making decisions about the shape of the nose on the actual day of surgery based on the most appropriate photograph. The methods of these four elements were covered in detail in Chap. 1.

The author utilized Microsoft Picture Manager® (Microsoft Corp., Redmond, WA, USA) to standardize the photograph. Microsoft PowerPoint (Microsoft Corp., Redmond, WA, USA) was used by copying and pasting pre-made points.

3.4 A Hands-on Analysis of a Deviated Nose Correction

3.4.1 Chief Complaint of the Patient

A 27-year-old female presented with a severely deviated nose. She wanted to improve her overall profile and function.

3.4.2 Discussions with Patients

She wanted surgery using autologous tissue and wanted to improve her natural profile simultaneously. She recognized her bony dorsum as a mild hump. She thought her nose was too short. She also desired increased projection, necessitating a substantial amount of cartilage for grafting. She planned to undergo a submucous resection (SMR) of the septum. She had a small nose; consequently, her septum appeared small on the CT scan. To prepare for the anticipated small amount of septum harvest during the surgery, the surgery was planned to use cavum concha and cymba concha cartilage together.

3.4.3 STCA Using 2D Photograph

3.4.3.1 Ideal Sellion

The position of the ideal sellion was maintained with almost no change. It was assumed that the height of ideal sellion (Si) would be slightly decreased by shaving the bony hump (Fig. 3.1).

3.4.3.2 Determination of the Length of the Nose: Ideal Subnasale

To determine the position of the subnasale, the point was marked where the stomion is divided into thirds. Afterwards, the point two-thirds below the Si and stomion was established. It was attempted to set Subi lower than this, but to ensure it stayed within the position of the alar, the aim was to be at the same level or 1–2 mm below. A goal was set to extend the subnasale downward to increase the length of the nose (Fig. 3.2).

3.4.3.3 Ideal Tip

The angle of the ideal tip was set at 105° from the perpendicular at the subnasale to the nasolabial angle. Special care was taken as the patient did not like the nose's appearance too upturned. The tip-lobular angle was set to 15° for a double break (Fig. 3.3).

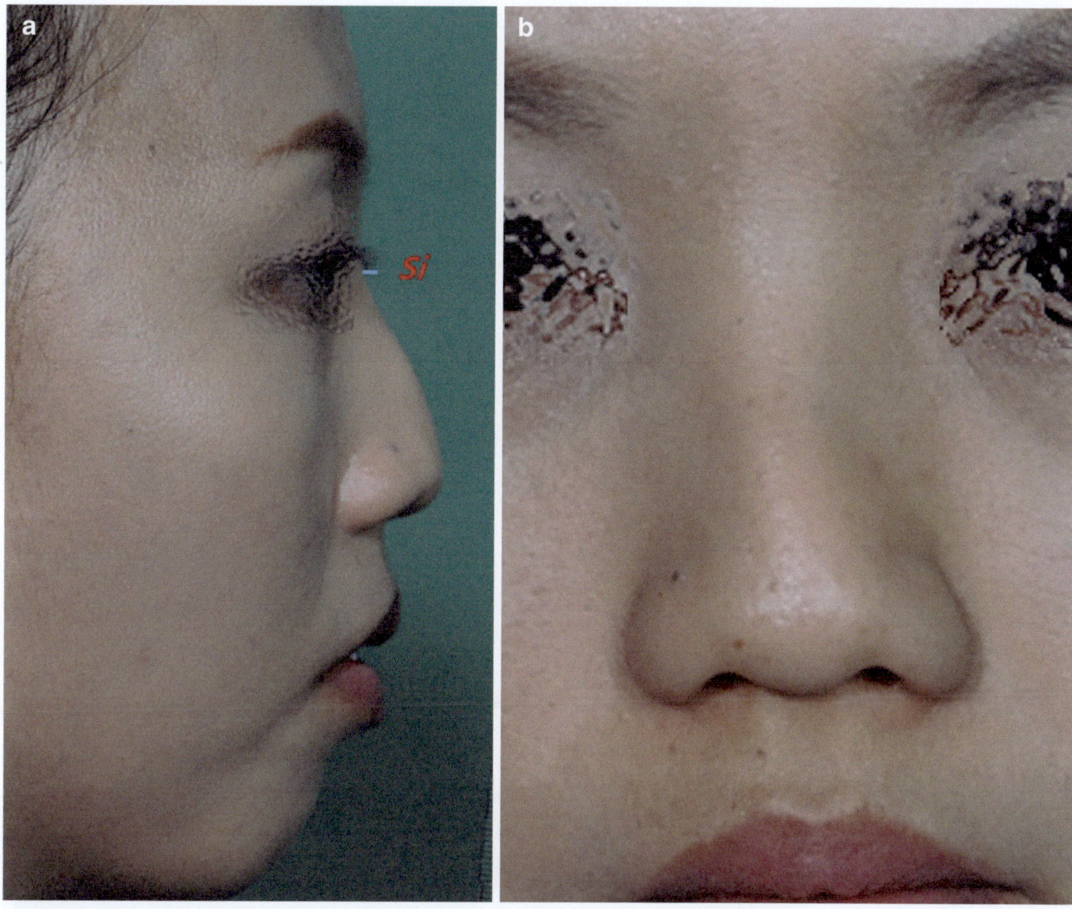

Fig. 3.1 Deviated and short nose. (**a**) Modified lateral view with Si. (**b**) AP view

3.4.3.4 Preparing the Autogenous Tissue

During the physical exam, the septum was found to be weak when pressed with a cotton tip, so additional cavum and cymba concha cartilages were prepared.

The cavum concha was prepared for tip plasty (Fig. 3.4).

3.4.3.5 Intraoperative Septal L-Strut Extension Graft

Two thin septal cartilages were used as anterior extended spreader grafts, and a folded cymba concha was utilized for a caudal septal extension graft (Fig. 3.5).

3.4.4 Long-Term Surgical Outcome

This is the improved profile of the nose after surgery. The patient was as satisfied with the improvement in the function of the nose as with its appearance (Fig. 3.6).

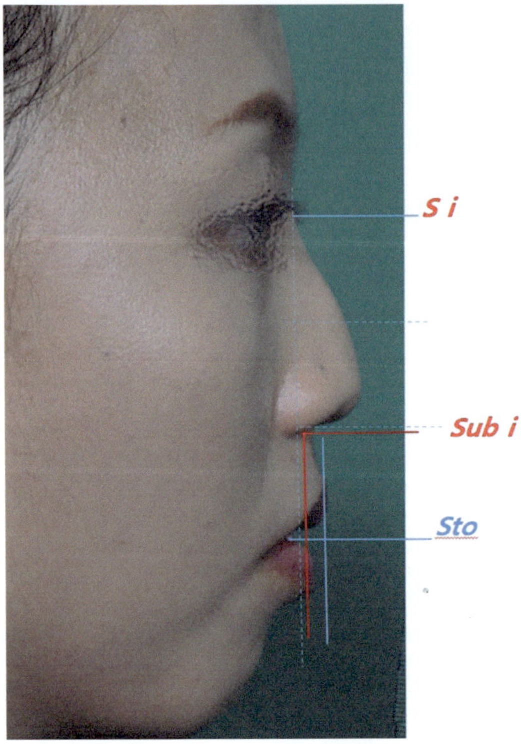

Fig. 3.2 Two STCA points: ideal sellion (Si) and ideal subnasale (Subi)

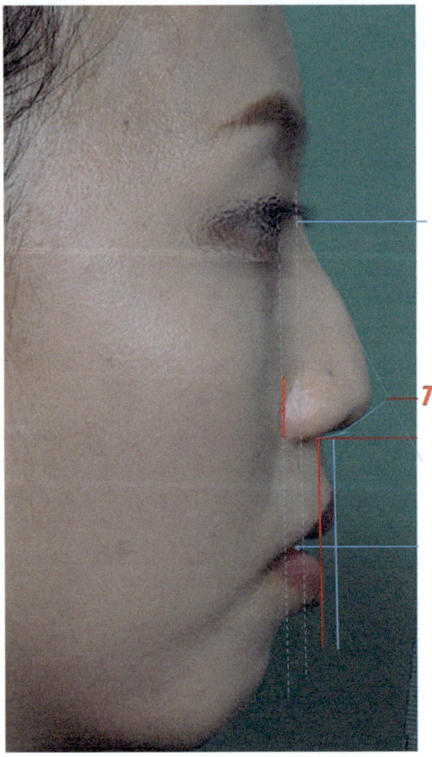

Fig. 3.3 Ideal tip (Ti)

Fig. 3.4 Preparation of autogenous tissue: septum, cymba, and cavum concha

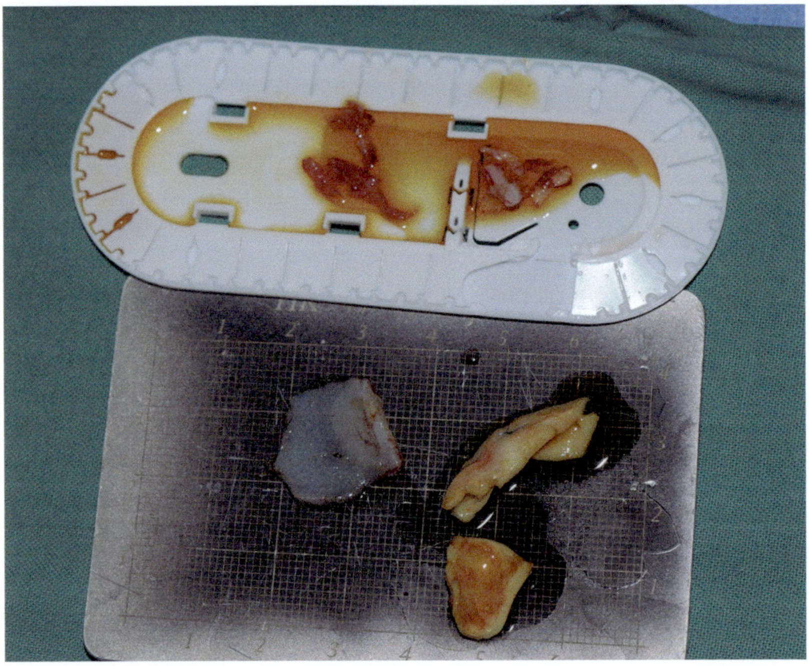

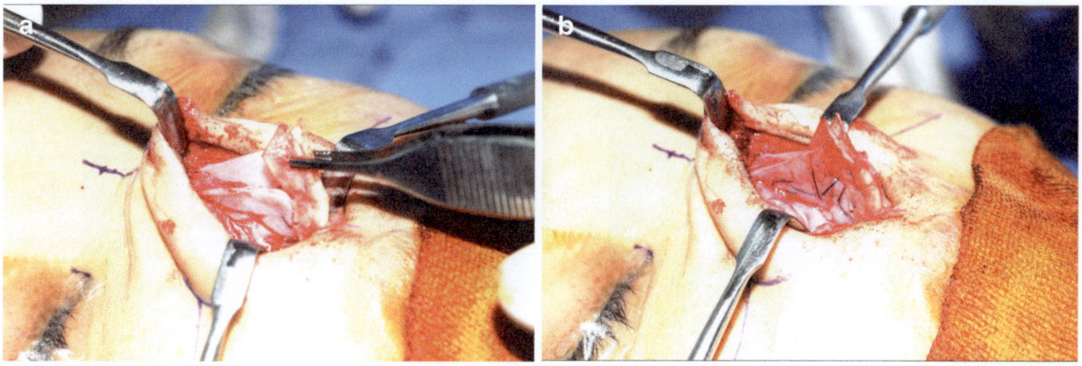

Fig. 3.5 Septal L-strut extension graft (SLEG). (**a**) Caudal septal extension graft with folded cymba concha. (**b**) Anterior extended spreader graft with septal cartilage

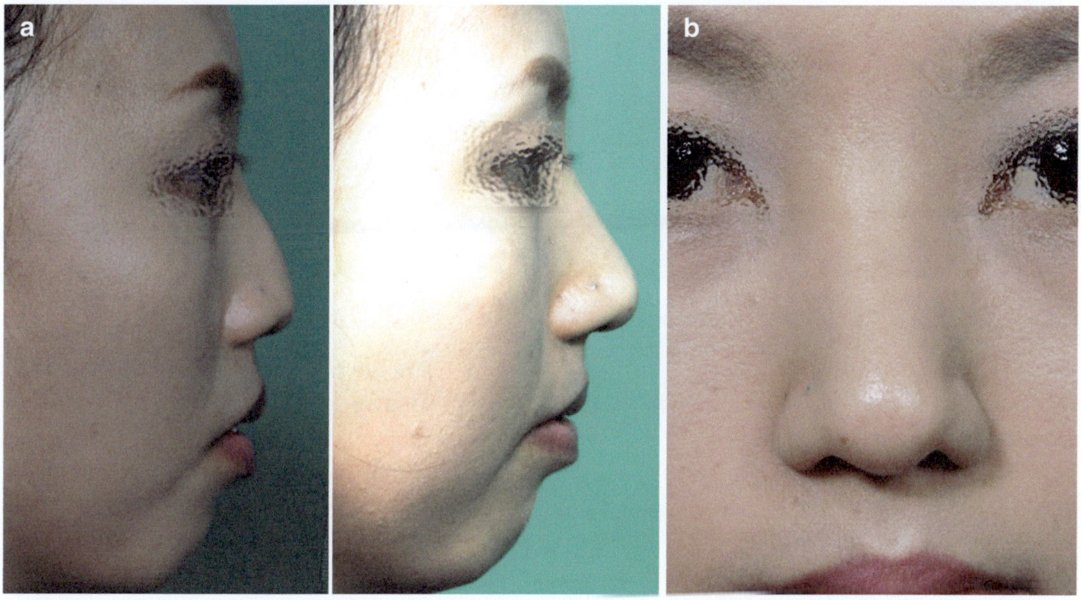

Fig. 3.6 Pre-and postoperative view. (**a**) Modified lateral view. (**b**) Postoperative AP view

3.5 A Hands-on Analysis of a Reduction-Anterior Augmentation Septorhinoplasty

3.5.1 Chief Complaint of the Patient

A 20-year-old male presented with a mild hump with a saddle nose. He wanted to improve his overall profile and entire lower two-third enhancement.

3.5.2 Discussions with Patients

He wanted a masculine, straight nose.

3.5.3 STCA Using 2D Photograph

3.5.3.1 Ideal Sellion and Dorsum

It was decided to perform a reduction from the ideal sellion to the hump. The area around the rhinion was to be rasped to remove a mild hump.

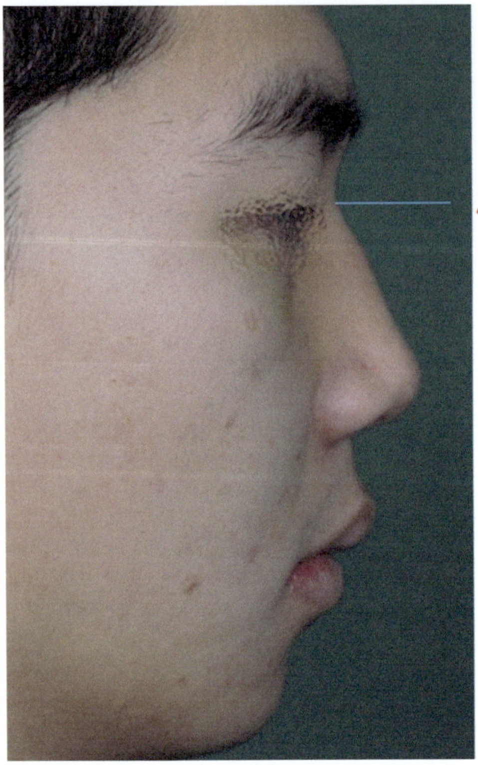

Fig. 3.7 Mild hump with saddle nose: ideal sellion (Si)

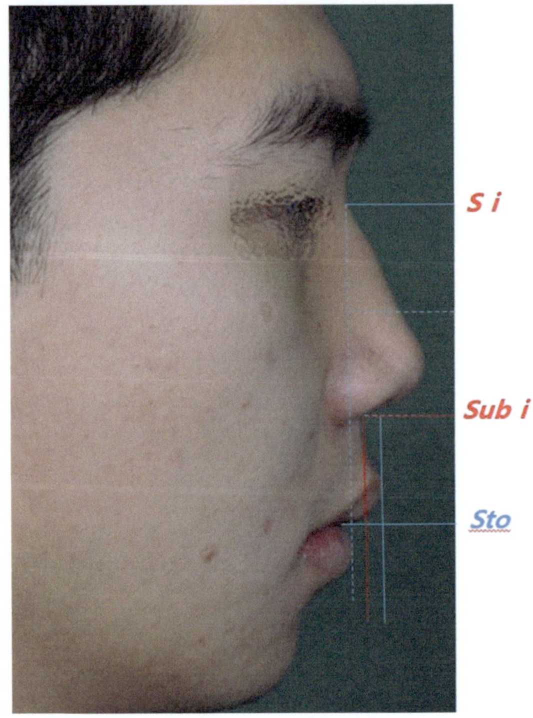

Fig. 3.8 Two STCA points: ideal sellion (Si) and ideal subnasale (Subi)

Enhancement of the anterior septum in the saddle area was also planned (Fig. 3.7).

3.5.3.2 Ideal Subnasale and Determination of the Length of the Nose

From the patient's frontal view, the midface displayed an appropriate height. In the lateral view, the length of the subnasale was ideally positioned at the lower two-thirds point between the sellion and the stomion (Fig. 3.8).

3.5.3.3 Ideal Tip

The ideal tip angle was set at 95° from the perpendicular of the subnasale to the nasolabial angle. The tip-lobular angle was set at 5° for a double break (Fig. 3.9).

3.5.4 Preparing the Autogenous Tissue

The septum and the cymba concha have been prepared. Additionally, the superficial mastoid fascia has been prepared for minimal dorsum augmentation (Fig. 3.10).

3.5.5 Intraoperative Septal L-Strut Extension Graft

The septal L-strut was augmented using an anterior extended spreader graft from the septum to enhance the cartilaginous dorsum. A caudal septal extension graft was applied using a folded cymba. Additionally, raftering grafts were performed to reinforce the anterior extended

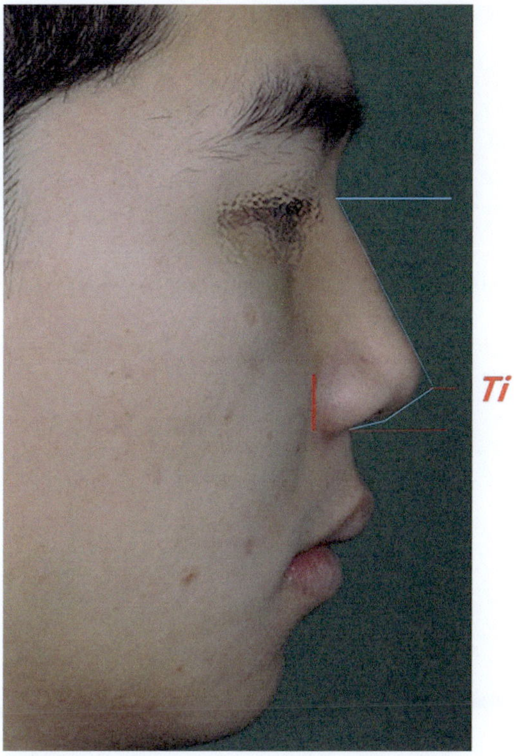

Fig. 3.9 Ideal tip (Ti)

spreader graft (AESG) and the caudal septal extension graft (CSEG). A small amount of superficial mastoid fascia was inserted for dorsal augmentation (Fig. 3.11).

3.5.6 Long-Term Surgical Outcome

The postoperative profile shows improvement, and the septum represents the cartilaginous dorsum (Fig. 3.12).

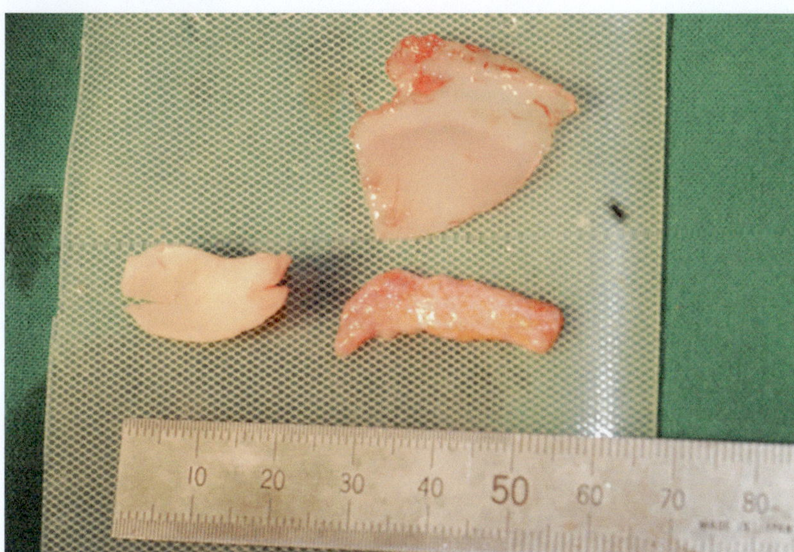

Fig. 3.10 Preparation of autogenous tissue: septum, cymba concha, and superficial mastoid fascia (SMF)

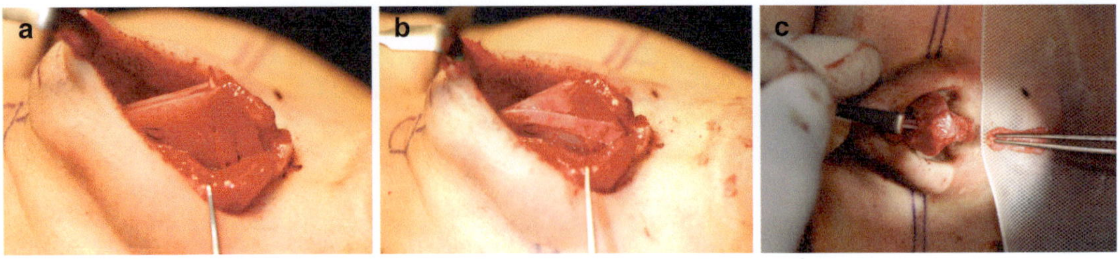

Fig. 3.11 Septal L-strut extension graft (SLEG). (**a**) SLEG, (**b**) raftering graft, (**c**) insertion of SMF

Fig. 3.12 Pre-and postoperative modified lateral view

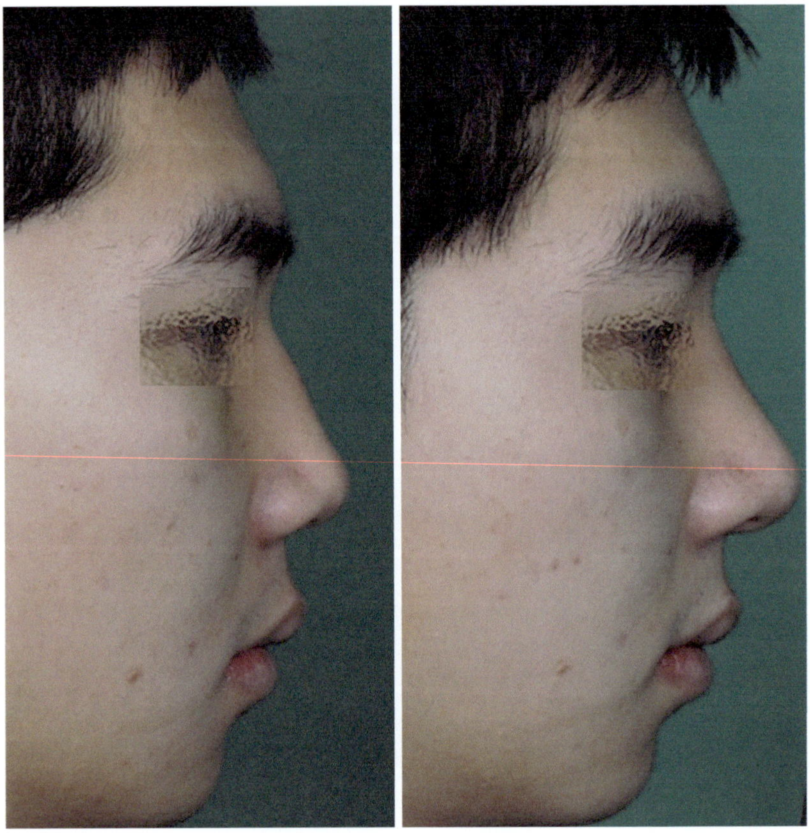

4 Adaptive Planning for Secondary Septorhinoplasty Using Soft Tissue Cephalometry Analysis (STCA)

It is important not to view a secondary rhinoplasty patient as just a single case but to understand the entire situation. When planning surgery, only realistic goals should be set. Before preparing this chapter, the author wants to mention the difficulties of Asian secondary rhinoplasty briefly. The challenges of Asian secondary septorhinoplasty are so significant that they cannot be generalized through patient analysis and surgery.

The burden is unimaginable compared to Western reduction rhinoplasty. Emphasizing that the mental state analysis of the patient is even more important than preoperative image analysis, it is crucial to recognize the significant suffering of these patients. Understanding them and identifying any mistakes made by previous physicians are essential in formulating a surgical plan.

4.1 Body Dysmorphic Disorder (BDD) in Aesthetic Rhinoplasty

Body Dysmorphic Disorder (BDD) is found in approximately 5% of individuals seeking cosmetic surgery. BDD is a type of obsessive-compulsive disorder characterized by the individual having a normal appearance but perceiving themselves as unattractive. Among those desiring rhinoplasty, the prevalence of BDD is reported to be around 20% in one report. Patients wishing for nasal surgery exhibit slightly different self-esteem characteristics than those seeking other cosmetic procedures. Another study from a decade ago found that approximately one-third of patients who undergo rhinoplasty for aesthetic reasons are found to suffer from body dysmorphic disorder (BDD) [1]. Another broadcaster's study found that also indicated that among patients undergoing rhinoplasty due to breathing difficulties, only 2% were diagnosed with BDD. In contrast, approximately 43% of patients who had the surgery for cosmetic purposes were found to suffer from BDD. Interestingly, a clear distinction is observed between patients who have achieved satisfactory outcomes from rhinoplasty without BDD and those with mild psychiatric symptoms of BDD who have yet to undergo the procedure [2].

Simplifying this, it appears, based on the author's experience, that deciding to undergo rhinoplasty requires a more significant commitment compared to other surgeries, possibly due to the nose's central facial position and the frequent encounters with one's reflection throughout the day, underscoring the procedure's gravity. Patients with BDD tend to exhibit higher levels of depression and anxiety. The author does not imply that all patients requiring secondary surgery suffer from BDD. Instead, the paradox lies in the fact that inappropriate prior surgery can lead to the development of BDD in patients.

E. S. Dhong, *Asian Septorhinoplasty*, https://doi.org/10.1007/978-981-96-6127-5_4

4.2 Multiple Surgical Histories in Secondary Rhinoplasty: There Always Is a "Black Hole" in a Particular Stage

Patients opting for secondary rhinoplasty may have higher expectations for perfection, demonstrate greater meticulousness, and exhibit increased sensitivity compared to those seeking other cosmetic surgeries.

Given the significant prevalence of BDD among individuals considering rhinoplasty, it is prudent to conduct a psychiatric assessment before surgery. However, in reality, the experience and intuition of the final rhinoplasty surgeon are the most important insurance policy. Consequently, the surgeon's expertise and intuition become the paramount safeguard against unnecessary procedures and ensure patient satisfaction.

Addressing the complex issues surrounding secondary patients, it is overly simplistic to attribute patients' mental distress solely to the worsening of BDD or other psychiatric conditions. The extent of secondary deformities frequently surpasses mere cosmetic dissatisfaction, reaching physical impairment.

Repeated unsatisfactory surgeries or the presence of deformities can lead to a progressive problem, pushing patients toward a detrimental path of doctor shopping and self-education. A significant challenge in cosmetic surgery lies within the variability of surgical outcomes, as the lack of standardized methods can perpetuate ongoing patient issues. The situation is further complicated when multiple surgeons offer divergent opinions, exacerbating the problem. Establishing rapport with these patients requires a level of psychiatric counseling that is altogether different.

Let's consider a hypothetical scenario involving a typical patient. This patient, seeking aesthetic improvement, has undergone multiple rhinoplasty procedures. The initial surgery was motivated by a desire for a more pleasing nasal appearance. However, dissatisfaction with the results led to a second surgery, which, instead of rectifying the issues, introduced new complications. And the materials and methods used were disagreeable.

Various alloplastic materials have been used, and with the advent of full-scale septal surgery, the scope of the operations has expanded. Surgery that damages the nasal framework was performed. Unfortunately, this procedure resulted in significant infection postoperatively, causing both functional and aesthetic impairments. The nose began to shorten, eventually making a third operation necessary.

Despite these setbacks, the patient pursued a third surgery, hoping to achieve the desired outcome finally. The operative notes were more common than the second method. As a result, the patient faced not only physical discomfort but also psychological distress, feeling compelled to seek further aesthetic improvement. The cumulative effect of these surgeries has exhausted the septal cartilage and both concha cartilages, requiring the harvest of the seventh rib from the right side.

The patient, now unable to live without wearing a mask, has quit the job and has been confined to their home for a year, suffering from severe depression and descending into social impoverishment. A settlement was reached with the hospital where the third surgery was performed, resulting in compensation that was double the cost of the surgery. However, legal proceedings against the hospital responsible for the final surgery are still underway. The surgeon's insurance company is negotiating a settlement that includes surgery costs.

This situation prompts critical questions: Who bears greater responsibility, the second or the third surgeon? Moreover, is the patient's suffering a consequence of body dysmorphic disorder (BDD), or does the surgeon hold accountability for the deformities that emerged post the third surgical intervention?

Complicating matters, each subsequent surgery increased the risk of complications and diminished the likelihood of a successful outcome. The patient's persistent pursuit of an ideal appearance, despite mounting challenges, raises questions about post-surgical psychological factors.

This scenario underscores the complexities of cosmetic surgery, highlighting the importance of thorough pre-surgical evaluations, including psychological assessments, to identify patients who may be at risk of adverse outcomes due to underlying mental health issues. It also emphasizes the need for clear communication between surgeons and patients about realistic expectations and potential risks associated with repeated surgeries.

However, the author's perspective differs slightly. It is inferred that the second surgery, which caused a critical impairment to the patient, likely had significant issues with the technique and materials used. The author, having encountered numerous such cases, concurs that there must be a "black hole"—a gap in the standard of care—among the intervening surgeons. Despite facing numerous lawsuits, these doctors continue to perform surgeries in the same manner or, in some cases, have moved their practices abroad, continuing to tarnish the nation's reputation.

4.2.1 Ambivalent Feelings: Resentment, Sympathy, and Self-Doubt

Even a brief history from two to three patients with severe deformities can be incredibly burdensome for a surgeon, consuming extensive time and effort. Moreover, a well-established rapport does not necessarily predict favorable outcomes. Maintaining a stable, disease-free state ultimately demands more objective and safer approaches.

Even if a surgeon succeeds in 100 secondary surgeries, a single failure can significantly tarnish their overall reputation, presenting an undue challenge.

Doctors tasked with correcting such adverse some doctor's outcomes often experience mixed emotions. Naturally, no one is compelled to take on such a challenge if they feel it is beyond their capacity due to the difficulty involved. However, the situation is different when my specialty is secondary rhinoplasty; in such cases, the responsibilities inherent to my profession come to the forefront.

From the standpoint of performing complex surgeries, one typically experiences two predominant emotions: resentment toward the previous surgeon and, more significantly, sympathy for the patient's condition. However, the predominant feeling in the medical field is self-doubt, questioning whether another surgery could make the patient happier and if the patient can endure the process while maintaining a good rapport until improvement is seen.

Surgeons, of course, operate with the best intentions, but there is always an element of uncertainty regarding the patient's mental state. This situation evokes the concept of "selective decision-making" from Eastern philosophy, often relying on the surgeon's intuition. The structure where the last surgeon bears all responsibility is problematic. Who will bear this challenging burden? A decade ago, criticizing a fellow surgeon's poor outcomes was unheard of, but the burden on the final surgeon has become excessively heavy. A shift toward holding the surgeon who performed the initial problematic surgery accountable is necessary, as they may continue using risky methods, rationalizing that the rare complications they cause are unavoidable incidents. This denial of responsibility for complications due to incorrect methods is concerning. It's essential to acknowledge the possibility of another surgeon having to perform a subsequent surgery and ensure that such a procedure remains feasible.

4.2.2 The Difficulty of the Analysis

Planning for secondary operations can be exceedingly challenging. Due to the myriad of potential variables, it is often only through direct observation during surgery that one can make an informed decision. It is essential to communicate to the patient that, despite any preliminary agreements, the surgical approach may vary based on the intraoperative findings, considering the numerous possibilities.

A critical decision involves determining whether to proceed with septal surgery or to opt against it. Following this, planning for the use of alloplastic materials is paramount. Should there be a need to remove an already implanted material, a comprehensive strategy must be in place to maintain or enhance volume and stability post-removal, incorporating various contingencies.

Since it is difficult to generalize these challenging patients, this chapter will focus on how implants change the analysis and the issues in determining Si and Subi, as mentioned in the previous chapter, using two patient cases as examples.

4.3 A Hands-on Analysis of a Foreshortened Nose

4.3.1 Chief Complaint of the Patient

A 42-year-old female presented with a foreshortened nose. Ten years before her visit, she had undergone surgery using silicone, and this was her fourth operation. She sought consultation as her nose appeared progressively shortening, and she complained of excessive visibility of her nostrils.

4.3.2 Discussions with Patients

She wanted surgery using autologous tissue and aimed to remove the dorsal implant. Her nose was very firm, and she was unaware of the specific type of silicone that had been inserted. Considering the expected difficulty of dissection and the presence of firm scarring, and given that the septum had already been utilized and was no longer available, a plan was made to use rib cartilage for a septal L-strut extension graft.

4.3.3 STCA Using 2D Photograph

4.3.3.1 Ideal Sellion

A lateral nasal X-ray showed that the sellion was below the nasion (Fig. 4.1). This displacement was caused by an L-type silicone implant, which contributed to the appearance of a shortened nose. The rib cartilage was repositioned to restore the sellion to its original location at the nasion.

Therefore, the silicone was removed to position the ideal sellion (Si) posteriorly and elevate it toward the nasion. This adjustment allowed the sellion to be positioned posteriorly relative to the most anterior point of the glabella (Fig. 4.2).

4.3.3.2 Determination of the Length of the Nose

Shortening of the nose was observed in both the frontal and lateral views of the patient. The subnasale was positioned higher than the lower two-thirds point between the sellion and stomion, and it was decided to lower it.

4.3.3.3 Ideal Subnasale

To increase the length of the nose, it was decided to extend the subnasale downward (Fig. 4.3).

4.3.3.4 Ideal Tip

The patient disliked the appearance of an overly lifted nose, so special attention was given to this concern. During dissection, care was taken to ensure that the columella-labial angle could achieve 105° within the possible limits. The tip-lobular angle was also set to 15–20° to facilitate a double break (Fig. 4.4).

4.3.4 Preparing the Autogenous Tissue

For slight dorsum augmentation, it was decided to use the diced rib cartilage and the rectus fascia to augment from the sellion to the supratip after removing the silicone.

4.3.5 Surgical Outcome

Rib cartilage was used for septal L-strut extension graft (SLEG), and the postoperative modified lateral view is as follows (Fig. 4.5).

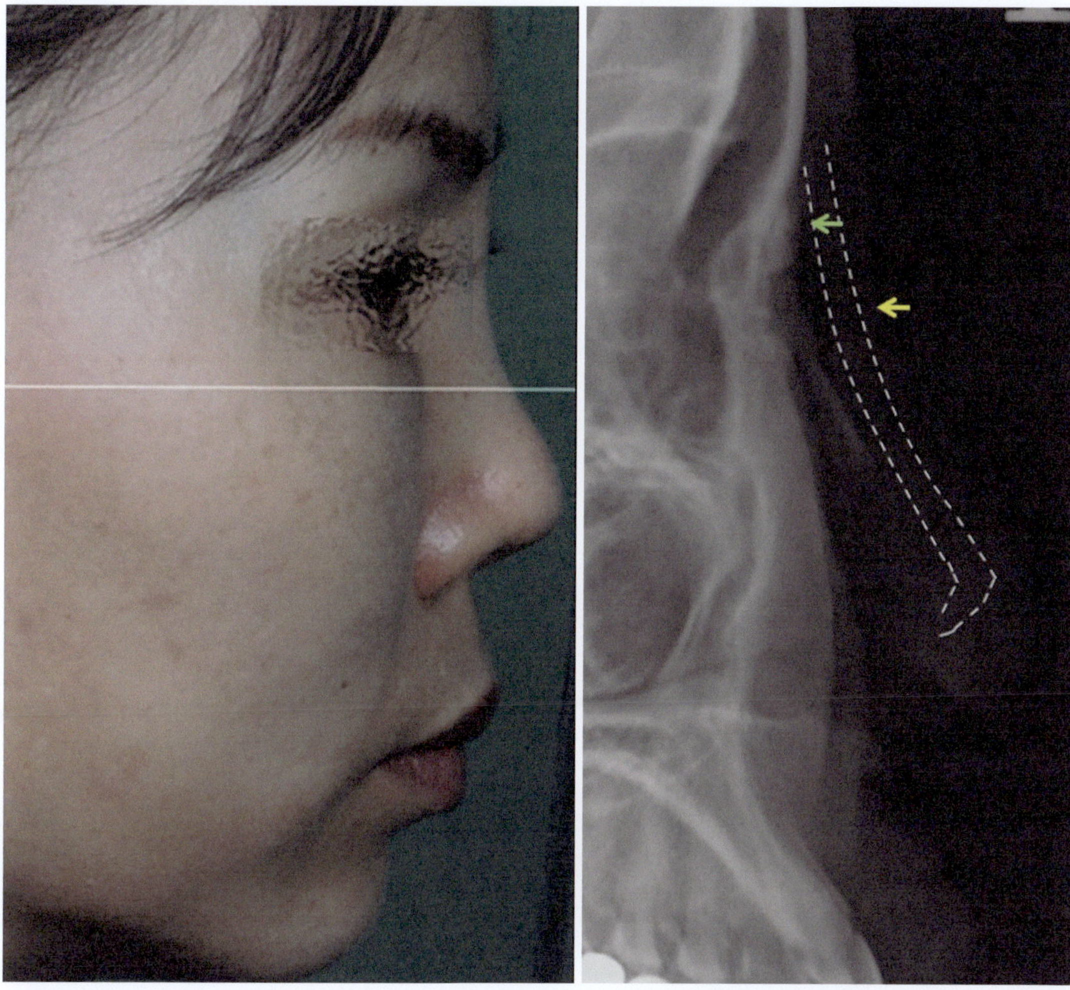

Fig. 4.1 Short nose deformity. (Left) Modified lateral view. (Right) X-ray shows an L-type silicone implant: nasion (green arrow) and sellion (yellow arrow)

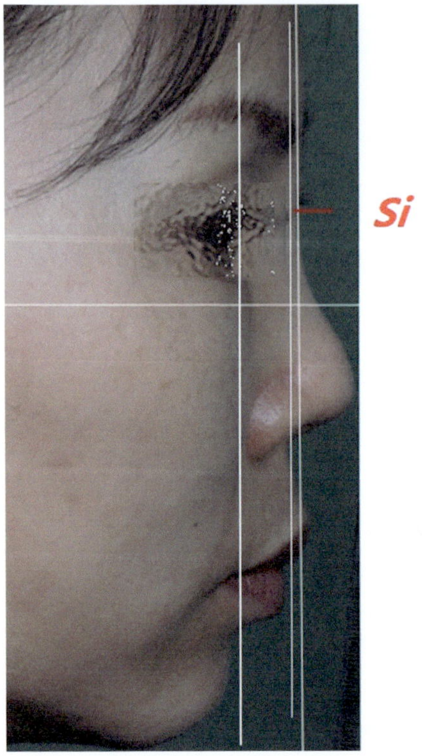

Fig. 4.2 Two STCA points: ideal sellion (Si)

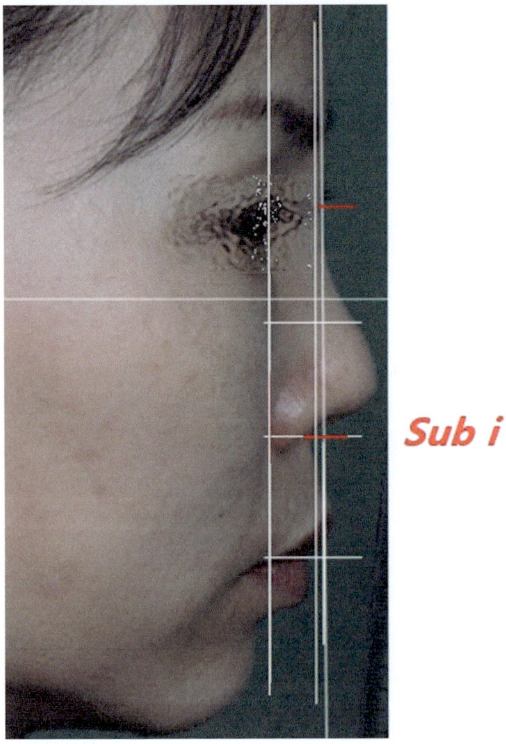

Fig. 4.3 Ideal subnasale (Subi)

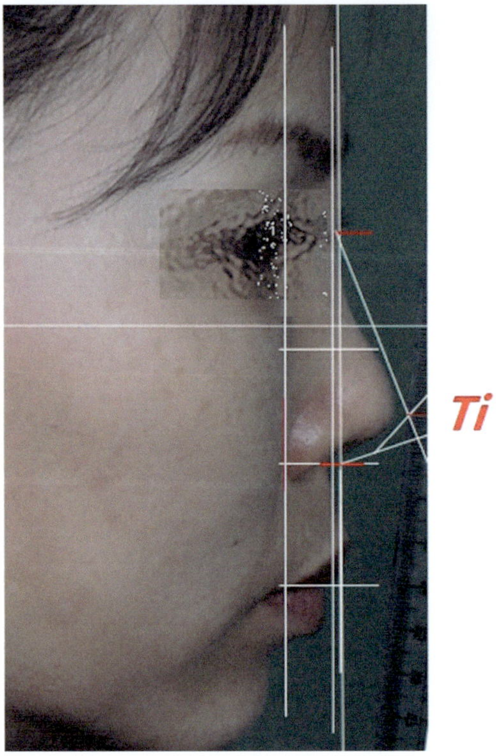

Fig. 4.4 Ideal tip (Ti)

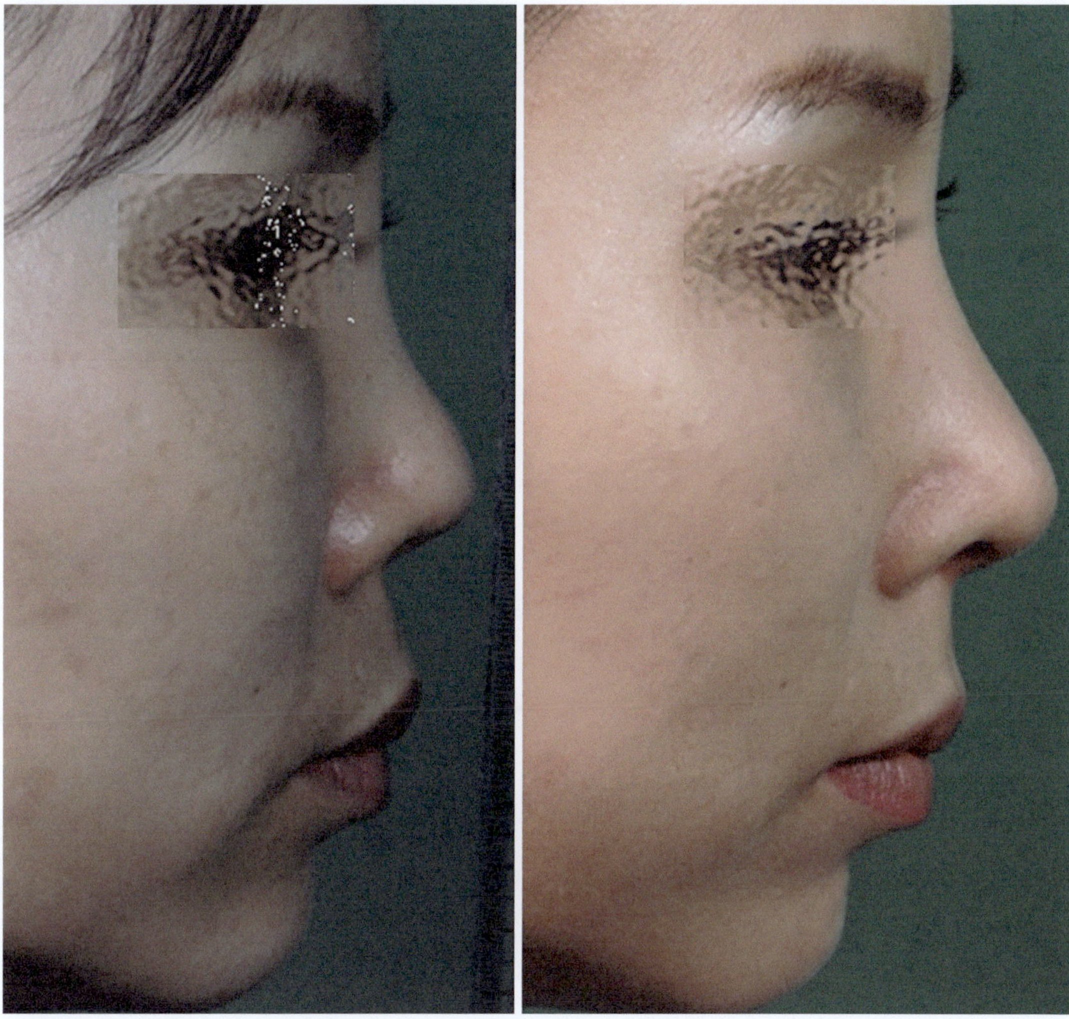

Fig. 4.5 Pre- and postoperative modified lateral view

4.4 A Hands-on Analysis of a Long Nose After Implantation

4.4.1 Chief Complaint of the Patient

A 50-year-old female presented with an aging nose and desired to improve her overall profile. She preferred a shorter nose. The patient reported undergoing rhinoplasty using silicone 25 years prior without any septal surgery. She desired a straightforward procedure and did not consent to using autologous tissue grafts from areas other than her ears.

4.4.2 Discussions with Patients

She wished to correct her elongated nose and desired increased tip projection to enhance the overall profile of the nasal tip.

4.4.3 STCA Using 2D Photograph

4.4.3.1 Ideal Sellion

The sellion was located superiorly compared to the existing nasion. The ideal sellion (Si) goal was set to 1–2 mm inferiorly (Figs. 4.6 and 4.7).

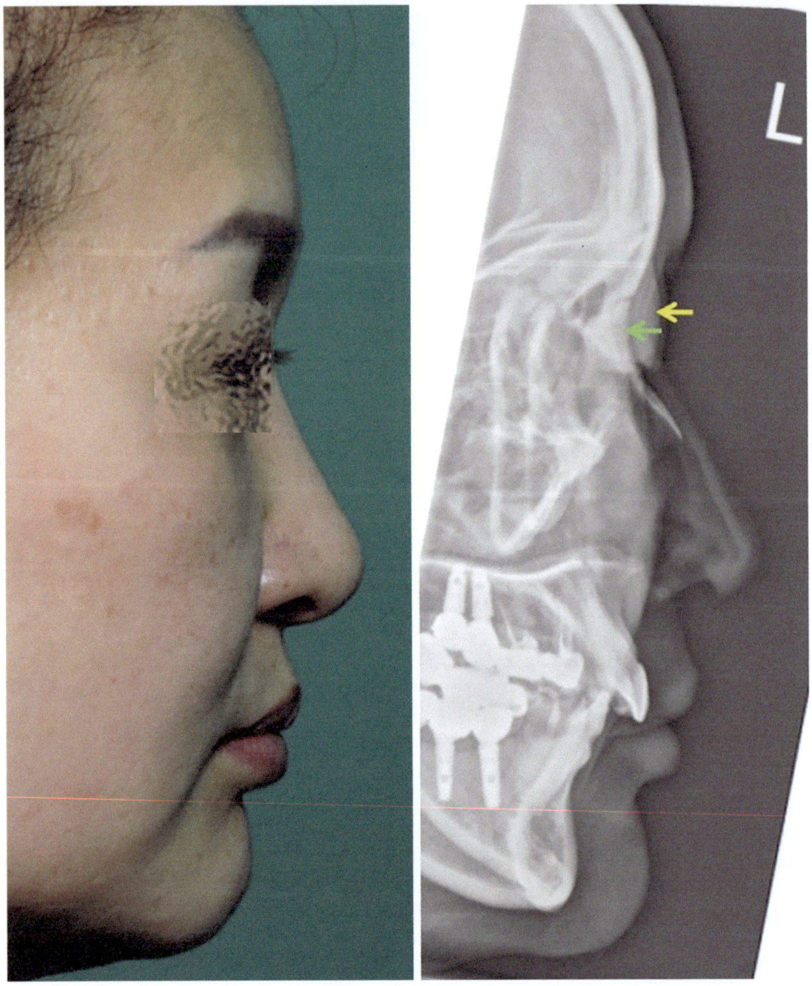

Fig. 4.6 Long nose deformity. (Left) Modified lateral view. (Right) X-ray shows an I-type silicone implant: nasion (green arrow) and sellion (yellow arrow)

4.4.3.2 Ideal Subnasale

The focus was on reducing the length of the nose while enhancing tip projection. Augmentation of the lower two-thirds of the dorsum was achieved through an extension of the cartilaginous septum, but it was decided to shorten the subnasale superiorly (Fig. 4.7).

4.4.3.3 Ideal Tip

The ideal angle for the tip was set at 105 degrees from the perpendicular of the subnasale to the nasolabial angle. Special care was taken as the patient disliked the appearance of an overly upturned nose. The tip-lobular angle was established at 25 degrees to allow for a double break (Fig. 4.8).

4.4.4 Preparing the Autogenous Tissue

For the dorsum, a 3 mm-thick silicone implant was decided on. An L-strut extension graft using cavum concha and cymba concha cartilage was planned for tip projection, followed by implanting on the dorsum. This case involves the removal and replacement of silicone with another silicone implant. When considering the insertion of silicone after a septal L-strut extension, the amount and angle of the implant should be adjusted according to the surgical goals. The use of an autogenous graft to define the tip remains unchanged.

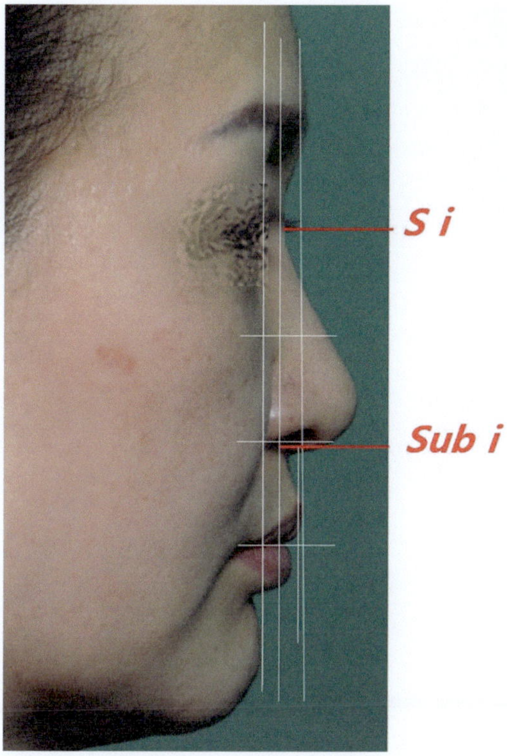

Fig. 4.7 Two STCA points: ideal sellion (Si) and ideal subnasale (Subi)

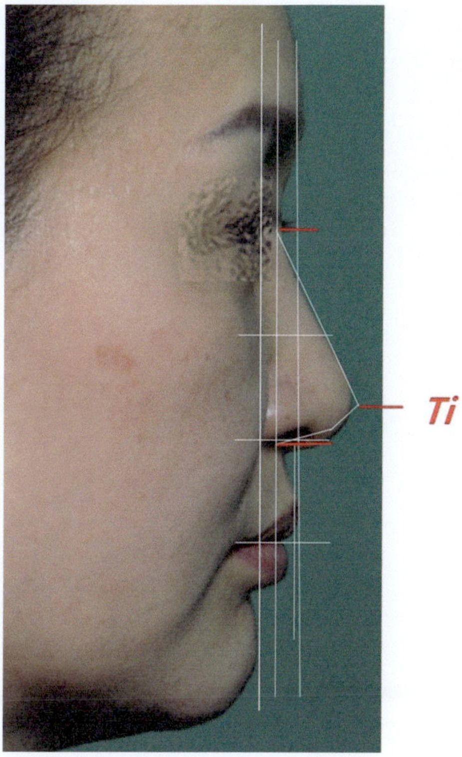

Fig. 4.8 Ideal tip (Ti)

This chapter focuses on the planning of the surgery. Detailed techniques will be described in subsequent chapters.

4.4.5 Long-Term Outcome

This is the modified lateral view after the surgery (Fig. 4.9).

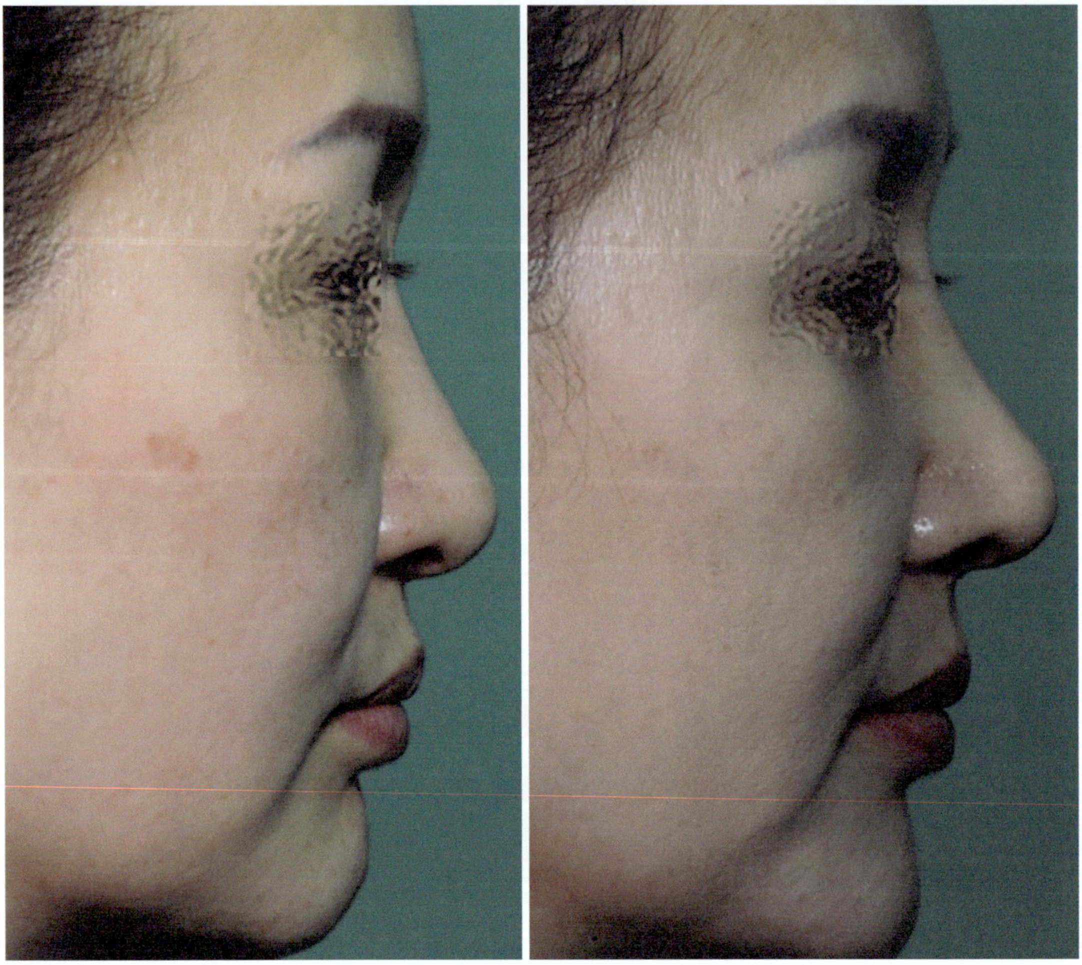

Fig. 4.9 Pre- and postoperative modified lateral view

References

1. Mr F, A GT, A FB, Sa N, A M. Body dysmorphic disorder in aesthetic rhinoplasty candidates. Pak J Med Sci Q. 2013;29:197–200.
2. Veale D, De Haro L, Lambrou C. Cosmetic rhinoplasty in body dysmorphic disorder. Br J Plast Surg. 2003;56:546–51.

Part II
Primary Nose

5 Asian Septoplasty: SMR with Caudal Swinging Door

Pearls

- Asian septal surgery encompasses two primary techniques: submucosal resection (SMR) for cartilage harvesting and the "swinging door procedure" to straighten the residual caudal septum.
- A critical consideration is determining whether a patient will benefit more from SMR despite the potential risk of compromising the structural integrity of the L-strut.
- Upon physical examination, patients exhibiting a soft nasal tip without detectable tip rigidity may indicate an overall underdeveloped cartilage structure.
- In small or short noses, the caudal end of the septal cartilage tends to be markedly short, rendering the expectation of substantial septal cartilage harvest from such noses unrealistic.
- When expecting too small quadrangular cartilage, it needs to be harvested with its junction to the ethmoidal perpendicular plate (EPP) intact.
- The integrity of the membranous septum is crucial for successful cartilage grafting, necessitating meticulous dissection to prevent mucosal tears.
- In applying a septal extension graft (SEG), beginning with bilateral reinforcement of the caudal septum is crucial to extend the L-strut effectively. Ensuring robust midline stability at this stage is essential for the success of the procedure.
- In secondary rhinoplasty, an explanting implant frequently reveals a masked saddle nose deformity, which may result from implant pressure and the prior septal harvest.

5.1 Asian Septoplasty: SMR with Caudal Swinging Door

In the early twentieth century, Dr. Freer and Dr. Killian pioneered the submucosal resection (SMR) technique to alleviate nasal obstruction by excising the protruding sections of the nasal septum. However, in Asian countries, this procedure is often performed not only for nasal obstruction but also to harvest cartilage for grafting purposes, regardless of the presence of obstruction.

When addressing septal deviation, the technique evolves with Dr. Metzenbaum's "swinging door" procedure, which builds upon the SMR approach. This advanced method involves preserving a portion of the septum post-SMR, specifically, the caudal part of the L-strut. The preserved caudal septum is then mobilized in a swinging door fashion to correct the deviation.

Supplementary Information The online version contains supplementary material available at https://doi.org/10.1007/978-981-96-6127-5_5.

E. S. Dhong, *Asian Septorhinoplasty*, https://doi.org/10.1007/978-981-96-6127-5_5

- Septal surgery in Asian contexts typically combines two key components: the SMR technique for cartilage harvesting and the caudal “swinging door” procedure for correcting any remaining deviation in the caudal septum, ensuring both functional and structural integrity of the nasal framework.

Dr. Cottle originally developed the conservative septoplasty technique, also known as septal reconstruction, to respond to the limitations associated with submucosal resection. Specifically, conservative septoplasty was introduced to address the issues of central mucosal contracture and the consequential saddle nose deformity, which are complications stemming from tissue retraction in traditional SMR procedures [1].

For most patients not seeking to alter the external nose morphology, Dr. Cottle’s technique, which emphasizes the preservation of the quadrangular cartilage and enhancing the cartilage’s natural shape through scoring and morselization, is ideally suited for addressing nasal obstruction. However, the primary motivation for Asian patients undergoing plastic surgery often lies in enhancing the aesthetics of the external nose, necessitating more complex procedures. The challenge in these cases stems from the need to maintain the structural integrity of the L-strut to ensure nasal strength while simultaneously harvesting septal cartilage for grafting purposes. If there’s a risk of weakening the L-strut, concurrent measures must be taken to reinforce it.

This chapter will delve into the methodologies for safely harvesting septal cartilage, the techniques for utilizing the harvested cartilage to reinforce the nasal structure, and the intricacies of septal surgery aimed at improving the anterior projection of the primary nose.

- The crucial consideration is determining whether a patient will benefit more than the risk of undergoing submucosal resection.

5.2 When Septal Cartilage Is Needed: Will SMR Benefit the Patient?

Thin septal cartilage offers limited utility. Its minimal contribution as a graft material also diminishes the support to the residual L-strut post-harvest. Weak quadrangular cartilage, besides being suboptimal for grafting, can compromise septal support, potentially jeopardizing the structural integrity of the nose. Therefore, patients with frail septal cartilage should consider SMR only in cases of significant nasal obstruction. Opting for ear cartilage as a substitute for septal cartilage is advisable, even in primary surgical procedures.

- Upon physical examination, patients with a soft nasal tip, characterized by a lack of palpable cartilage stiffness, often indicate weak cartilage, including the septal cartilage.
- A method to assess cartilage flexibility involves using the tip of a freer elevator or swab to gently probe the nasal cavity through the opposite nostril, observing for any flutter of the cartilage.
- In small or short noses, the caudal end of the septal cartilage tends to be very short, making it unrealistic to expect a significant amount of septal cartilage to be harvested from the EPP junction.
- Determining the exact size of the septal cartilage through CT imaging can be challenging, complicating pre-surgical planning.

5.3 Post-SMR Strategies: Balancing Nasal Obstruction Correction with Aesthetic Considerations and Caudal Septal Support

Submucosal resection invariably compromises the septum’s residual structural support. Following the septal harvest, a strategy for reinforcing the weakened L-strut is essential.

In cases where a caudal swinging door procedure is applied to the remaining L-strut post-SMR, particularly in patients with a deviated nose or columellar tilt, the integrity of the entire L-strut depends on the structural support provided by the connection between the anterior nasal spine (ANS) and the keystone area. As such, careful planning is required to reinforce and preserve the remaining L-strut's strength.

- Submucous dissection for SMR is ideally performed unilaterally, ensuring that it remains connected to an L-strut with some mucoperichondrium intact. While it is feasible to harvest septal cartilage after extensively removing the mucosal flap on both sides, such detachment significantly reduces the strength of the remaining L-strut.
- Regarding the dimensions of the L-strut, a conservative approach is to retain a width of at least 12 mm, which enhances safety by preserving structural integrity. However, this raises the question of whether the remaining 12 mm yields sufficient graft material.

The septal size in Asian populations is generally smaller than in Western counterparts, which naturally limits the dimensions of the harvested septal cartilage. Traditionally, even when preserving a width of 10 mm or more for safety, the actual size of the harvested septal cartilage often needs to be 20 x 20 mm [2]. Consequently, as this book outlines, a septum measuring around 15 mm in length is insufficient for use as a spreader graft or an extended spreader graft.

- Masked saddle nose deformity, frequently discovered incidentally during secondary rhinoplasty following implant removal, is attributed to the septal harvest during the initial surgery.
- The weakening of the caudal region, observed after the caudal swinging door technique post-harvest, warrants attention. Reinforcing the area between the posterior septal angle and the anterior nasal spine often proves challenging with sutures alone. Therefore, considering even a minimal graft is advisable to ensure adequate structural support.

5.4 Submucous Resection Attaching with EPP

The septal L-strut extension graft (SLEG) technique described in this book necessitates cartilages sized with a minimum length of 20 mm for practical application. Consequently, the author's primary approach involves harvesting septal cartilage to ensure the acquisition of a length that meets or exceeds this requirement.

- Measurement of the distance from the caudal margin to the ethmoid perpendicular plate (EPP)—quadrangular cartilage junction is essential intraoperatively.
- Preoperative CT imaging is essential to assess the thickness of the EPP and the extent of osteogenesis.
- Consider the scenario where the quadrangular cartilage is harvested with its junction intact to the EPP. In such cases, a small oscillating saw will be suitable for safe cutting through the dense EPP.
- If the EPP found on CT is thin, the McCollough elevator can harvest the connected septum without a significant fracture of the EPP.

If the quadrangular cartilage and the EPP are harvested independently, their utility diminishes, and the subsequent repair process becomes time-consuming. It is crucial to approach the harvesting process with precision from the outset. Multiple drill holes should be created in the harvested EPP to aid in future repairs (Fig. 5.1).

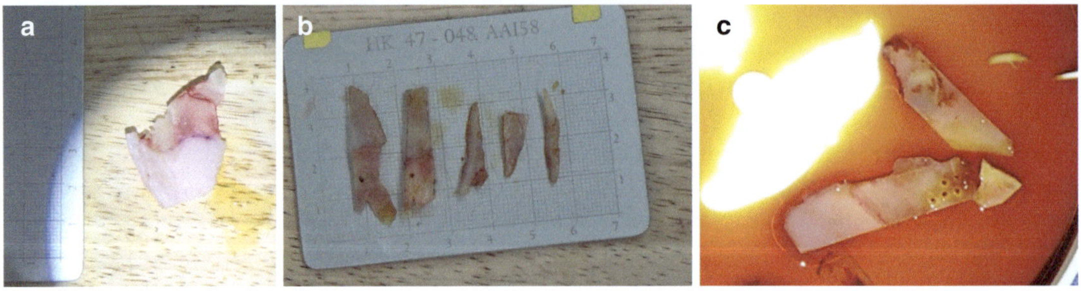

Fig. 5.1 Quadrangular cartilage harvested with EPP. (**a**) Quadrangular cartilage harvested in connection with EPP. (**b**) A single drill hole is made to a thick EPP for repair at the keystone area. A small wedge was made to fit in the caudal border of the nasal dorsum. (**c**) Multiple drill holes for future repairs

5.5 Caudal Swinging Door Technique: One Figure of "8" Suture Is Not Sufficient for Asians

The approaches to reinforcement can be bifurcated into a figure of the "8" procedure and the septal batten graft. The choice between implementing both techniques concurrently or opting for a singular approach is influenced by the stability and the planned extension method.

Furthermore, the batten graft's configuration can be delineated as unilateral or bilateral. This distinction is based on the posterior septal angle's orientation and the adequacy of its contact with the ANS for support.

Suppose the caudal septum is aligned with the midline above ANS but exhibits convexity or concavity. In that case, it is unnecessary to compromise its stability by conducting a swinging door procedure. Under such circumstances, one viable approach is to apply a batten graft to the concave side.

Suspected overgrowth of the quadrangular cartilage may warrant a caudal swinging door procedure, mainly if the caudal and inferior septal cartilage displacement to one side is observed with ANS and the maxillary crest. Furthermore, reliance on a singular figure-of-eight suture may prove insufficient when aiming for enhanced tip projection. Implementing bilateral caudal batten grafts is a beneficial strategy in such cases. This context underscores the utility of the caudal septal extension graft (CSEG), a technique extensively discussed within this book, offering a valuable surgical adjunct.

5.5.1 Septum and Inferior Turbinate as One Unit

The nasal septum and inferior turbinates function as a cohesive unit. Patients reporting nasal obstruction exhibit swelling or enlargement of the inferior turbinate on the concave side. Removing septal cartilage to rectify this curvature can exacerbate the issue by rendering the swollen turbinate problematic. This phenomenon elucidates why corrections for turbinate hypertrophy typically necessitate concurrent surgical interventions on the inferior turbinates.

Consideration of inferior turbinate surgery as a complementary procedure to septal surgery is prudent. The author advocates for the conservative pursuit of external turbinate fractures and coblation, which can be effectively performed within a few minutes. The mucoperiosteum covering the inferior turbinate is distinguished by its composition of loose connective tissue and a surface layer enriched with inflammatory cells. Beneath this layer lies the cancellous bone, characterized by a fibrous, columnar structure that encases the turbinate artery. Given this anatomical configuration, the efficacy of submucosal turbinectomy may be limited, as the primary target for reduction should be the mucosa.

When comparing radiofrequency-assisted inferior turbinoplasty (RAIT) with microdebrider-assisted inferior turbinoplasty (MAIT), the choice of technique is contingent upon computed tomography (CT) scan findings. The author prefers out-fracture techniques for medial enlargement of the inferior turbinate, whereas RAIT is favored when overdevelopment of the lamina propria is identified. In cases where both conditions coexist, a combined approach of out-fracture and RAIT is employed to achieve optimal outcomes.

5.5.2 Low Dorsum with Septal Deviation

Regardless of the dorsal height, a septal deviation can often be observed, which is mistakenly overlooked because the dorsal profile is not apparent. In short, deflecting the nasal septum poses a more significant challenge in the low nasal dorsum.

Septal surgery is generally not advised for patients with a small nose who do not experience nasal obstruction. Discrepancies between the cartilaginous and bony axes can be addressed by implementing a unilateral spreader graft alongside a lateral nasal osteotomy on one side, followed by the placement of a dorsal implant.

However, the stability of the bony framework and the spreader graft beneath the implant must be substantiated. The outcomes may not significantly differ from those achieved by merely inserting an implant with cosmetic camouflage. Moreover, the benefits may not justify the effort involved.

- Evidence supporting the stability of the bony framework and the spreader graft beneath the implant is limited. Indeed, the effectiveness of such a complex dissection may not proportionately match the effort expended.

If the nose is low, small, and short, the skin pocket for implanting can be very tight. It is advisable to perform an extensive pocket dissection and select an implant with a greater width to ensure coverage beyond the implant's edges. When placed in a constricted pocket, a longer implant may conform more noticeably to the floor's incline, appearing more curved.

5.6 Techniques of SMR and Caudal Swinging Door

5.6.1 The Directions in Septoplasty

The sudden focus on defining the direction of the septum, frequently used throughout this book, is critical for understanding septal surgery. Misalignment during the procedure can lead to significant misunderstandings. The term "high septum" typically refers to the anterior portion of the septum. Conversely, descriptions extend into the cephalocaudal axis for the remaining sections, positioning them posteriorly relative to the anterior segment. It's noteworthy that several textbooks differentiate chondrotomy techniques into "posterior chondrotomy" and "inferior chondrotomy," as highlighted in subsequent discussions. However, this text maintains a consistent terminology across different readers to avoid confusion. It's important to clarify that its placement in a postero cephalic direction renders the term "inferior" inappropriate for describing septal directions. However, in this book, inferior chondrotomy refers to a chondrotomy performed on the vomer side, while posterior chondrotomy refers to a chondrotomy performed on the EPP junction (Fig. 5.2).

5.6.2 Anesthesia: Hydrodissection of Mucosal Flap

Adequate local anesthesia is crucial for septal surgery, necessitating 5–8 precise infiltrations on one side of the septum, ideally with a spinal needle or a similarly long needle. Optimal infiltration is pivotal for facilitating meticulous mucosal dissection. While there are differing viewpoints regarding the use of local anesthesia directly on the septum, the author advocates for its application. For infiltration, the spinal needle must be carefully prepared. To ensure that only the mucosa is penetrated by the obliquely angled needle tip, it should be slightly bent and inserted following the orientation. This technique prevents the needle from passing to the opposite side, causing unintended perforations.

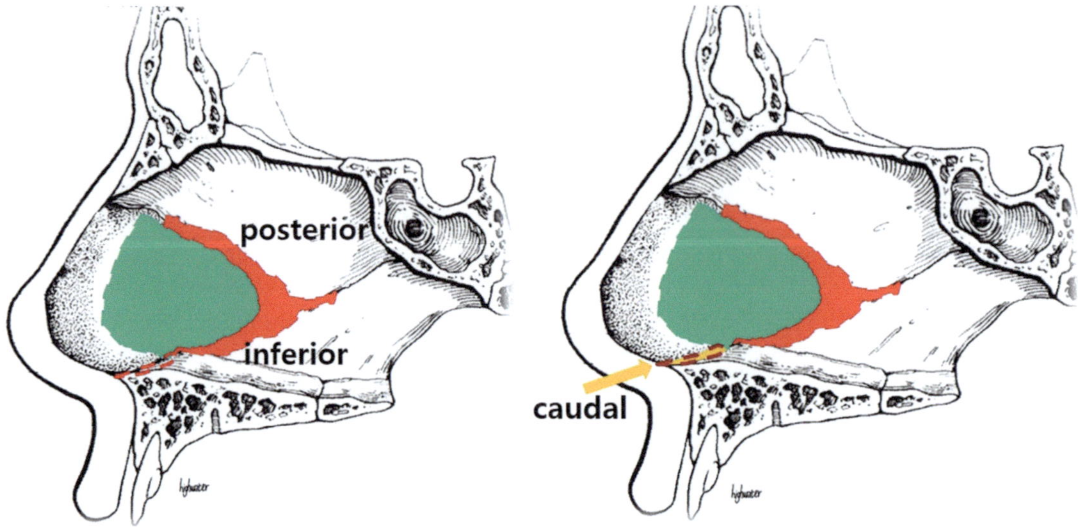

Fig. 5.2 Directions of chondrotomy. (Left) Posterior chondrotomy vs. inferior chondrotomy. (Right) Caudal swing door procedure in yellow, chondrotomy and chondrectomy in red, and SMR in green

The author favors general anesthesia over local anesthesia for septal surgery and in cases of septorhinoplasty lasting more than 3 h. The anesthesia protocol includes the administration of primary anesthesia using two specific types of anesthetic agents, followed by secondary anesthesia administered 10 min before making the incision. This approach ensures adequate hydrodissection for optimal surgical conditions.

- First solution: 0.5% Lidocaine + 1:200,000 Epinephrine + Hyaluronidase < 30 U/mL containing solution
- Second solution: 0.5% Marcaine + 1:100,000 Epinephrine + Hyaluronidase < 30 U/mL containing solution

Multiple anesthetic blocks are placed in the anterior and posterior areas of the septum to block the anterior ethmoidal nerve, nasopalatine nerve, and anterior superior alveolar nerve.

5.6.3 Approach: Open Rhinoplasty Approach

The Killian approach or the modified Killian incision has a limited scope of application. It is suitable for a subset of patients undergoing exclusively septal surgery without the need for open rhinoplasty. However, as discussed in this book, its utility for applying the SLEG technique is nearly impractical. While endonasal spreader grafts are possible, achieving the extended definition of the nose's dorsum and tip through soft tissue release, a central aim of this text, presents significant challenges.

Transfixion incisions are rarely used in Asian rhinoplasty. Their application is mainly confined to cases requiring shortening a long nose.

Selecting a nasoscope with the appropriate width and length facilitates the entire septoplasty. If the width is too broad or the size is too short, it will cause much discomfort during septal surgery (Fig. 5.3).

- The membranous septum is critical for cartilage grafting. Therefore, it is imperative to avoid mucosal tearing during the dissection. A mucosal tearing at the columellar base can be meticulously repaired using 6.0 Vicryl sutures from the inside.

Care should be taken to prevent the invagination of the epidermis during the repair process.

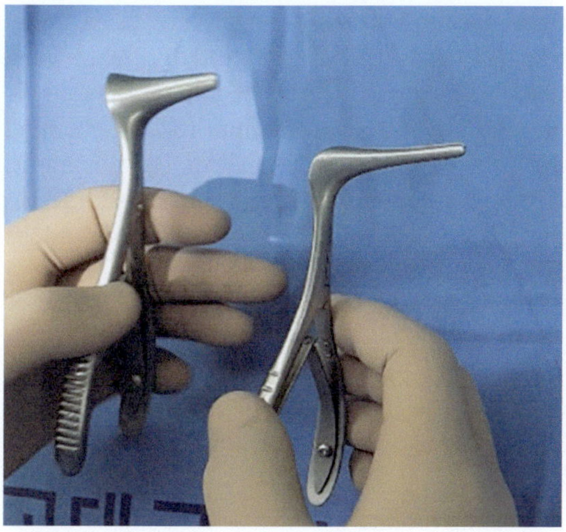

Fig. 5.3 Selection of appropriate nasoscope

5.6.4 Finding Caudal Margin of Septal Cartilage

The caudal margin of the septum can be readily identified by gently spreading and sliding the nasoscope between the bilateral lower lateral cartilages (LLCs). At this juncture, a No. 15 scalpel blade may be utilized to carefully scrape the caudal margin, facilitating the removal of the slippery perichondrium. This step enhances the visibility and accessibility of the caudal end, making subsequent surgical interventions more precise (Video 5.1). Interestingly, locating the caudal end, which typically takes less than a minute in primary procedures, emerges as one of the most challenging aspects of secondary septorhinoplasty. Therefore, this step should be particularly appreciated during primary septorhinoplasty.

For right-handed surgeons, the dissection process is often more comfortable when initiated from the patient's left nasal cavity, leading to the first dissection of the left mucosal flap of the septum. A blunt Freer elevator may be employed at this stage, ensuring that the mucosal flap includes all perichondrial layers and that the septal cartilage is meticulously dissected bare. Achieving a pure subperichondrial dissection is confirmed by the absence of a slippery sensation when the area is gently scraped with a sharp elevator. It is crucial to remain vigilant for the potential presence of one or two additional perichondrial layers and to carefully separate the mucoperichondrium starting from the areas with the most texture (Video 5.2).

5.6.5 Mucosal Flap Elevation: Separation Between ULC and Septum

If the mucosal dissection is carried out cephalically on one side, the perpendicular plate of the ethmoid bone should be readily encountered. Following this, the upper lateral cartilage (ULC) must be detached from the septum. This separation should proceed from the inferior aspect upwards to ensure the preservation and careful peeling of the mucosa (Video 5.3).

In other surgical videos, you might observe scalpels or fine scissors used to directly detach the ULC from the septum. However, this approach risks damaging the anterior portion of mucosa between the septum and ULC. Therefore, once the correct submucosal plane is identified, it is advisable to employ a slightly blunt Freer elevator for dissection, starting from the inferior aspect and moving upwards.

When harvesting a section of the ethmoid perpendicular plate, the Cottle septum elevator or McCollough elevator can effectively fracture and remove the desired amount of thin EPP. In cases where the EPP is thick, cutting the bone with an elevator or scissors may prove challenging. Under such circumstances, osteotomizing the EPP with an oscillating microsaw and a reciprocating microsaw can facilitate more extensive peeling.

5.6.6 Posterior Chondrotomy

Direct dislocation or chondrotomy at the junction between the quadrangular cartilage and the ethmoid perpendicular plate must be executed precisely. It is crucial to avoid disrupting the connection at the rhinion to prevent breakage. Since septal surgery typically precedes osteotomy, understanding the ethmoid perpendicular plate positioning relative to the medial osteotomy on both the left and right sides is essential for maintaining structural stability.

Dissect the EPP with a contralateral dissection for later resection or realignment of the EPP. A portion of the mucosal flap is detached to create a tunnel (Video 5.4).

5.6.7 Inferior Chondrotomy

To achieve sufficient volume for the planned submucous resection, dislocate the quadrangular cartilage from the maxillary crest and liberate the septal cartilage by connecting it to a suitable inferior chondrotomy. Following this procedure, remove any protruding bony spurs from the maxillary crest on both the left and right sides using an appropriate osteotome or Jansen-Middleton forceps (Video 5.5). Removing an excessive amount of the crest may lead to postoperative tingling or paresthesia in the incisors. Any bone bleeding that occurs in this area must be cauterized. In cases where bleeding is difficult to control, it must be effectively managed using bone wax or similar methods.

After performing an inferior chondrotomy, the cartilage should be harvested with care. If there are sites where the cartilage remains attached, these should be meticulously debrided. Applying excessive force during this process could result in unintended breakage.

5.6.8 Remodeling of Bony Deformity

Correcting the convexity of the ethmoid perpendicular plate can be achieved using scissors or by removal with Jansen-Middleton forceps (Video 5.6). However, removing bone should be approached conservatively to avoid compromising the stability of the bony dorsum. The EPP plays a minimal role in nasal physiology. Nasal obstruction typically originates from the anterior inferior site; therefore, excessive osteotomy in this area should be avoided. Applying too much force during fracturing can, in rare cases, cause trauma to the skull base and lead to cerebrospinal fluid (CSF) rhinorrhea. Precision in osteotomy is preferred over manual fracture for straightening the EPP to mitigate the risk of complications. Accurate osteotomy is preferred, and straightening by manual fracture of the EPP should be avoided [3].

5.6.9 Dissection Around the Anterior Nasal Spine (ANS)

Dissecting around the ANS is challenging due to the complex interweaving of the maxillary periosteum and the septal perichondrium. Therefore, it is safer to begin by dissecting the periosteum of the nasal floor and proceeding in an upward direction. This approach helps to navigate the intricate anatomical structures more effectively and reduces the risk of mucosal laceration. This region is particularly susceptible to tearing during surgery, with mucosal tears commonly occurring along the maxillary crest. During the learning phase of septal surgery, lacerations in this area, especially bilateral lacerations of the maxillary crest, are most likely to result in postoperative perforations. It is crucial to clearly understand the attachment relationship between the periosteum and the perichondrium to minimize such complications.

- Since the periosteum is located deeper than the perichondrium, forcefully dissecting from the quadrangular cartilage to the anterior nasal spine (ANS) can be challenging. Attempting to dissect this area from the anterior to the posterior direction can easily result in tearing at the decussation site by beginners (Video 5.7).
- If the patient has previously experienced a dislocation with a laceration due to past trauma and has been asymptomatic, such a mucosal defect might only be discovered during the dissection process.

Even in a bilateral laceration, repairing the mucosa at the membranous septum is relatively straightforward, whereas repairing deeper lacerations poses more difficulty. Repair is not always necessary unless there is a risk of perforation due to a bilateral laceration; if the mucosa remains intact on one side, it may be left as is. However, in cases where bilateral mucosal tears occur in the same area without any mucosal defect, efforts should be made to repair at least one side.

For extensive defects, reconstructive flap surgery on one side, the placement of a wide interposition cartilage graft, or cartilage + perichondrial graft may be recommended to block perforation on both sides and prevent a posterior enlargement. The choice of intervention depends on the size of the mucosal defect. If the defect is minor, silastic sheets should be placed on both sides before nasal packing to prevent the enlargement of the perforation due to the packing. Typically, healing is observed within 3–5 days post-dressing.

5.6.10 Swinging Door Procedure and Fixation of PSA (Posterior Septal Angle)

Secure the PSA and ANS with a figure-of-eight suture. This step marks the beginning of the posterior caudal septal extension repair and must be performed carefully. Conserving some of the periosteum and mucosa surrounding the ANS is crucial. While 4.0 PDS sutures are commonly employed, one or two nonabsorbable sutures might be considered for enhanced stability (Video 5.8).

Directly repairing PSA and the periosteum around the ANS is usually sufficient. However, during secondary surgeries, if only scar tissue remains around the ANS, or if the ANS is exposed following Medpor removal, the periosteum may be completely absent, compromising the stability of the figure-of-eight suture.

When the ANS is significantly deformed, an osteotome may be used on the ANS. Alternatively, if the periosteum and mucosa around the ANS are absent, stability can be achieved by drilling holes on both sides and passing a Keith needle through them [4]. However, threading through bilateral drill holes can be particularly challenging in Asian patients due to the smaller size of the ANS, the thickness of the soft tissue, and the difficulty of creating parallel drill holes. Using too large drill may risk fracturing the ANS before it is repaired. The preferred approach is to retain as much of the periosteum as possible for the repair. Combining the PSA and ANS with a figure of "8" suture is the starting point of the posterior caudal septal extension and should be repaired securely.

5.6.11 Remodeling of Intrinsic Property of Septal Cartilage: Does the Scoring Straighten the Septal Cartilage?

It has been suggested that incising the cartilage and scoring it on the concave side can lead to straightening during the healing process. This technique leverages the inherent tension within the cartilage, allowing it to realign as it heals, potentially correcting deviations or irregularities [5]. In cases of a weakened L-strut following SMR, I have observed that the septum does not straighten on its own if an implant or a tight pocket in the dorsum exerts pressure. In such situations, it invariably necessitates using a batten graft on at least one concave side to ensure proper straightening and stabilization of the septum. There is no expectation that the scored septum will stretch as it heals, overcoming the tight pressure of the dorsum and soft tissue envelope.

5.6.12 Transfixion Suture for Septal Support

Following cartilage harvest, securing the transfixion suture to the septum is as crucial as nasal packing in preventing postoperative complications. This technique is particularly effective in minimizing the risk of hematoma, surpassing even the early coaptation of the mucosal flap in efficacy. Due to the prohibition of Catgut thread in Korea, a 4.0 Vicryl suture with a straight needle is commonly employed for this purpose.

Typically, this suture is applied in two groups: one located in the posterior portion of the columella and the other in the area of the septal harvest. This dual-site approach ensures comprehensive support and stabilization, aiding in the healing process (Video 5.9).

5.7 Packing and External Dressing

5.7.1 Packing

Nasal packing and its effectiveness are subjects of considerable debate within the medical community. The author advocates for its use, initially incorporating gauze with antibiotics, but later discontinuing it. It's important to note that even minor mucosal injuries can lead to mucosal synechiae following the removal of the packing.

A soft sponge material is favored for its ease of removal, offering a gentler alternative to blunt instruments. Products such as Merocel (Medtronic, Xomed, USA) or polyurethane foam (Nasopore, Stryker, Kalamazoo, MI) are preferred. Nasopore notably causes less in situ discomfort, nasal pressure, pain, or bleeding upon removal and exerts less pressure during the packing process.

In Asian practices, using the entire length of the packing material as a single piece is often unnecessary. Therefore, cutting it in half and applying double packing anteriorly, both above and below, is advisable for optimal results.

Before packing, a 2 mm wide penrose drain should be inserted bilaterally at the incision site and left in place for 24 ho before removal. This method is highly effective and advantageous for controlling bleeding, particularly when the patient is recovering from general anesthesia.

5.7.2 External Dressing

The external dressing is just as important as the packing. Particularly when employing an osteotome on the bony dorsum, it's crucial to apply continuous compression from the outside toward the inside. The infracted bone fragment tends to dislocate outwardly during nasal packing. Moreover, paper taping of the skin plays a vital role. Taping is essential for shaping the overall appearance and maintaining skin tension to prevent unwanted stretching.

Following this, aquaplast or thermoplast is shaped into a nasal splint, softened in hot water, and then applied to ensure proper nasal contouring. Applying an aluminum splint is then necessary to sustain external pressure, achieving a balance between the inward force of the packing and the outward force of the external dressing.

Septoplasty procedures may result in the nose appearing lifted or shortened post-packing, which could be an optical illusion caused by immediate post-surgical edema. To counteract the potential counterclockwise tension that may arise immediately after surgery, the author recommends extending a long skin tape from the cephalic side of the aluminum splint down to the cheek. This approach might be particularly unique in Asia, where extensive skin flap dissection and efforts to lengthen the nose are prevalent (Video 5.10).

References

1. Subramaniam V, Basheer M, Hosagadde R. Evolution of correction of the deviated nasal septum—A historical overview. Arch Med Health Sci. 2018;6:293. https://doi.org/10.4103/amhs.amhs_129_18.
2. Kim J-S, Khan NA, Song HM, Jang YJ. Intraoperative measurements of harvestable septal cartilage in rhinoplasty. Ann Plast Surg. 2010;65:519–23.
3. Soni RS, Choudhry OJ, Liu JK, Eloy JA. Postoperative cerebrospinal fluid leak after septoplasty: a potential complication of occult anterior skull base encephalocele. Allergy Rhinol. 2013;4:e41–4.
4. Becker DG. Surgical management of nasal obstruction: facial plastic surgery perspective. Saunders; 2009.
5. Kim B-H, Kim J-Y, Park JS, Kang S-H, Lim DJ, Yu MS. Combined use of scoring incisions and 2-octylcyanoacrylate adhesive during endonasal septoplasty to correct cartilaginous deviations. Am J Rhinol Allergy. 2014;28:209–13.

Septal L-Strut Extension Graft (SLEG)

6

Pearls

- The septal L-strut extension graft (SLEG) has a broad spectrum of primary and secondary septorhinoplasty applications.
- In primary septorhinoplasty, the SLEG is a physiological graft optimally suited for patients with a reasonably structured bony dorsum and a hypoplastic lower two-thirds of the nose. This grafting technique utilizes the septal structure to facilitate the cartilaginous dorsum and tip formation.
- SLEG proves particularly advantageous in projecting the cartilaginous portion of the dorsum without necessitating augmentation of the bony dorsum. This is especially relevant in primary pseudo-hump or mild saddle nose deformities.
- SLEG offers a strategic approach to achieving anterior projection while managing nasal deviation.
- SLEG is universally recommended in secondary septorhinoplasty cases requiring nasal framework reconstruction. This underscores the technique's versatility and utility in addressing various nasal deformities and reconstructive needs.
- The long-term follow-up shows minimal changes in the shape of the cartilaginous dorsum, including the supratip, likely due to orthotopic cartilage grafts in the septum.
- Functionally, SLEG improves the nasal airway, at least at the site of obstruction. SLEG is a suitable technique for Asian autogenous-only septorhinoplasty, which makes the entire nose dependent on the septum.

Supplementary Information The online version contains supplementary material available at https://doi.org/10.1007/978-981-96-6127-5_6.

6.1 Typical Features in Asian Septorhinoplasty

The approach to Asian rhinoplasty encompasses two types: primary rhinoplasty and secondary rhinoplasty, each requiring distinct planning and surgical techniques. As detailed in Chap. 1, primary rhinoplasty in Asian patients can be systematically analyzed using frontal and lateral views. From the lateral perspective in Asian rhinoplasty, patients can be classified into three primary groups: those requiring reduction, those necessitating augmentation, and those who benefit from a combination of both reduction and augmentation procedures. Additionally, from the frontal perspective, cases are classified into deviated and non-deviated noses.

Secondary rhinoplasty requires a tailored approach based on each case's unique circumstances. Although it can be broadly categorized into several types, these classifications serve as a general guide. While the techniques may share similarities with those used in Western rhinoplasty, the specifics often differ significantly due to distinct anatomical and aesthetic considerations.

E. S. Dhong, *Asian Septorhinoplasty*, https://doi.org/10.1007/978-981-96-6127-5_6

6.1.1 Characteristics Indicating the Reduction Techniques

- Generalized hump nose
- Localized hump nose
- Long nose

6.1.2 Indications for Augmentation Techniques

- Small nose
- Short nose
- Saddle nose
- Deviated nose
- Contracted nose

6.1.3 Implementing Reduction and Augmentation Techniques

- Fair bony dorsum with hypoplastic lower 2/3 nose
- Pseudo-hump nose
- Secondary nose (contracted nose)

6.1.4 Generalized Nasal Hump, Localized Nasal Hump, Long Nose Deformity

This is a category where many of the textbooks and techniques published in Western society can be applied. Asian does not require any different methods.

It is essential to acknowledge that the cartilage in the Asian septum is generally less robust than that found in Western populations.

6.1.5 Small Nose, Short Nose

There are two approaches to concealing the septal framework in Asian rhinoplasty with structural correction and without. Reconstructing the entire septal framework in primary surgery is uncommon, particularly in Asian rhinoplasty, where emphasis is often placed on tip refinement. The dorsal aspect, by contrast, is typically augmented using alloplastic materials.

The popular technique has become grafting at the nasal tip combined with silicone augmentation extending from the nasion to the supratip. A contentious point is the advisability of performing SMR for a cartilage donor in cases with limited quadrangular cartilage, often seen in small or short noses. Techniques described in Western textbooks may not be suitable for these scenarios.

Many short noses also present with a low nasion, necessitating careful evaluation before septoplasty. The potential for loss of structural support post-SMR and the value of the harvested small septal cartilage warrant serious consideration. For patients with a septal deviation, this concern is mitigated. In situations where septal surgery is necessitated by obstruction or deviation, this aspect becomes a relatively minor concern, given its indispensability.

While quadrangular cartilage and one concha cartilage harvests are generally acceptable, extensive harvesting, including both sides of conchae, requires careful contemplation.

Rib cartilage grafting at primary rhinoplasty is not preferred in young female patients due to their aversion to scarring and the extensive nature of the surgery. Moreover, mixing donor sites of septum and rib, or concha and rib, is rare and unusual.

The author advises against combining autogenous cartilage with donated rib due to the unpredictability of outcomes and the challenges in achieving precise sculpting with donated rib cartilage. For optimal results, a simpler, more homogeneous donor source is preferable.

The donor choice should always be made concerning the alloplastic implant entering the dorsum.

- When employing a dorsal implant, the authors prefer to limit donor material to one or two ear cartilages, except in cases of septal deviation, to preserve options for potential future revisions.
- SMR should always be executed with utmost effectiveness to maintain the integrity of the L-strut.

- Should the need for rib cartilage arise in primary procedures, it is advisable to conserve ear and septal cartilage for future use.
- The author no longer uses donated rib cartilage due to the risks of resorption and fracture.

6.1.6 Fair Bony Dorsum with Hypoplastic Lower 2/3 Nose

In this book, the author focuses on a patient cohort that exhibits characteristics commonly seen in Asian populations, notably a significantly low nasion. However, the keystone area's dorsal profile is usually high to some extent. Often, these patients present with underdevelopment of the lower two-thirds of the nose, coupled with a desire for enhanced tip projection. Clinically, these cases may manifest as pseudo-hump noses or mild saddle noses with or without deviation, encompassing a substantial segment of the patient population we address.

In primary cases, many Asians can be augmented only at the lower two-thirds of the nose, altering the overall nasal profile. This approach allows for achieving a septum-dependent formation of the remaining dorsum and tip, offering a significant advantage (Fig. 6.1).

Only the segment from the nasion to the rhinion may require dorsal onlay grafting, with the rest of the nasal dorsum constructible through the nasal framework. This method provides a distinct benefit, particularly in addressing the common occurrence of deviated noses, which often exhibit a lower cartilaginous dorsum than the bony dorsum in lateral views. Similar post-septal surgery strategies can be applied to reinforce the lower two-thirds of the framework for both functional and aesthetic concerns.

6.1.7 Secondary Cases

In secondary rhinoplasty, using autologous tissue frequently becomes essential for reconstruction. The SLEG technique, which utilizes autologous tissue for reconstructing the nasal framework, is particularly well suited for such scenarios. However, cases that involve extensive dissection followed by the insertion of

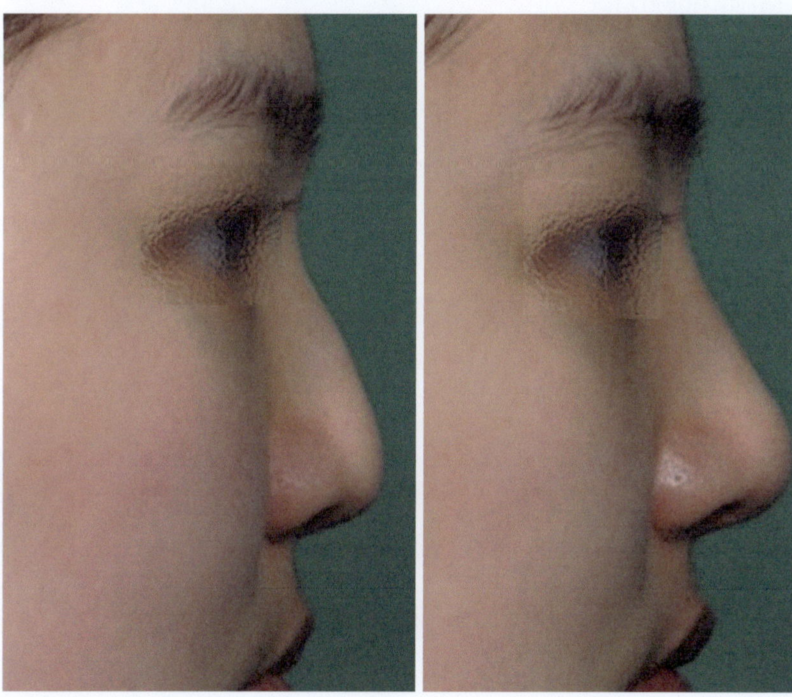

Fig. 6.1 Septal L-strut extension graft (SLEG): Bony dorsum is high, but the lower 2/3 is low in the patient. (Left) Preoperative modified lateral view. (Right) After SLEG surgery

allografts or alloplastic materials often experience stability issues. These situations can lead to severe inflammatory responses, which may result in contractures and significant deformities (Fig. 6.2). Solely placing an implant in the dorsum and bypassing septal surgery can also be the solution; preserving the septum simplifies potential sequelae and often yields promising outcomes. However, complications arising from complex post-septal surgeries cannot be overcome by that camouflage.

Drawing on this evidence, the impetus for writing this book was to outline strategies that mitigate such risks. The proposed solution involves utilizing all available grafting options to construct a robust framework, thereby minimizing the necessity for dorsal implantation and focusing on salvaging the septum. This approach aims to solve the septal problems and improve the overall success rate of secondary rhinoplasties.

6.2 Indications for Septal L-Strut Extension Graft (SLEG)

6.2.1 Indications of SLEG in Primary Surgery

- Every nose with hypoplastic lower 2/3
- Severely deviated nose
- Deviated nose with an under-projected tip
- Saddle nose with an under-projected tip
- Short nose and a small nose

6.2.2 Indications of SLEG in Secondary Surgery

- Contracted nose
- Patients in need of nasal framework reconstruction for functional issues
- Antero-caudal septal defect resulting from previous surgery

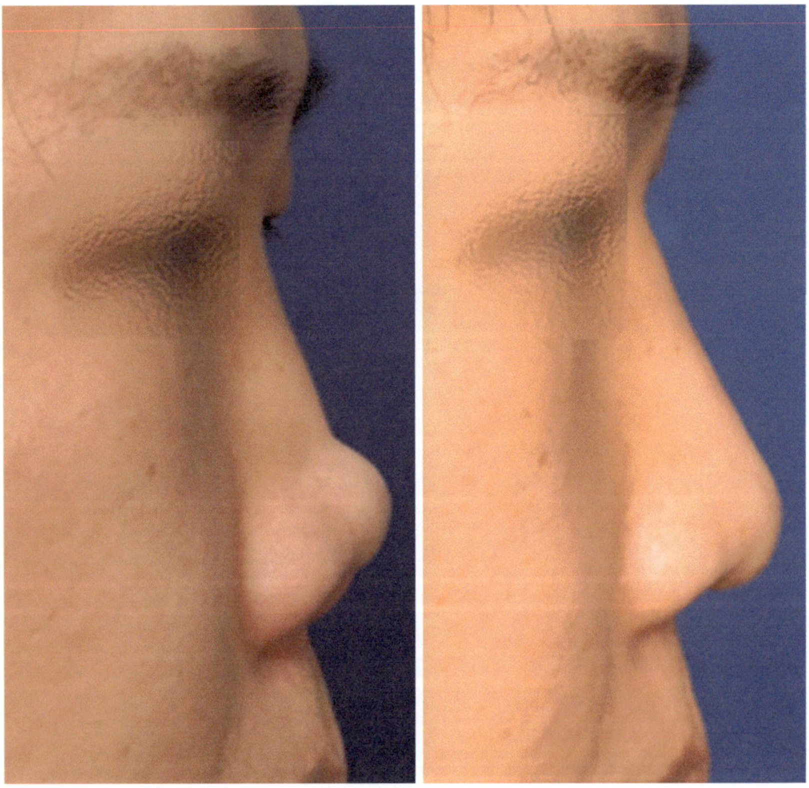

Fig. 6.2 Severe destruction of the septal framework due to multiple failures. (Left) Contracted nose deformity. (Right) After SLEG surgery

6.3 Techniques

6.3.1 Preparation of Graft

In preparing grafts for rhinoplasty, meticulous attention is devoted to crafting the caudal septal extension graft (CSEG) and the anterior extended spreader graft (AESG). The dimensions of each graft are crucial, as they are tailored to achieve the desired height of the nasal tip and the overall length of the nose. Specifically, in the context of the Asian demographic, where the lower two-thirds of the nasal structure is a common focal point, the graft sizes differ by gender. For men, the AESG typically requires a length of 20–25 mm and a width of at least 8–10 mm, while in female patients, the required length and width are slightly reduced. The width and length of grafts are based on the author's experience, emphasizing the need for more precision in lowering the ideal subnasale position and enhancing the dorsal profile of the lower two-thirds. It is noted that a width of AESG exceeding 10 mm in the high septum area can extend toward the inferior part of the nasal roof, which might reduce the volume of the nasal cavity, leading to complaints of nasal obstruction.

When preparing septal cartilage, a minimum length of 20 mm is essential to ensure adequate structural support. When the available length is insufficient, parts of the ethmoid perpendicular plate (EPP) might be necessary, albeit cautiously. Preoperative planning with computed tomography scans to assess the thickness of the EPP is advised, as harvesting from a thick EPP can be challenging.

It is preferable for CSEG to have a length and width smaller than AESG. Considering the most commonly used dimensions of a folded cymba, the length should be within 20 mm, and the width should be about 5–7 mm to ensure a stable batten.

For conchal grafts, one side of each slice should invariably contain perichondrium, and reinforcing the graft by folding it from concave side, face-to-face folding is recommended. When preparing rib cartilage, crafting the graft such that both cortical layers are included in a single slice is advantageous for structural integrity.

Chapter 7 elaborates on these methodologies and their specific applications and advantages, offering detailed guidance for achieving optimal outcomes in rhinoplasty.

6.3.2 Combinations of Graft

AESG and CSEG can be created by combining multiple cartilages. The possible combinations are as follows.

- AESG (septum) + CSEG (septum)
- AESG (septum) + CSEG (cymba or cavum)
- AESG (rib) + CSEG (rib)
- AESG (cavum) + CSEG (cymba)
- AESG (cymba) + CSEG (cavum)
- AESG (cymba) + CSEG (other cymba)

The most commonly used combination is the AESG (septum) and CSEG (cymba) when performing primary septorhinoplasty; each combination is described in detail in Chap. 7.

6.3.3 Caudal Septal Extension Graft (CSEG)

The caudal septal extension graft (CSEG) is designed to reinforce the entire length of the caudal septum, particularly emphasizing the enhancement at the junction between the anterior nasal spine (ANS) and the posterior septal angle (PSA), acting as a batten graft (Fig. 6.3; Animation 6.1). This concept introduces the extension of the caudal septum, essentially creating a new anterior septal angle. However, achieving stability can only be challenging with at least 3–4 well-overlapped contact points between the CSEG and the caudal septum. By adjusting these contact points, the angle and height of attachment for the CSEG can be determined, as well as the degree of rotation needed to establish the position of the de novo anterior septal angle. In Asian rhinoplasty, cases requiring the ideal subnasale to be positioned more than 3–4 mm caudally are rare,

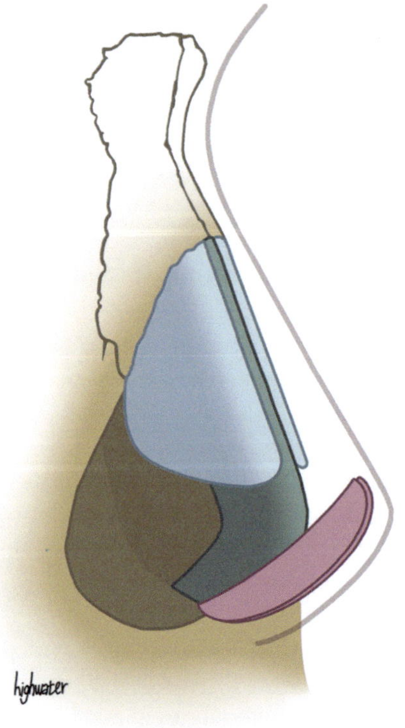

Fig. 6.3 Fig. 6.3 Caudal septal extension graft: bilateral batten at ANS (illustration from Kim et al. [4])

excluding secondary cases, making folded cymba conchal cartilage an excellent material choice. The idea follows Dr. Kridel's introduction of the "tongue-in-groove" technique for lower lateral cartilages (LLC) in septorhinoplasty, adapting it to a "tongue-in-batten" format for reinforcement from both sides [1].

However, supporting the junction of the ANS and PSA down to their inferior parts, enhancing strength, is particularly pertinent to Asian septorhinoplasty. This foundational support for the L-strut is critical. Around the ANS, three methods are commonly employed for repair:

1. A "figure of 8" suture at the junction of the ANS and PSA, including the periosteum around the ANS and the cartilaginous margin of the PSA.
2. Creating a drill hole in the ANS for passing a needle or attaching it with non-absorbable sutures.
3. Passing through the ANS to create a deep periosteal pocket toward the maxillary crest, inserting a small rim of the CSEG into the pocket.

If a small stalk of the ANS and PSA remains or the periosteum is intact, there's no need for bone tunneling or suture anchoring. However, in secondary surgeries where the ANS is absent or affected by procedures like a Lefort I osteotomy, which can sometimes damage the ANS, using bone screw anchoring or plate screws is possible. Still, due to long-term concerns about scarring and potential exposure of plates or anchoring screws, these methods are generally avoided.

6.3.4 Anterior Extended Spreader Graft (AESG)

The essence of SLEG is that tip projection is achieved with CSEG, while the lower two-thirds of the nasal dorsum is represented with AESG. This highlights the importance of the stability of the anterior portion of the framework (Fig. 6.4; Animation 6.2).

When inserting AESG, a small wedge can be made on both sides of the cephalic AESG, offering stability during the repair process. Stable caudal nasal bone enables this method, and after the graft, the dorsal line along the AESG must be refined with a No. 11 scalpel.

Inserting flat septal cartilage or laminated rib is relatively easy. However, insertion methods for the cavum concha or cymba concha involve folding these cartilages and embedding them into the anterior portion of the existing septal cartilage (Fig. 6.5; Animation 6.3). Preoperative measurement of the patient's ear size is crucial to ensure sufficient length of the folded cavum, as not all patients will have cartilage of uniform length. Insufficient length may lead to challenges in supporting the area from the rhinion, resulting in an inability to create a smooth line across this gap.

In secondary surgeries, the instability of the keystone area at the rhinion necessitates a different level of preparation. Costal cartilage may be used, creating a small wedge to fit into the key-

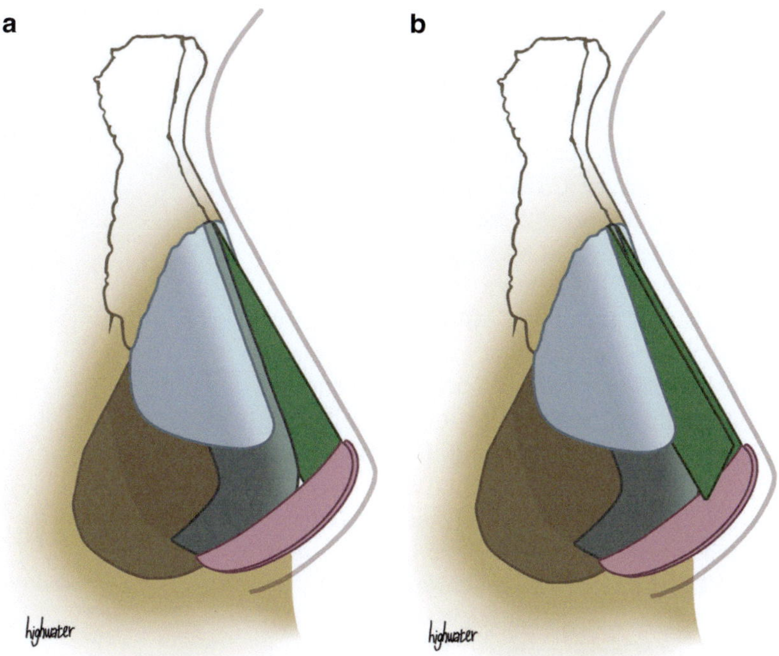

Fig. 6.4 Anterior extended spreader graft. (**a**) AESG at the left side of the high septum. (**b**) AESG at the right side of the high septum (illustration from illustration from Kim et al. [4])

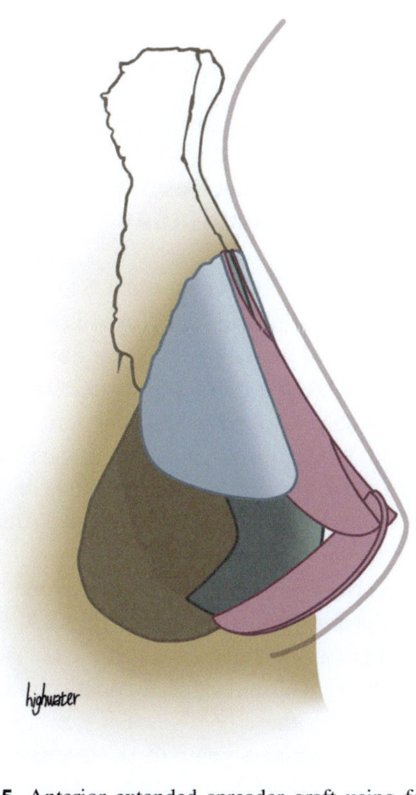

Fig. 6.5 Anterior extended spreader graft using folded concha cartilage

stone for stability during and after the repair with trimming. The initial fixation of the AESG with 4.0 Vicryl can enhance stability, followed by repairs using 4.0 PDS or 5.0 PDS for multiple sutures. Sometimes, one or two non-absorbable sutures may be necessary to secure the AESG.

Limiting the mucoperichondrial dissection to just enough to fit the AESG can prevent the graft from sinking downward. Traditionally, during SMR, one mucoperichondrial flap is preserved on the septum, with only anterior dissection sufficient for inserting the spreader graft, maintaining a 2–3 mm attachment during high septal dissection. The right-handed author typically performs this dissection on the patient's left nasal cavity, applying this technique when creating the pocket in the right high septum. This method facilitates the insertion of the extended spreader graft.

In patients with severe deviation, bilateral AESG may not adequately control the deviation. In such cases, preparing and inserting an additional layer of AESG can help achieve a straighter dorsal line on the desired side; multiple layers of AESG can assist in obtaining a straight dorsum line.

6.3.5 Sequence of SLEG

6.3.5.1 The Method of First Placing the CSEG and Then the AESG

Determining the sequence for implementing the AESG and the CSEG is crucial in septorhinoplasty. Suppose there is stability at the ANS and the PSA, allowing for a stable fixation of the CSEG above the ANS. In that case, placing the CSEG first, followed by the AESG, is advantageous. In secondary surgeries, if the septum's alloplastic material needs to be removed or there is a breakage at the rhinion, making it difficult to attach the EPP to the septal cartilage, it becomes challenging to apply an AESG first. In such instances, building the L-strut foundation on the CSEG is essential for achieving stability. The advantage of starting the L-strut construction above the ANS, rather than from the rhinion, is due to the continual gravitational pull on the AESG during surgery, which can complicate the repair process.

6.3.5.2 The Method of First Placing the AESG and Then the CSEG

In cases where the AESG is placed first, it typically involves situations where the high septum remains intact, a scenario more common in secondary surgeries.

The approach of inserting the AESG before the CSEG is considered when the ANS is missing, when solid fixation around the ANS is unachievable, or when the graft is better inserted through subperiosteal pocket dissection. This technique allows the AESG to provide the necessary support for the subsequent placement of the CSEG.

The method of first performing the AESG bilaterally, followed by inserting the CSEG, has been introduced in Dr. Guyuron's "tongue and groove" technique (Fig. 6.6). There might be concerns about stability if there isn't a firm fixation around the ANS. In that case, it can be snugly fitted between the bilateral spreader grafts, with the caudal portion of the CSEG inserted in the middle. However, there are instances where long-term subnasale contracture may reoccur, which is not considered an ideal outcome. Restoring a weakened or lost ANS and subsequently extending the subnasale can be exceedingly challenging in such patients.

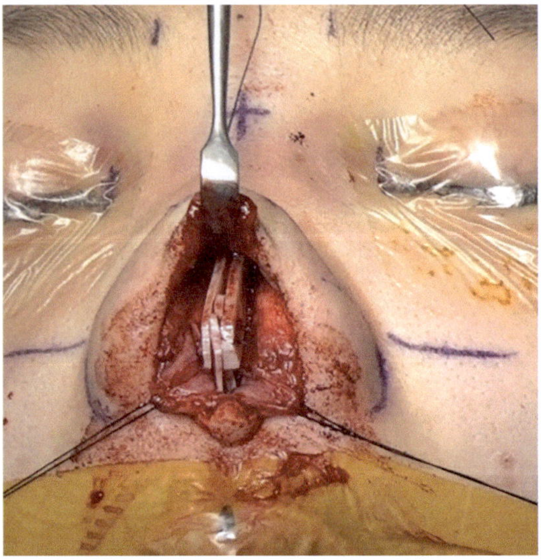

Fig. 6.6 Tongue and groove technique for caudal septal extension graft

6.3.6 Creating De Novo Anterior Septal Angle (ASA)

The connection between the CSEG and the AESG facilitates the creation of a de novo anterior septal angle (ASA). The construction of this new ASA using septal cartilage from the dorsum and folded cymba concha from the caudal side poses challenges, particularly in terms of thickness. This issue becomes more pronounced when costal cartilage is utilized.

When two layers of CSEG meet two layers of AESG, forming a quadruple-layered ASA, there's a risk of excessive thickness, potentially narrowing the internal nasal valve area. One approach to relieve the thickness involves using an appropriate raftering graft, which will be described later. If a raftering graft is not feasible, one alternative is to trim one side of the CSEG to reduce its thickness.

6.3.7 Raftering Graft

For robust support between CSEG and the AESG, the use of one batten or interposition grafts significantly aids in the creation of a de novo ASA instead of forming quadruple-layered coaptation. Supporting each other obliquely prevents the bilateral internal nasal valve walls from becoming too thick. The narrower the width of the raftering graft, the less stable it becomes, but there is less concern about thickening. Due to the complexity of this task, ear cartilage may not be suitable, making this technique more applicable when utilizing a small piece of flat cartilage (Fig. 6.7).

6.3.8 Approximation of LLCs: Creating Tip

After the de novo ASA creation, the LLCs and ULCs are approximated (Animations 6.4 and 6.5). For effective elevation of the LLC through interdomal suturing, thorough dissection around the cartilage is required. If lifting the sides of the LLC easily positions them correctly, no special measures are needed. However, if tension occurs during lifting, it indicates insufficient dissection. Begin with a cephalic trim to release the attachment between the LLCs and the ULCs. In primary rhinoplasty, this method usually achieves the desired projection. More extensive dissection is necessary for secondary surgeries, especially between the scroll area. Further loosening or cutting at the hinge area may be required if the release is still inadequate.

Elevate the LLCs to the appropriate position and temporarily secure them with a needle. The first suture applied is the interdomal suture. Achieving the correct position with the first interdomal suture is crucial for setting the projection and rotation. The next suture is the lateral crural spanning suture, which plays a vital role in spanning the LLCs while positioning the lateral crura, aiming for a beautiful right angle between the lateral and middle crura. If the desired angle is not achieved, consider suturing to adjust the convexity of the lateral crus, with the lateral crural mattress suture being commonly used. Sutures are less effective for controlling concavity, so small batten-type onlay grafts for balance may be better.

The decision to anchor the interdomal suture directly to the high septum depends on the amount of projection. If a straight dorsal line without a supratip break is desired, direct fixation to the AESG is advantageous and can minimize the supratip break.

The SLEG method's beauty lies in its ability to rely directly on the high septum to determine

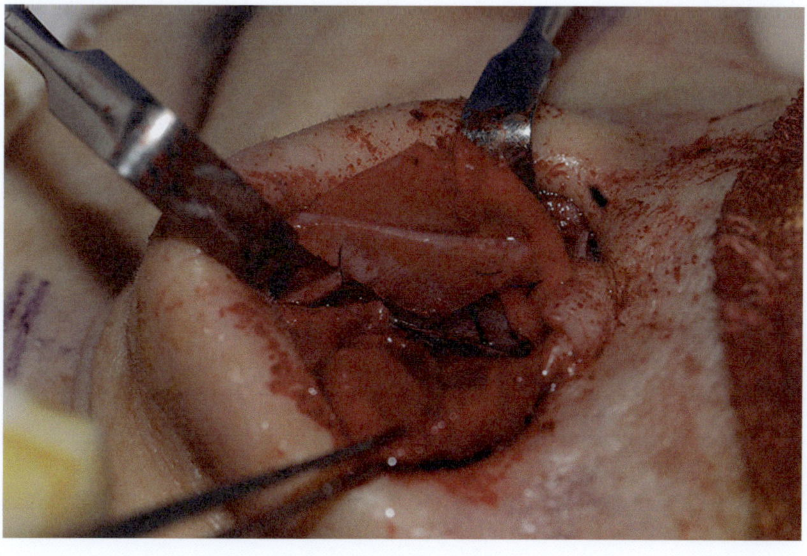

Fig. 6.7 Raftering graft: connecting the AESG and CSEG

the tip position. It is considered the only method that shapes the dorsum through the high septum while supporting the tip (Animation 6.6).

Furthermore, the AESG, as a physiological graft, shows less long-term change than derotation grafts or lateral crural spanning onlay grafts. The author attributes this stability to the graft's orthotopic placement, positing that adequate mucoperichondrial blood supply enhances the overall graft survival rate.

6.3.9 Nasion Graft: Creating Dorsal Aesthetic Lines

After constructing the cartilaginous dorsum in the lower two-thirds of the nose, augmentation is carried out from the nasion through the rhinion, shaping the entire nasal dorsum. The AESG minimizes the need for additional grafting thanks to the already projected cartilaginous dorsum. When employing costal cartilage, either carved costal cartilage blocks or laminated slices are utilized. For a smoother dorsal aesthetic line or secondary surgeries with skin and soft tissue issues, adding dermal layers or costal perichondrium can prevent demarcation along the aligned AESG.

Considering absorption rates, creating a smooth line from the nasion to the supratip may require more grafting, ensuring a seamless transition along the nasal dorsum.

6.4 Specific Considerations

6.4.1 Lifting the Upper Lateral Cartilage

Releasing the ULC adjacent to the bone allows for mobility. This includes detaching the perichondrium underneath the ULC near the nasal bone, the area adjacent to the lateral maxillary process, and the pyriform ligament, facilitating considerable movement.

The scroll area of the ULC, compared to the cephalic portion, is surrounded by relatively more movable soft tissue, enhancing its mobility. However, the ULC does not move as freely as the LLC. The amount by which the anteriorly extended high septum can "catch up" is limited, resulting in cases where the ULC does not coapt to the high septum. Nonetheless, lifting the ULC as much as possible can aid functionally. Even if the upper end does not directly touch the high septum, repair with 4.0 PDS is attempted. A forceful repair can have the adverse effect of pulling down the high septum, lowering the anterior septum.

Protruding AESGs are not palpable and do not cause significant issues during healing, possibly due to the thicker skin and soft tissue envelope typical in Asian patients. However, a layer of soft tissue graft is applied in cases with thin dermis where demarcation is anticipated. Techniques like spreading out remaining diced cartilage or small soft tissue pieces to fill spaces with a sidewall graft are also explored without significant issues.

The author has rarely encountered situations where the two upper ends of the AESG are visibly protruding. In secondary surgeries, if an extremely thin skin flap remains and the ULC is visible through the skin, a soft tissue onlay graft may be necessary to cover it.

6.4.2 Lifting the Internal Nasal Valve

The most significant benefit of this surgery, the lift of the internal nasal valve, is made possible by repositioning the LLCs to a newly projected high septum. Tip projection is relatively straightforward, and as mentioned earlier, the suture of the LLC with high septum using lateral crural spanning sutures allows for the lifting of the entire internal nasal valve. Analyzing the functional improvement before and after the surgery in patients is complex. There are reports on using spring grafts and upper lateral splay grafts for nasal obstruction [2, 3], but no reports exist on grafts that can lift the entire LLC along with the ULC.

Without a lift in the parts that do not catch up after creating tip projection, the roof of the internal nasal valve abruptly decreases. However, the

SLEG technique avoids this drawback by simultaneously lifting the ULC and LLC.

Since the surgery addresses the complex causes of nasal obstruction, including hypertrophy of the inferior turbinates and nasal septal deviation, determining the effect solely based on the internal nasal valve lift is challenging. The author is continuously monitoring the effects through ongoing follow-ups [4].

6.5 Long-Term Results

6.5.1 Aesthetic Perspectives

One of the significant drawbacks of autogenous tissue-only septorhinoplasty is the difficulty in predicting the extent of resorption. This is especially true for onlay grafts placed on the bony dorsum from nasion to rhinion, where the amount of resorption can vary significantly depending on the type of graft used. Reports have highlighted this variability, and further details are expected to be published. A review suggests that the resorption rate of soft tissue is relatively high, continuing up to 18 months post-surgery.

- The long-term augmentation effect of the rolled SDF in the same area is around 3 mm; the absorption rate is 40–50%.
- The effect of long-term augmentation of diced cartilage wrapped with SMF depends on the amount of packed cartilage, but the augmented amount should be planned with an absorption rate of 30–40% [5, 6].

However, the cartilaginous dorsum of the lower two-thirds, constructed from cartilage, exhibits less resorption. Therefore, it allows for the long-term maintenance of the desired aesthetic lines (data in publish).

6.5.2 Functional Perspectives

In the author's recent study on the functional outcomes of the SLEG, The nasal obstruction symptom evaluation (NOSE) scale was utilized to assess patient-reported nasal function, both preoperatively and 3 months postoperatively. The analysis revealed a significant reduction in NOSE scale scores post-surgery, indicating improved subjective nasal symptoms [4].

- Aesthetically, SLEG reduces the amount of graft needed for dorsal aesthetics. In long-term follow-up, there were minimal changes in the shape of the cartilaginous dorsum, including the supratip, likely due to the use of orthotopic cartilage grafts.
- Functionally, SLEG improves the nasal airway, at least at the site of obstruction. SLEG is a suitable technique for Asian autogenous-only septorhinoplasty, which makes the entire nose dependent on the septum.

However, it is a challenging method that requires a significant amount of cartilage and demands control over the patient's microbial condition during the graft's integration. It requires time-consuming efforts, and before integration, an autogenous graft is merely a graft susceptible to infection, thus presenting challenges with antibiotic therapy in the immediate postoperative period. Nonetheless, the surgery should be completed in one session, especially in cases of secondary septorhinoplasty, where it becomes one of the necessary approaches when seriously considering what benefits the patient in the battle against alloplastic materials.

References

1. Kim HR, Jeong SH, Han SK, Dhong ES. Folded cymba concha: is it large and stable enough for caudal septal extension graft in Asian rhinoplasty? Aesthet Surg J. 2021. https://academic.oup.com/asj/article-abstract/41/7/NP737/6131996
2. Guyuron B, Michelow BJ, Englebardt C. Upper lateral splay graft. Plast Reconstr Surg. 1998;102:2169–77.
3. Sen C, Iscen D. Use of the spring graft for prevention of midvault complications in rhinoplasty. Plast Reconstr Surg. 2007;119:332–6.
4. Kim S-B, Baik S-H, Lee K-I, Dhong E-S, Jeong S-H, Han S-K. Functional evaluation of septal L-strut extension graft in east Asians. J Plast Reconstr Aesthet Surg. 2024;94:178. https://doi.org/10.1016/j.bjps.2024.05.010.

5. Dhong E-S, Na M-W. The resorption: the hurdle for autogenous-based Asian rhinoplasty. In: Dhong E-S, Na M-W, editors. Asian septorhinoplasty: conundrums and solutions. Singapore: Springer Singapore; 2021. p. 77–89.
6. Lee T-Y, Lee K-I, Dhong E-S, Jeong S-H, Kim D-W, Han S-K. Long-term resorption rate of autogenous onlay graft in east Asian rhinoplasty: a retrospective study. Plast Reconstr Surg. 2022;149:360–71.

7 Fragile Framework: Various Combinations of Septal L-Strut Extension Graft (SLEG)

Pearls

- Asian septorhinoplasty often involves "reduction-augmentation" techniques, where surgeons may use implants to enhance the dorsal profile, even in cases with a hump.
- The framework's weakening primarily results from excessive reduction of the nasal structure, particularly the bone and septum.
- Excessive reduction compromises the nose's stability and integrity, potentially leading to long-term complications.
- Silicone and Gore-Tex offer an easy dorsal line. Still, the true art lies in using autogenous grafts for a natural look and safety. This highlights the need for a paradigm shift in Asian rhinoplasty away from mere implant replacement, especially in secondary septorhinoplasty.
- Strategic graft placement ensures stability and addresses deviations in septal L-strut extension graft.
- The cartilaginous dorsum is enhanced by elevating the anterior septal extension graft (AESG) to the desired height. At the same time, the stability of the AESG is secured through the fixation of the caudal septal extension graft (CSEG).
- AESG and CSEG can be crafted from various cartilage combinations, with a septum and cymba concha common in primary rhinoplasties. This reflects the author's experience and emphasizes flexibility in cartilage selection based on the shape for optimal outcomes.
- Achieving a seamless aesthetic line from the nasion to the tip post-SLEG challenges due to graft resorption.
- Strategic overcorrection, employing soft tissues for dorsal refinement, or, in cases of thin skin, diced cartilage wrapped in fascia or laminated or solid rib grafts, accompanied by meticulous perichondrium management, may be necessary.

7.1 Preoperative Considerations for Septal L-Strut Extension Graft (SLEG) Candidates

The chapter critically examines the complexity of Asian rhinoplasty, pointing out the excessive dependence on synthetic implants for nasal enhancement and advocating for reconsidering adopting a septal L-strut extension graft. It draws attention to the unique challenges in revision surgeries due to scar tissue, which is less prevalent in Western procedures. It debates the suitability of modern rhinoplasty trends in Asia due to anatomical distinctions. The text favors targeted reduction techniques over general hump removal and disapproves of the overuse of synthetic materials for augmenting the lower two-thirds. It also discusses the risk of surgical complications and emphasizes the need for careful dorsal implanting over a fragile framework.

It urges a significant shift toward reconstructing the nasal framework and a deeper compre-

E. S. Dhong, *Asian Septorhinoplasty*, https://doi.org/10.1007/978-981-96-6127-5_7

hension of Asia's unique anatomical and aesthetic characteristics, pushing for more complex techniques requiring many grafts.

- Besides surgery, what are the perspectives of Asian rhinoplasty on the dorsum? Are we too complacent and assume that an alloplastic implant is the only answer?

Should the tip be higher to match the dorsal height?

The author is most at ease when dealing with primary reduction rhinoplasty patients. On the contrary, there is always a sense of pressure and frustration when performing secondary rhinoplasty.

- The previous surgeons should bear the burden, but the final surgeon shoulders all the responsibility in real life.

Although we share many aspects with Asians and other ethnicities in secondary rhinoplasty, we should have a different perspective on the overall aesthetics, not just the anatomical size and thickness differences of cartilage and soft tissue. In Western rhinoplasty, many publications have expressed concern about visible grafts on the tip under thin skin, even for three decades [1, 2].

Why is preservation rhinoplasty, which has recently become a new trend in Western society, not commonly performed in Asian rhinoplasty? [3]. In the West, we know that there are many complications from too much excision. The problem is that the Asian view is too different.

Component reduction is the method of choice and should be emphasized [4]. There are still some surgeons who perform en bloc hump reduction and cover the defect with an alloplastic implant (Fig. 7.1).

When the desired nasal dorsal height exceeds the height of the hump, the choice is to leave the hump in place or perform augmentation over it [5]. However, many Asian surgeons prefer to create a flat implant base. If dorsal implantation is desired, excision of the platform is better not recommended.

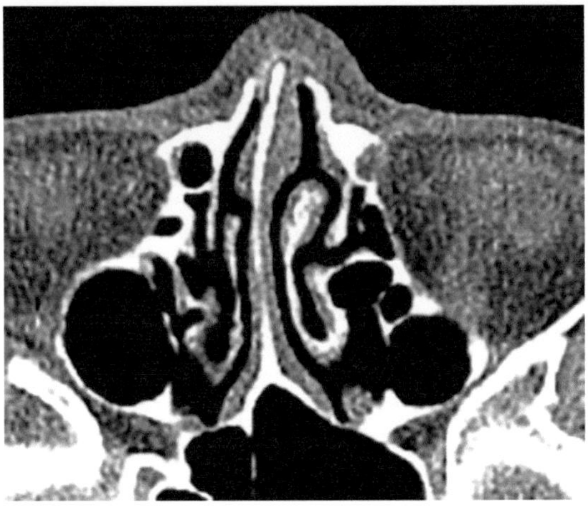

Fig. 7.1 Open roof deformity at the bottom of a silicone implant

A simple camouflage operation using alloplastic implanting is performed frequently in many patients with proper bony dorsal height but underdeveloped lower two-thirds. This often results in an imbalance of nasal implants—simple implanting after rasping the bony hump results in high sellion or high rhinion deformities. Camouflage is easy, but the longevity of alloplastic materials is short, so proper selection must be made. All Asian rhinoplasty is focusing on tip surgery. Tip extension and tip projection are the main focus, and the dorsum is neglected except for onlay.

This is not a cause-and-effect statement but rather evidence based on the history of many complicated patients who have had such surgery when followed up. The extrinsic cause of deformity in Asian secondary septorhinoplasty is the alloplastic materials applied in the primary surgery. The intrinsic cause of deformity in Asian secondary septorhinoplasty is caused by inappropriate septal reduction, resulting in a characteristic unstable nasal deformity, mainly due to a collapsed septum.

- Many problems are caused by surgical site infections or late-onset inflammation after humpectomy or medial and lateral osteotomy when torn mucosa jeopardizes the implant in the nasal dorsum.

7.1.1 Paradigm Shift

Achieving the dorsal aesthetic line that silicone or Gore-Tex provides is easy. However, a conceptual shift is needed to realize that autogenous grafts are the wise way to achieve a natural aesthetic line, especially in secondary surgery. Above all, they are safe, which is the most significant advantage.

- Many Asian rhinoplasty surgeons still consider secondary rhinoplasty an implant-changing surgery, which is why this book is meaningful.
- The SLEG is not a new idea but rather an effort to recognize camouflage's limitations and solve problems by framework reconstruction.

It cannot be emphasized enough that Asian rhinoplasty should be approached from a different perspective than Western one [6, 7].

7.2 Common Issues Encountered in Camouflage Techniques

7.2.1 Excessive Resection at the Bony Dorsum

One of the distinguishing features of Asian septorhinoplasty is the concept of "reduction-augmentation rhinoplasty." Even in patients with a generalized hump, many surgeons opt to insert an implant to achieve a desirable dorsal line (an artificial nasal contour). Silicone implants offer a quick solution to attain an aesthetically pleasing line. However, numerous issues arise during the process of reducing the underlying structure to accommodate the implant, as it cannot be adequately positioned without reducing the hump.

Over time, subsidence or settling of both the bony and cartilaginous parts of the nasal dorsum can lead to significant problems. Similarly, surgeries for pseudo-humps often follow this approach, where after minimal hump removal, the overall nasal shape is easily corrected with an alloplastic implant. While patients may go 10–15 years without issues, many eventually present with problems due to minor trauma or inflammation within the nasal cavity.

An alternative method to overcome these drawbacks is to carve the underside of the implant, particularly where it meets the bony dorsum. This involves reshaping the implant's undersurface to match the nasal platform after humpectomy (Fig. 7.2).

Recent advancements in 3D printing technology and the concept of cartilage molding are being explored to address these challenges. Silicone implants can now be produced using 3D printing, significantly altering their shapes (Fig. 7.3). According to the manufacturer, these implants can either be customized based on the patient's CT scans to fit the specific shape of the nasal dorsum or be newly created using 3D printing techniques.

The various shapes of silicone implants are merely a desperate measure to address the irregularities of the implant's lower platform mentioned above (Fig. 7.4). It is impossible to insert an implant that fits perfectly into the pocket, and I have never seen a patient with an implant placed precisely on top of the nasal bony pyramid.

Simple rhinoplasties that involve merely inserting an implant without septal surgery might be understandable within a perfect theoretical framework. Still, even in these cases, the extent of surrounding tissue recruitment and pocket dissection can vary, leading to unpredictable outcomes. In most patients undergoing septal surgery, it is easy to observe that the platform where the planned implant will be placed changes during the septal surgery. Therefore, it is emphasized that the above method is useless except for surgeries that merely create a pocket for inserting the silicone implant and then closing it.

7.2.2 Dead Space at the Supratip Area

The design of most nasal implants resembles a boat shape, featuring a slender supratip region. While numerous efforts have been made to refine the implant's shape by augmenting the supratip

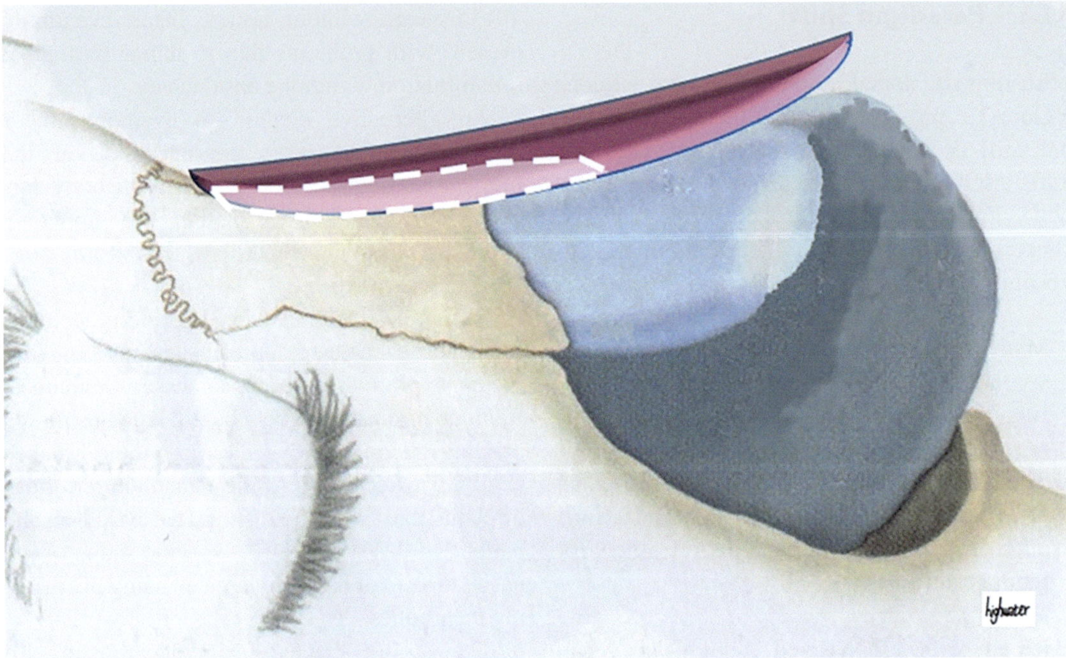

Fig. 7.2 Undersurface carving of a silicone implant

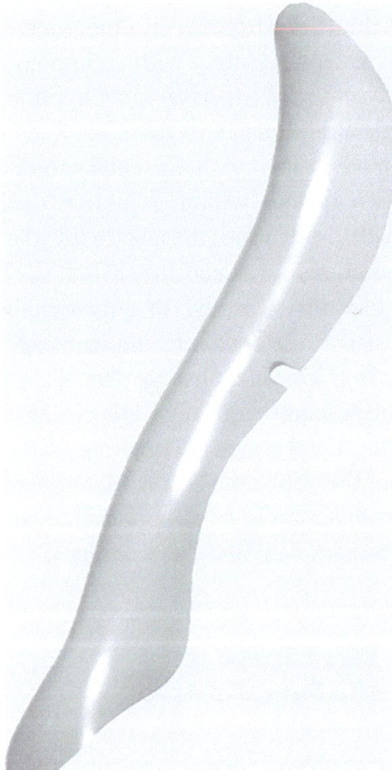

Fig. 7.3 3D manufactured silicone implant

area to enhance its overall contour, many surgeons have observed skin thinning following sustained pressure on the implant's tip for extended periods. Consequently, reducing the implant's lower portion or delicate tip carving is often employed.

Recognizing that supratip grafts are generally utilized as concealed grafts to reinforce the dead space beneath the implant. Placing a cartilage graft on the supratip above the implant carries a risk of demarcation, so it is mostly placed underneath, while the dorsal line is done with silicone. Dead space formation in the supratip region is a well-acknowledged issue among surgeons experienced in Asian rhinoplasty. Advanced three-dimensional manufacturing techniques have been developed to either increase the thickness of the implant in the supratip area or to augment the region to eliminate the dead space strategically. However, this approach does not typically reflect the natural anatomy of the nose, which possesses a significant volume of soft tissue overlaying the cartilaginous structures of the LLC. As previously

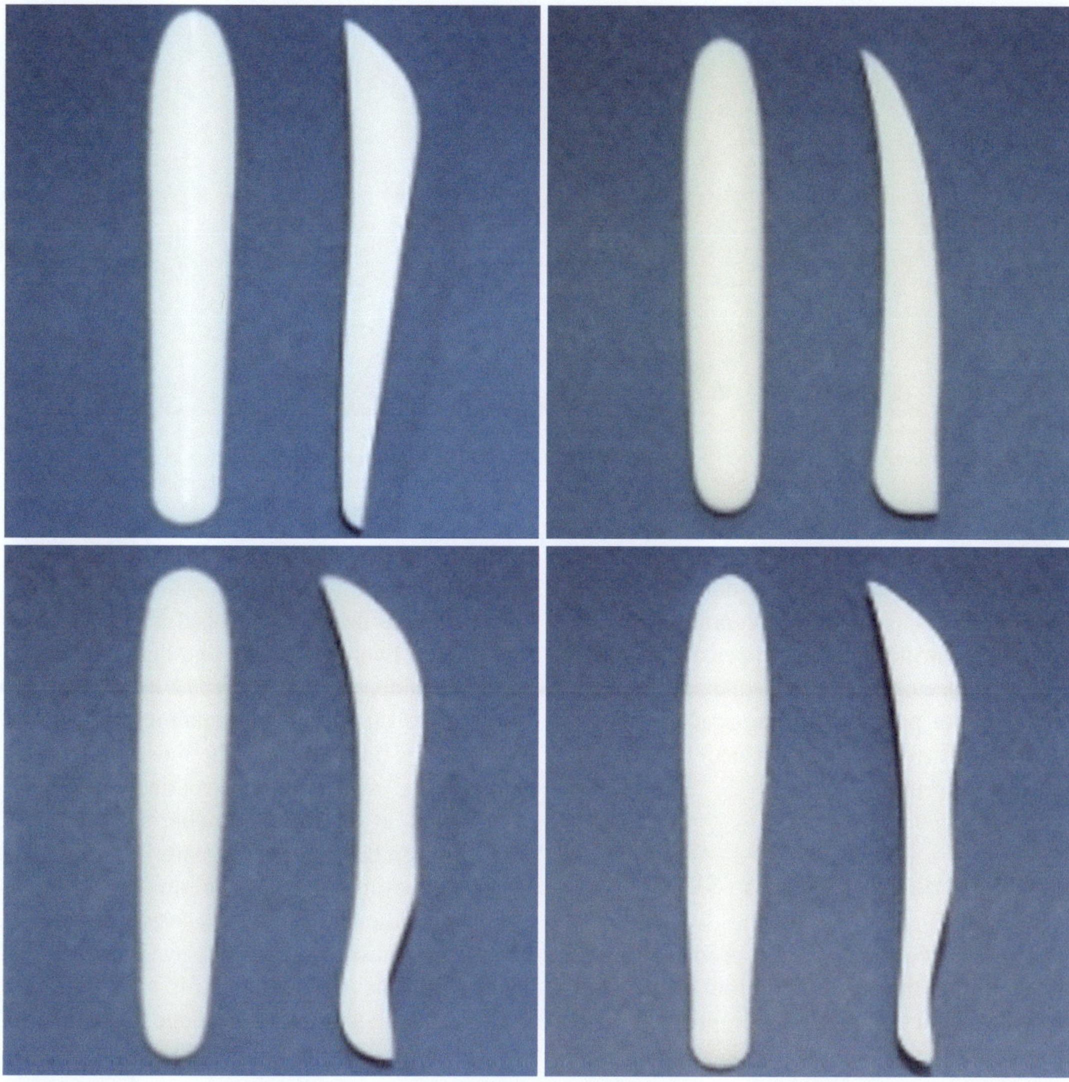

Fig. 7.4 Various types of silicone implants: The nasion and supratip features vary

mentioned, the absence of the high septum is considered an inherent limitation of Asian secondary rhinoplasty. Under such circumstances, crafting an aesthetically pleasing dorsal line largely relies on camouflage, presenting a unique challenge within nasal aesthetic surgery.

Placing numerous grafts in the supratip area typically leads to a stratified stacking effect. While this can aesthetically enhance the dorsal profile, the resulting accumulation of scar tissue, as indicated by axial scans, may become a source of discomfort over time (Fig. 7.5).

7.2.3 Dead Space at the Nasion

In many patients, a notably low nasion is a common finding, particularly among Asian populations. This characteristic feature often results in a profile that resembles a hump nose, necessitating augmentation of the low nasion to harmonize the overall facial contour.

Recent advancements in implant design have aimed to provide enhanced augmentation, specifically in the nasion region (Fig. 7.4) However, achieving an exact match still needs to be achieved. Consequently, the use of implants

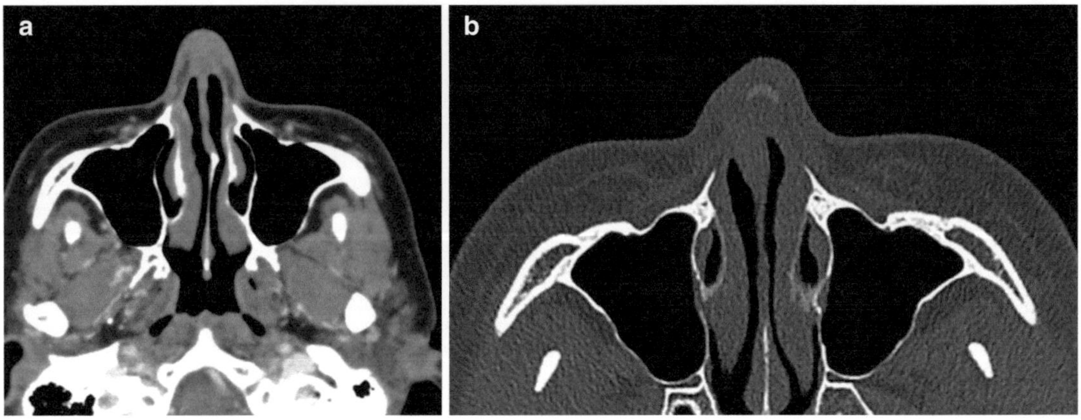

Fig. 7.5 Excessively grafted supratip. (**a**) The dorsal profile is smooth, but there is a tightly filled scar between the high septum and skin envelope. (**b**) There is a lot of soft tissue shadow in the space between the silicone implant and the nasal roof

necessitates specialized grafting techniques for the nasion void area to address this discrepancy. Dead space in the nasion and supratip areas significantly contributes to the propensity for excessive humpectomy. This underscores the importance of precise, location-specific grafting as a more effective strategy for achieving optimal aesthetic outcomes.

7.3 Preparation for the SLEG

The SLEG requires proper preparation and harvesting of the needed amount of material. For the primary operation, the preferred first choice is cymba concha for a caudal septal extension graft (CSEG) and septal cartilage for an anterior extended spreader graft (AESG).

7.3.1 Preparing Septal Cartilage for SLEG

Harvesting as much of the septal quadrangular cartilage as possible, more than 20 mm in length, and as much as is safe to operate on for AESG, even if it is less in width. Since most cartilage is harvested in a pentagonal shape, a long axis of more than 20 mm or more can be obtained by preparing it in an oblique direction when dividing it into smaller pieces.

Inserting two AESGs parallel to each side of the existing septum is usually stable. Still, correction of severe deviation requires two AESGs on one side or two on one side and one on the contralateral side, so it is essential to prepare the appropriate amount. The remaining pieces are reserved for tip plasty. For the most effective tip surgery, the author almost routinely performs three grafts at the tip: columellar strut grafts, a subdomal graft, and a shield graft.

The subdomal graft is the smallest piece to achieve middle crus symmetry, so even the smallest septal cartilage should be saved, not thrown away [8]. The columellar strut also does not require a large amount of cartilage. Small pieces of cartilage in combination with a shield graft are three combinations that can be used to create a harmonious tip.

- The success of the SLEG is determined by the ability to project the robust AESG to the desired height anteriorly.

7.3.2 Septal Cartilage Harvesting, Including EPP-Cartilage Junction

If the quadrangular cartilage is too small to achieve the desired 20–24 mm dimension, it should be harvested to include the EPP-quadrangular cartilage junction. During this procedure, repairing the AESG can be challenging, and the EPP on the anterior aspect is often thickened. Despite this, osteotomy at the EPP may be feasible using a sharp septal Freer elevator at harvest time. Multiple drill holes should be made on the bony aspect to facilitate future repair with the existing septum. Caution is advised to prevent drilling huge holes, which could compromise the integrity of the EPP contact area. It is preferable to position the EPP segment at the keystone area, where the bony aspect aligns with the rhinion, and the junction for repair with the CSEG will involve the cartilaginous portion (Fig. 7.6).

7.3.3 Preparing Ear Cartilage for SLEG

7.3.3.1 Cymba Concha

The cymba conchae, when folded, is the ear cartilage most frequently utilized for the caudal septal extension graft (CSEG). Based on the author's experience, the average length and width for folded cymba conchae in men and women are 24.2 [±3.9] mm by 7.8 [±1.9] mm and 22.4 [±3.7] mm by 7.2 [±1.9] mm, respectively. These measurements indicate that optimal harvesting should aim for a minimum length of 22 mm and a folded width of approximately 7 mm, irrespective of the patient's gender. This rationale underpins the author's preference for the anterior approach. The anterior ear approach for harvesting becomes particularly advantageous when it is challenging to achieve a CSEG length of 20 mm or more, as it complicates the surgical procedure. To prevent unsightly anterior incisional scars post-surgery, meticulous attention to the dissection plane is crucial. While alternative techniques have been employed in some instances, they have often resulted in less satisfactory scars or postoperative outcomes, as per the author's observations.

- An anterior incision is more accessible for obtaining a more considerable amount of conchal cartilage.
- If the cymba concha is harvested through an anterior incision, the perichondrium should be left attached to the anterior skin flap.
- The perichondrium should be attached to the posterior convex surface of the cymba concha. Fold the anterior surface (concave side) of the cymba concha face-to-face with each other (Fig. 7.7).

The above gave the best results. In the author's opinion, the reasons for this are as follows.

- The dead space left after harvesting the cymba concha is vulnerable to contracture, so the perichondrium should remain on at least one flap to maintain stability.
- In the case of the concave side face-to-face, it is directly in contact with the cartilage, so integration is better when inserting the tongue-in-groove caudal septal cartilage in between.
- The perichondrium attached to the convex side should face outward and have a favorable external blood supply to facilitate rapid engraftment of the cartilage.

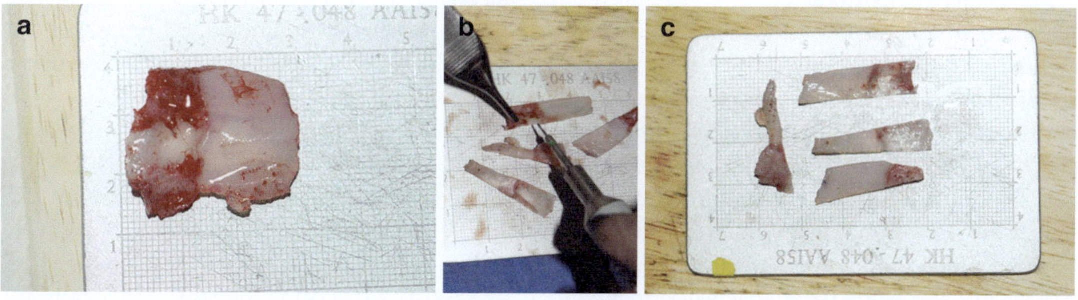

Fig. 7.6 Quadrangular cartilage harvested in conjunction with EPP. (**a**) The cartilaginous portion is less than 20 mm. (**b**) Creating a drill hole. (**c**) The two pieces are prepared for AESG, and the rest is used for tip plasty and other purposes

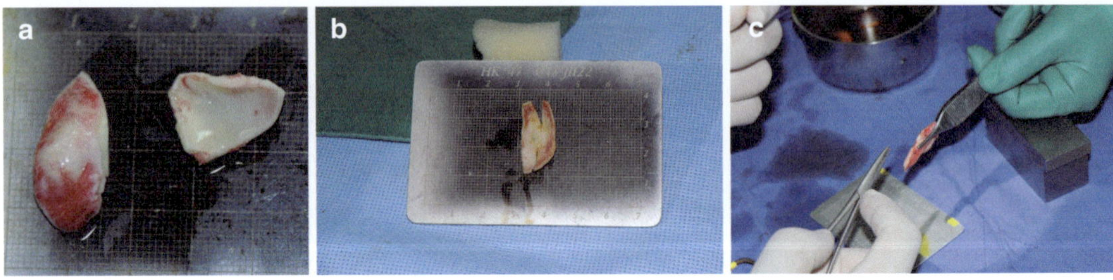

Fig. 7.7 Folding the cymba concha. (**a**) Cymba and cavum conchas attached perichodrium at the convex side. (**b**) Longitudinal chondrotomy preserving the midportion. (**c**) Folding the cymba concha

Fig. 7.8 Folding the cavum concha

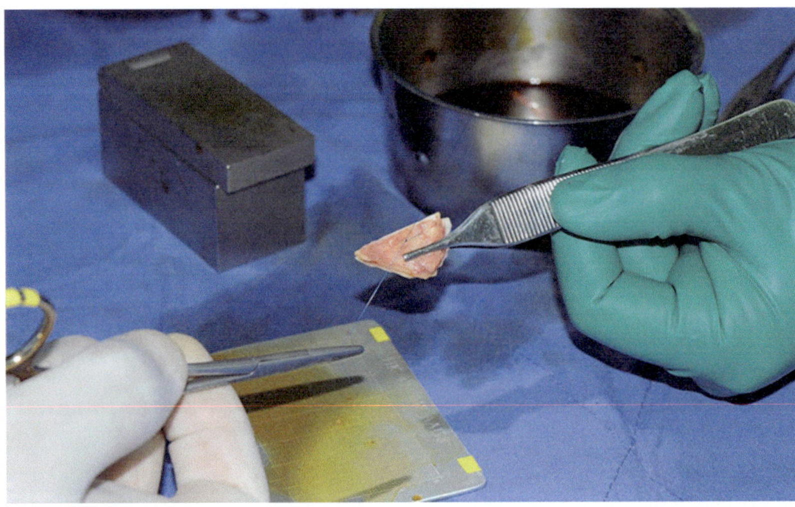

When folding with a repair, it is more advantageous to perform the folding with a partial attachment in the middle of the entire lengthwise direction to maintain stability and folding force. Folding after a complete longitudinal resection is more complicated (Fig. 7.7).

7.3.3.2 Cavum Concha

If additional lengths of cartilage are required in addition to the cymba concha, the cavum concha is harvested and folded in the same manner to prepare it. The incision for harvesting the cavum concha is also at the anterior side. Similarly, the perichondrium is left attached to the anterior skin flap. After harvesting, a longitudinal chondrotomy is applied to fold it. At this time, the center part should also be partially attached to maintain strength during folding. Depending on the shape of the patient's ear, the folded cavum is 2–4 mm shorter in length and 2–3 mm wider than the cymba concha when folded (Fig. 7.8).

7.3.4 Tragal Cartilage

It is sometimes used when septal cartilage is unavailable, when cymba concha and cavum concha are small and insufficient after harvesting both, or when an additional raftering graft is needed. It is very small but beneficial when a small cartilage graft is needed.

7.3.5 Preparing Costal Cartilage for SLEG

The seventh rib is often the most convenient for constructing laminated cartilage slices. The dimensions needed for AESG typically span more than 22–25 mm in length and 7–10 mm in width for contracted noses. Crafting a slice that simultaneously encompasses the anterior and posterior cortex of the rib is crucial. While utilizing rib cartilage may raise concerns about screw-like deformation due to three-dimensional warping, a slicing technique that includes both cortices tends to provide a balanced approach and mitigate this issue. This theory was introduced more than five decades ago, and instead of imagining a complex cross-section, consider how the laminated slice includes the cortex at both long edges.

For preventing later warping and solving many problems encountered with solid bloc grafts, the laminated rib has the advantage of applying SLEG [9].

7.4 Various Modifications of Septal L-Strut Extension Graft (SLEG)

7.4.1 Combinations of Graft

AESG and CSEG can be created by combining multiple cartilages. The possible combinations are shown below. Combining the septum and cymba concha is the easiest in most primary rhinoplasties. It is simply based on the % frequency of the author's clinical cases. Of course, more heterogeneous cartilage combinations are not included in the combinations below. Any other combinations are possible depending on the shape of the cartilage, so the following descriptions are only a snapshot of my experience. You can use any combination if you have flat, straight cartilage.

7.4.2 AESG (Septum) + CSEG (Septum)

If the nose or the quadrangular cartilage is sufficiently large, it may be feasible to use septal cartilage for both grafting purposes. However, finding an adequate amount of septal cartilage for the CSEG is often challenging after the AESG with the septum. This approach may be viable if the required caudal extension is minimal and the stability of the ANS and posterior septal angle (PSA) is preserved. Yet, according to the authors' clinical experience, employing this method in Asian septorhinoplasty accounts for less than 10% of all cases. The occurrence is even lower in secondary procedures, at merely 3%.

7.4.3 AESG (Septum) + CSEG (Cymba)

For maximizing the length, septal cartilage is commonly employed for spreader grafts, while the more elastic cymba concha is preferred for the CSEG. This is the most frequently utilized combination, with 67% of primary and 12% of secondary operations employing this method. It is considered the ideal combination for maintaining the appropriate elasticity of the nasal tip and creating the desired shape of a high septum. However, this combination is significantly less common in secondary operations, as the septal cartilage has often already been utilized in previous procedures.

7.4.4 AESG (Cavum) + CSEG (Cymba)

When using auricular cartilage exclusively for the SLEG, it's important to note that the length of the folded cavum concha is generally shorter than that of the folded cymba concha. However, the greater thickness of the folded cavum often makes it a more advantageous choice, especially in situations where the opposite cymba is less favorable. Due to its thickness, the folded cavum can be particularly beneficial for the AESG. In most cases of secondary surgery, the anterior margin of the septum is often destroyed, making the relatively wider width of the folded cavum more advantageous (Fig. 7.9).

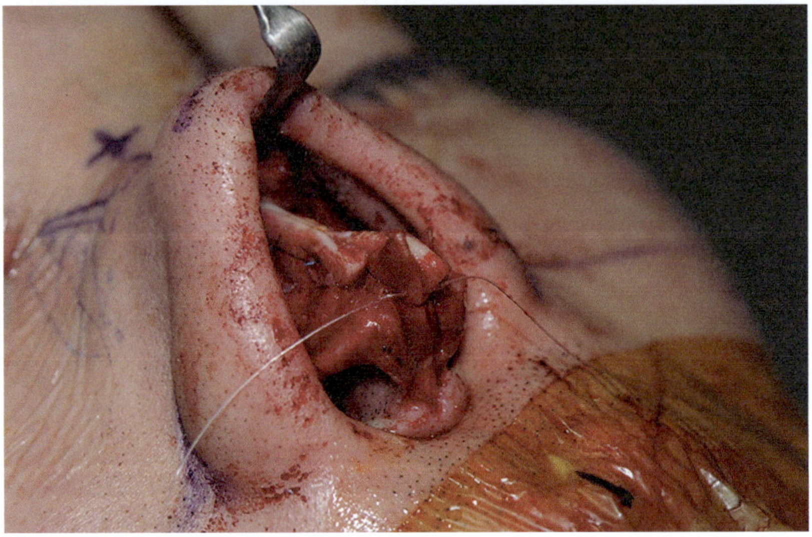

Fig. 7.9 Folded cavum concha as AESGs: folded cymba concha as CSEG

7.4.5 AESG (Cymba) + CSEG (Cavum)

This combination is a rare example of its application in secondary surgery. It depends entirely on the ear's size and the cartilage's shape to determine how it is used after harvest. This is the case when the cavum concha is long enough when folding.

7.4.6 AESG (Cymba) + CSEG (Cymba)

Many surgeons still prefer the posterior approach to auricular cartilage harvesting, so patients often come in after having cavum concha harvested in a previous surgery. It is even possible to see patients with bilateral cavum harvested. This is why it is sometimes necessary to harvest bilateral cymba to make every possible effort to achieve a SLEG.

7.4.7 AESG (Rib) + CSEG (Rib)

A SLEG using costal cartilage is the answer in most severe secondary cases. It is the best choice in secondary cases because it avoids the complicated combination of ear cartilage and shortens the operation time. It has the advantages of obtaining abundant perichondrium from the harvest site and creating an aesthetic line of the dorsum with a laminated piece.

7.5 Various Dorsal Onlay Grafts for Aesthetic Line

After performing a septal L-strut extension graft (SLEG), augmenting the bony dorsum from the nasion to the rhinion is a significant concern. This area poses a challenge despite the potential use of cantilever or solid rib grafts. Achieving a smooth, continuous aesthetic line extending to the nasal tip ideally involves incorporating a small aesthetic graft. However, the main challenge with autogenous grafts is their susceptibility to resorption, which is a considerable concern.

The use of alloplastic materials on the dorsum to maintain this line indefinitely goes against the fundamental philosophy of this book, which advocates for using a high septum to define the dorsum without relying on alloplastic implants. It is crucial to address the resorption issue thoroughly and plan for the necessary overcorrection.

Employing diced cartilage wrapped with fascia (DCF) may be necessary to amend the dorsum's smooth aesthetic line or address thinned skin in secondary surgeries. Additionally, in cases with a thicker soft tissue skin envelope or when a rib has been harvested, using a solid or laminated rib graft with appropriate perichondrium coverage or application to the undersurface can be a practical approach.

7.5.1 Soft Tissue Graft

Several types of soft tissue can be used. The author prefers the superficial mastoid fascia or sacral dermis in that order, expecting more than 30–50% resorption each, and overcorrect as a rule.

7.5.2 Superficial Mastoid Fascia (SMF)

For subtle 1–2 mm augmentations, utilizing multiple layers of superficial mastoid fascia can effectively enhance the nasion or bony dorsum. This technique is precious for achieving a smooth dorsal aesthetic line and correcting any unwanted irregularities in the SLEG area after shaving. Employing SMF is advantageous for its simplicity and does not require the patient's position to be changed during surgery if the area has been adequately prepared [10].

The choice between superficial mastoid fascia and deep temporal fascia (DTF) often comes down to personal preference. Each material has unique advantages, and the decision to use one over the other is not a matter of inferiority but rather of the surgeon's taste and the specific procedure needs.

7.5.3 Sacral Dermis

When anticipated conditions include significant thinning of the skin envelope or a need for augmentation exceeding 3 mm, it is advisable to harvest the sacral dermis under local anesthesia in preparation for rhinoplasty. The sacral dermis can be prepared as a double layer or rolled, depending on the desired thickness, and it's beneficial to include a small portion of fatty tissue in the preparation. There are two methods for rolling a single layer of sacral dermis: dermis-in rolling, where the dermal side is internal, and dermis-out rolling, where the dermal side is external.

In cases where the skin envelope is thin or uneven, utilizing the dermis-in rolling technique, with the fatty tissue facing outward, offers the advantage of achieving a smoother, more aesthetically pleasing line [11].

7.5.4 Diced Cartilage Wrapping with Fascia: DCF

The author has investigated the absorption rates of diced cartilage wrapped with fascia, reporting better long-term outcomes than other dermis grafts such as sacral dermis or superficial mastoid fascia. This study found that the resorption rate of diced cartilage wrapped with fascia is the lowest [12]. However, a 30% resorption rate must still be considered, necessitating an equivalent level of overcorrection.

The common practice for preparing the fascia, especially with SMF, is to thin the SMF by placing it in a cartilage crusher and flattening it with a mallet. This technique cannot be applied to the sacral dermis. Although the author does not use it, deep temporal fascia is another option.

In cases where a rib is harvested, the rectus fascia may be used, and Scarpa's fascia could be considered if necessary. However, its utility may be limited due to its tendency to perforate easily.

7.5.5 Diced Cartilage Without Wrapping, with or Without Fibrin Glue Mixing

Surgeons who have revisited patients with diced cartilage previously inserted without any wrapping material understand how this approach can complicate subsequent surgeries. This is not about using subtle grafts for augmenting depressions or employing less than 2 cc of a fibrin glue mixture to correct the dorsal aesthetic line. When the previous operator has used a significant amount of finely diced rib cartilage for augmentation, the next surgeon is often faced with a considerable mass of scar tissue.

Recent reports suggested that free diced cartilage may result in a lower revision rate than diced cartilage wrapped in fascia (DCF), indicating its potential utility. This finding highlights the importance of evaluating the long-term outcomes and revision rates associated with different cartilage grafting techniques [13]. The volume of dorsal augmentation applied in Asian procedures often significantly exceeds that used in Western operations, making direct comparisons of efficacy challenging. While the author agrees and finds it highly beneficial to mix diced cartilage with fibrin glue for fine-tuning dorsal irregularities, subtle depressions, or flattening sidewalls, extensive experience has shown that widespread implantation of finely diced cartilage across the dorsum can lead to uniformly formed scar masses, especially as the dicing becomes finer. This can complicate flap dissection in secondary surgeries, making the process more difficult. In cases where removing the entire grafted cartilage becomes necessary, the difficulty level can be exceptionally high, akin to the challenges faced when removing paraffinomas.

Given the drawbacks of not maintaining appropriate volume without wrapping and the increased difficulty of secondary surgeries, the author does not utilize this method. There is a critical need for more in-depth evidence on this approach's long-term pros and cons for individuals who have undergone such dorsal augmentation procedures. The author does not endorse this method due to these significant scar formations.

7.5.6 Laminated Rib Graft with the Perichondrium Vs. Solid Rib Graft

Solid rib graft has several problems in the long term. Warping is the biggest problem, followed by demarcation. It is expected to observe dorsal vasculogenesis with solid rib; the thinner the dorsal skin, the more severe the condition. It is similar to vascular hyperplasia around a long-standing silicone capsule. Once healthy circulation reaches the rib and stabilization occurs, hypervascularity will disappear. However, this process takes more than 2 years. Further research is needed to understand the underlying causes fully, but it is hypothesized that the reaction of the dorsal skin may be due to poor circulation. While warping can be corrected through revision surgery, treating vascular hyperplasia of the dorsal skin is considerably more challenging, necessitating caution when using solid rib grafts.

The author believes harvesting the perichondrium and the rib, particularly from the anterior side, is beneficial. A suitable amount of perichondrium attached to the undersurface of the solid rib can significantly contribute to integration with the underlying bone. Dr. Toriumi's technique of using a perichondrial interface is highly effective, and his micro fat-infused soft tissue augmentation approach offers an active solution to issues such as skin thinning [14].

Using laminated rib involves utilizing single or multiple layers of rib laminates at an appropriate thickness. An ongoing debate exists about the risk of three-dimensional warping with laminated rib grafts. The author resolves the issue of augmentations of around 3 mm using a laminated rib covered with perichondrium. For augmentations exceeding this thickness, solid rib grafts are employed. Even when using a septal L-strut extension Graft (SLEG), the need for a long graft extending to the cartilaginous dorsum is lessened, thus favoring the use of a laminated rib. For achieving a smooth dorsal line and addressing a thin skin envelope, a perichondrial cover is necessary, as reported by several authors recently [15].

Since the amount of perichondrium that can be harvested is limited, it is helpful to harvest as much perichondrium as possible when using rib.

References

1. Tebbetts JB. Shaping and positioning the nasal tip without structural disruption: a new, systematic approach. Plast Reconstr Surg. 1994;94:61–77.

2. Daniel RK. Rhinoplasty: open tip suture techniques: a 25-year experience. Facial Plast Surg. 2011;27:213–24.
3. Saban Y, Daniel RK, Polselli R, Trapasso M, Palhazi P. Dorsal preservation: the push down technique reassessed. Aesthet Surg J. 2018;38:117–31.
4. Rohrich RJ, Muzaffar AR, Janis JE. Component dorsal hump reduction: the importance of maintaining dorsal aesthetic lines in rhinoplasty. Plast Reconstr Surg. 2004;114:1298–308. https://doi.org/10.1097/01.prs.0000135861.45986.cf.
5. Jin HR, Won T-B. Rhinoplasty in the Asian patient. Clin Plast Surg. 2016;43:265–79.
6. Toriumi DM, Swartout B. Asian rhinoplasty. Facial Plast Surg Clin North Am. 2007;15:293–307, v.
7. Lam SM. Asian rhinoplasty. Semin Plast Surg. 2009;23:215–22.
8. Guyuron B, Poggi JT, Michelow BJ. The subdomal graft. Plast Reconstr Surg. 2004;113:1037–40; discussion 1041–3.
9. Swanepoel PF, Fysh R. Laminated dorsal beam graft to eliminate postoperative twisting complications. Arch Facial Plast Surg. 2007;9:285–9.
10. Hong S-T, Kim D-W, Yoon E-S, Kim H-Y, Dhong E-S. Superficial mastoid fascia as an accessible donor for various augmentations in Asian rhinoplasty. J Plast Reconstr Aesthet Surg. 2012;65:1035–40.
11. Dhong E-S, Na M-W. The resorption: the hurdle for autogenous-based Asian rhinoplasty. In: Dhong E-S, Na M-W, editors. Asian septorhinoplasty: conundrums and solutions. Singapore: Springer Singapore; 2021. p. 77–89.
12. Lee T-Y, Lee K-I, Dhong E-S, Jeong S-H, Kim D-W, Han S-K. Long-term resorption rate of autogenous onlay graft in east Asian rhinoplasty: a retrospective study. Plast Reconstr Surg. 2022;149:360–71.
13. Kreutzer C, Hoehne J, Gubisch W, Rezaeian F, Haack S. Free diced cartilage: a new application of diced cartilage grafts in primary and secondary rhinoplasty. Plast Reconstr Surg. 2017;140:461–70.
14. Toriumi DM. Dorsal augmentation using autologous costal cartilage or microfat-infused soft tissue augmentation. Facial Plast Surg. 2017;33:162–78.
15. Robotti E, Leone F. The SPF-SPLF graft: building the ideal dorsum in revision rhinoplasty. Plast Reconstr Surg. 2020;145:1420–4.

8 Septal L-Strut Extension Graft (SLEG) for Deviated Nose in Asians

Pearls

- Accurately identifying the nasal midline is very important. It helps understand patient perceptions and consider facial asymmetries and occlusal planes for a balanced surgery.
- For patients whose true nasion is hidden due to fillers, it is necessary to dissolve the fillers before surgery to determine how low the actual nasion is or if the deviation of the bony axis was hidden.
- Caudal septal extension graft (CSEG), using folded cymba cartilage, offers enhanced tip support and stability for correcting deviated caudal septum.
- Anterior extended spreader graft (AESG), applied to the concave side of the septum, is key for aligning the septal axis to the midline.
- AESG with unilateral or bilateral applications tailored to patient deviations. AESG using concha or costal cartilage enhances nasal stability and symmetry, addressing challenges in septal deviation and dorsal aesthetic deficiencies.
- Correcting the bony axis follows septal alignment, utilizing conservative methods like bone shaving and targeted osteotomies to address nasal humps and sidewall convexities.
- Correcting the bony axis is tailored to individual anatomical variations, ensuring stability and symmetry. Careful consideration of intranasal packing is also used to maintain postoperative bony alignment.

Supplementary Information The online version contains supplementary material available at https://doi.org/10.1007/978-981-96-6127-5_8.

8.1 The Deviated Nose Correction: Septal L-Strut Extension Graft (SLEG)

The objective of using SLEG for septal axis correction is to display the dorsum through a rebuilt septum. This method simultaneously represents the anteroposterior projection of the dorsum and the cephalocaudal length. A spreader graft not only aids in improving nasal obstruction but also serves as a visible graft, directly representing the cartilaginous dorsum. The process is not about flattening the base to insert alloplastic material. In low-profile noses, some surgeons may opt for camouflaging the external nose without correcting the septal deviation.

Maintaining the structural integrity of the nasal support L-strut while correcting nasal obstruction is crucial to enhance functionality and aesthetic appearance, even in low-profile noses.

It is more sophisticated to consider the bony and septal axes separately, initially aligning the expected axis of the anterior septum as close to the midline as possible, followed by aligning the bony axis.

E. S. Dhong, *Asian Septorhinoplasty*, https://doi.org/10.1007/978-981-96-6127-5_8

A different strategy is required in patients with severe deflection in the keystone area. Patients with a severely deviated high septum at the rhinion, along with the entire EPP shifting to one side, necessitate efforts to create a new keystone midline, as the already deviated keystone's bony dorsum can hardly be centrally positioned through EPP remodeling alone. It is appropriate to perform EPP correction conservatively.

While there is a method of remodeling to reposition severely convex EPP through transverse osteotomy, recurrence is common. Therefore, the author generally removes EPP that encroaches on the midline but preserves the keystone area (the high portion of EPP). This means the high EPP is preserved and camouflaged, and only the posterior EPP is removed.

The reverse swing door technique may be helpful for a crooked and depressed bony dorsum [1]. Suppose the nasal bone is to be covered as a lid is movable. In that case, one can experience the bony axis being corrected merely by the movement of the nasal bone, even if the deviation of the EPP is not entirely reversed. This method is akin to the reverse of letting down the nasal bone lid in preservation rhinoplasty.

8.2 Bony Axis Vs. Septal Axis

8.2.1 The Midline

The nasal axis deviation should be examined by referring to the lateral photographs in conjunction with the AP photographs of the face mentioned in Chap. 1. If the patient's nose is small or the ANS is lopsided, the patient may not have an accurate perception of their nasal axis because they are used to the illusion of their reflection in the mirror. Most often, when patients complain of a unilateral nose deviation, they describe it as a C-shape or reverse C-shape.

- Observe the patient's eyebrows to determine if they are drawn correctly with the medial canthus.
- Check the position of the ANS and its relationship to the center line of the cupid's bow.
- Have the patient smile to check the relationship with the center of the central incisor.

If a patient is aware of their midline, it is beneficial during the consultation to ask them how they perceive their deviation and to show them a mirror for reassurance. Chapter 1 explains the patient's head-tilting habit, and consideration should be given to the patient's preferred head position when adjusting the roll of the photo to determine the midline (Fig. 8.1).

To demonstrate the patient's occlusal plane, it is helpful to have them bite a tongue depressor using their bilateral molars. It is also essential to make them aware of overall facial asymmetry if occlusal canting or one side of the jaw is smaller. After complex explanations, in cases of severe facial asymmetry, it is wise to determine the midline at a reasonable compromise between reality and the ideal, as a "normal" midline may not exist.

In the operating room, the midline should be referenced by marking the center of the nasion and the center of the cupid's bow on the patient's face, and goals should be set by comparing with the preoperative plan.

- In the operating room, the midline should be determined using the center of the bilateral brow, the center of the bilateral medial canthus, and the center of the cupid's bow as reference points. The target axis to be created after surgery should be determined in advance by referring to the target points from the preoperative analysis.
- The patient should be operated with the perspective of the compromised midline.
- You should refer to artificial eyebrow tattoos or hair grooming.

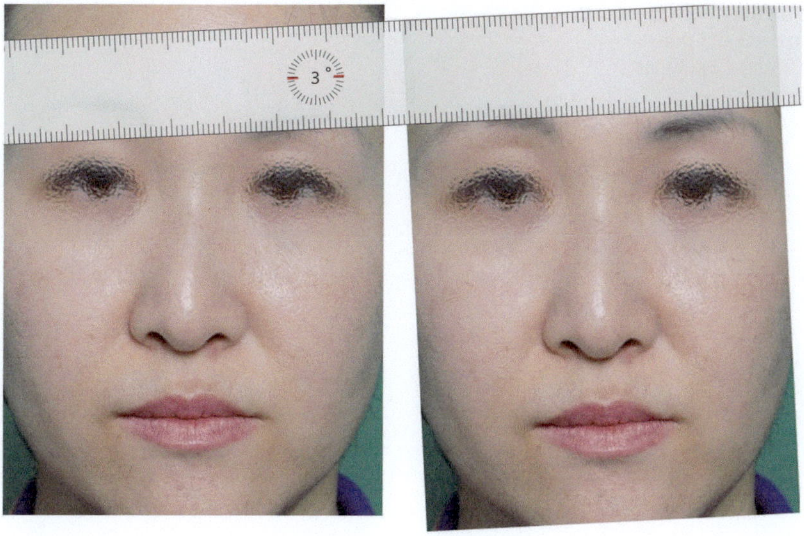

Fig. 8.1 Controlling rolling in AP view. (**a**) Original AP view: Patient's natural head position. (**b**) Rolling control by rotating the photo −3°

8.2.2 The Filler

In patients with a low nasion or a low bony dorsum, it is common for the actual nasion to be masked with filler upon consultation. Since the true nasion can be accurately assessed after dissolving the filler, it is advisable to dissolve it with hyaluronidase 1–2 weeks before surgery and then re-consult.

When using local injections, mix hyaluronidase at less than 50 U to prepare for patients who may not accurately disclose their history of filler injections.

8.2.3 Small Nose and Low Dorsum

When the bony or cartilaginous dorsum is low, diagnosing and planning for axis deviation can be challenging due to its less pronounced nature. It necessitates an effort to correlate the degree of deviation expressed on the external nose by checking the convexity and concavity of the septum through intranasal inspection and referencing CT findings.

In cases where the nose is small and low, and camouflage is attempted solely with an alloplastic implant if the pocket dissection is extensive, it might initially appear that the dorsal axis is straight due to the dead space beneath the implant. However, as the edema subsides and the pocket tightens, the reduction in dead space causes the implant to adhere closely to the platform, thereby revealing any deviation.

8.2.4 Septal Deviation: Nasoscopic and Endoscopic Inspection

Inspect the nasal cavity to determine the degree of deviation of the nasal septum by comparing decongestion and congestion. Observe the shape of the adjacent inferior turbinate. Observe the appearance of the internal nasal valve. Verify that the patient's NOSE scale is consistent with the findings.

- Anatomical findings and patient symptoms are not always the same.
- If an anatomical deviation is found, the doctor will try to correct it, but the surgery should be based on the patient's subjective symptoms.
- Suppose the deviated septum is removed, and the remaining posterior margin and the swinging door of the EPP are in good condition. In that case, surgery is planned for the inferior turbinate at the obstructive site.
- Acoustic rhinometry is performed to obtain an overview of the preoperative and postoperative conditions.

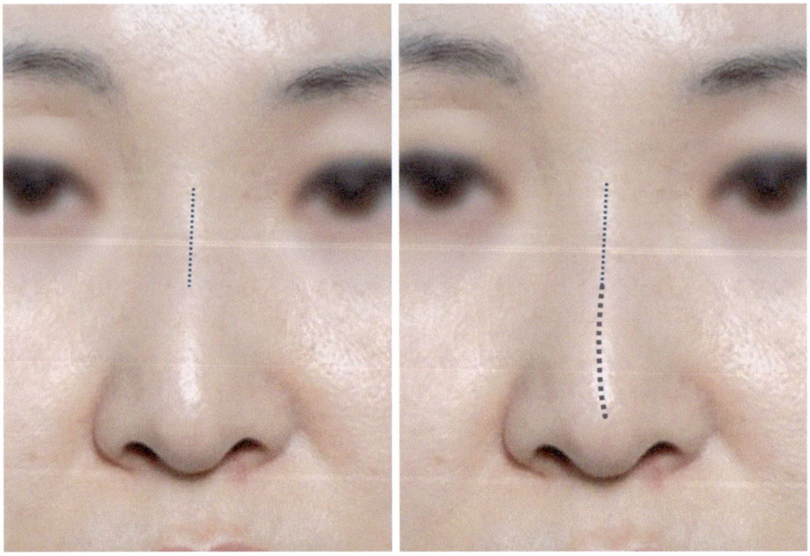

Fig. 8.2 Two different axes. (Left) Bony axis. (Right) Cartilaginous axis

8.2.5 The Difference Between the Bony Axis and the Septal Axis

The entire bony axis and septal axis are connected. Deviations involving both axes can be divided into C-shape and reverse-C shape. If there is no bony axis deviation, it can be divided into left or right septal tilt.

From the side, it can be seen that the tip position is low in cases of severe septal tilt and deviation from C-shape or reverse C-shape. This is because the anterior septal angle is displaced to one side, which is why SLEG is used to overcome this problem. The author prefers to approach the two axes separately and correct the septal axis first (Fig. 8.2).

8.3 The Sequence of the Operation

There is an order to correct the deviation. If the osteotomy is performed before the completion of SLEG, the integrity of the keystone area may be lost, which may cause instability and ruin the entire operation.

The order of operations below is the author's preferred and is meant to be used as needed, picking and choosing from each section, not all.

8.3.1 Hump Shaving

When the dissection is complete, and the nose's soft tissue skin envelope is elevated, the first step is typically to shave any existing hump of the bone. Shaving before septal dissection allows for the removal of the targeted amount of protrusion. After dissection in the keystone area, hidden cartilaginous spurs may be discovered, and the upper lateral cartilages (ULC) may be palpable in a swollen form, necessitating caution.

8.3.2 Caudal Septoplasty with or Without Graft

The following method is used to locate the caudal septum at the desired midline. In conjunction with septal dissection, perform SMR if necessary and position the posterior septal angle at the midline using the following method.

- Caudal septal swinging door suture between ANS and PSA
- Reshaping (scoring incision)
- Translocation to opposite side
- Batten graft
- Caudal septal extension graft (CSEG)

8.3.3 Anterior Septoplasty with Graft

The anterior septum is targeted for midline positioning after correcting the caudal septum. Depending on the situation, this can be done using one of the following methods:

- Unilateral spreader graft (invisible graft)
- Bilateral spreader graft (invisible graft)
- Asymmetric spreader graft (invisible graft) (Fig. 8.3)
- Unilateral anterior extended spreader graft (AESG, visible graft)
- Bilateral AESG (visible graft)
- Asymmetric AESG (visible graft)

8.3.4 Sidewall Shaving

The bony axis will be more noticeable if the septal axis is aligned with the midline. First, excessive convexity of the lateral wall is removed by rasping or burring, which makes the lateral osteotomy easier.

8.3.4.1 Medial Osteotomy

- Medial oblique osteotomy (low nasion and small nose) (Fig. 8.4)
- Paramedian osteotomy (big nose)

8.3.4.2 Lateral Osteotomy

- Intermediate osteotomy
- High to low to high osteotomy (Fig. 8.4)
- Double osteotomy

8.3.4.3 Transverse Osteotomy

- It is required when merging paramedian osteotomy and low-to-low osteotomy.

8.3.5 Tip Plasty

Various sutures and grafts are used to shape the tip. The sutures the author performs on all patients are the interdomal and the lateral crural spanning sutures.

Afterward, the necessary grafts are performed. For Asians with a low absolute amount of cartilage, the subdomal graft, columellar strut graft, and shield graft are helpful ways to create a middle crus with a small amount of cartilage.

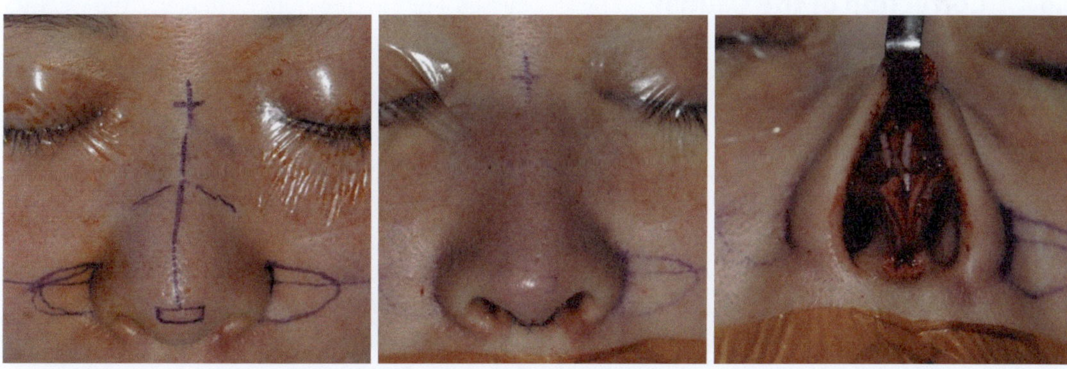

Fig. 8.3 Controlling the cartilaginous axis by applying a spreader graft. (Left) Preoperative design. (Middle) Immediate postoperative status. (Right) Asymmetric AESG, invisible graft

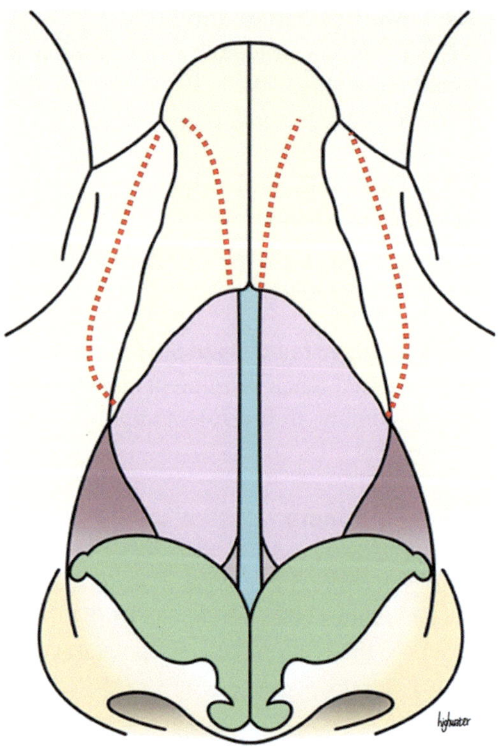

Fig. 8.4 Medial oblique osteotomy and lateral high-low-high osteotomy

8.4 Correction of the Caudal Septum: Caudal Septal Extension Graft (CSEG)

In this paragraph, amidst various methods, we will discuss the advantages of applying the CSEG technique to a deviated nose, which is the center of this book. The most suitable combination for CSEG involves the use of folded cymba cartilage for the following reasons:

In the caudal swing door technique, the reduction in tip support can be reinforced with bilateral batten-type grafts. While the figure of the "8" suture between the anterior nasal spine (ANS) and the posterior septal angle (PSA) can also strengthen the weakened support, its effectiveness is often limited.

During the primary correction of a deviated nose, the soft tissue around the ANS is mostly preserved, making it easier to insert a spread-out folded cymba concha in a tongue-in-groove fashion and repair it to the surrounding periosteum. Initiating the suture with a 4.0 Vicryl can aid in achieving stability.

Most patients with a deviated nose also desire an aesthetically pleasing tip projection, necessitating projection from the caudal septum. In such cases, the transplanted CSEG can be extended to reach the mid crura of the LLC, utilizing it in the form of a midcrural extension graft (Fig. 8.5).

A tip created with only a columellar strut and interdomal suture may find that the tip drops below the original plan in the long term if an excessive amount of SEG is performed, a problem that many rhinoplasty surgeons can relate to [2]. As mentioned, extending the folded cymba concha to reach the midcrural alleviates concerns about long-term tip drooping. As discussed in a previous chapter, the CSEG technique starts with the idea of repairing the caudal end of the quadrangular cartilage using a concave side face-to-face method, where perichondrium exists only on the convex side to facilitate rapid blood supply.

There is sufficient evidence from revision surgeries of patients who used this method, showing well-integrated folded cymba at the caudal end, which supports the effectiveness of this technique in providing long-term stability and reducing the risk of tip drooping.

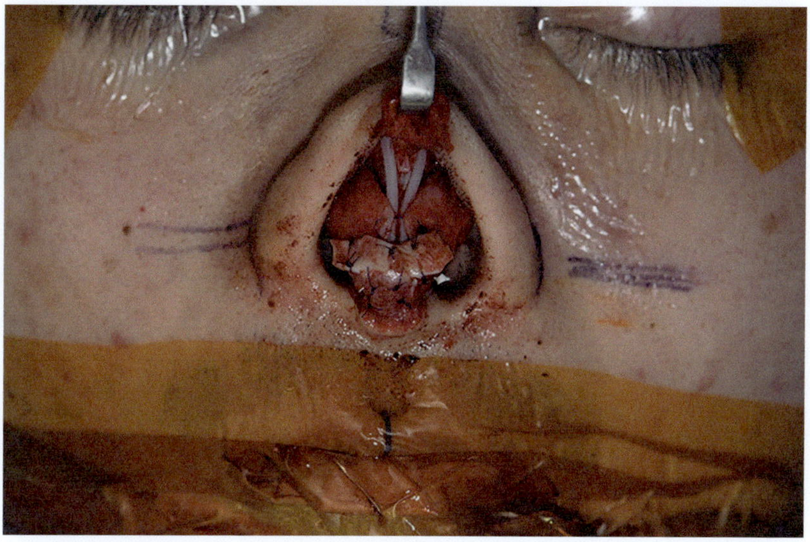

Fig. 8.5 Midcrural extension graft applying the CSEG using folded cymba

8.5 Correction of the Septal Axis: Anterior Extended Spreader Graft (AESG)

8.5.1 Unilateral AESG at the Septal Concave Side

A strategy is needed to bring the septal axis to the midline using AESG. There is debate about whether the spreader graft applied to one side should be on the convex or concave side. However, the author prefers to do it on the concave side [3–5].

Some authors prefer to do a unilateral spreader graft on the convex side [6]. However, the author disagrees. While improvements in the septal axis can be observed during the repair with AESG, it may be pointless to establish a uniform principle.

While bilateral application relative to the central septum is the preferred method, it should be applied according to the patient's deviation, not as a rule.

8.5.2 Bilateral AESG Using Cavum Concha

When AESG is applied to both sides of the anterior septum, facing the concave side of the cavum toward each other is not problematic. Care should be taken to ensure that the repair increases stability as much as possible due to its short length. The entire length should be represented as the anterior septum as much as possible by creating the midline with multiple repairs. This method is among the most technically challenging introduced here. If the cartilage is small or brittle, starting with rib cartilage can save time and increase the success of the surgery.

8.5.3 Bilateral AESG Using Costal Cartilage

Using laminated rib cartilage that has been soaked in Adam's solution for at least an hour is a common practice. Still, even if there is no three-dimensional warping at the time of repair, it is not entirely immune to potential warping that may occur later. However, repairing with the concave sides facing each other can also help mitigate this issue. In the author's practice, laminated rib is always used for bilateral grafting to ensure symmetry and reduce the risk of warping postoperatively.

8.5.4 Asymmetric AESG and Septal Rotation Suture

A helpful method for rotating the AESG in the desired direction involves a septal rotation suture between the AESGs. Alternatively, repairing it

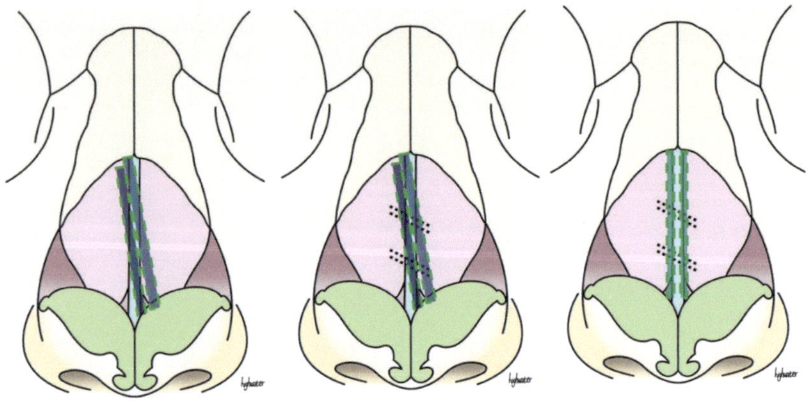

Fig. 8.6 Septal rotation suture. (Left) Two AESGs are tilted. (Middle) Applying two septal rotation sutures. (Right) After the coaptation

with the ULC facilitates axis rotation [7] (Fig. 8.6). The upper lateral cartilage must be repaired in conjunction with the spreader grafts to correct deviation. Although the spreader graft serves as an invisible graft or an anterior septal strut, it is transplanted on the concave side to straighten the anterior septum.

In septal L-strut extension graft (SLEG), the AESGs are usually visible grafts representing the cartilaginous dorsum. The author adds a graft layer on the deficient concave side or one side where the dorsal height remains deficient. In cases where a single layer of AESG does not control the deviation, the author may insert two layers of AESG on the concave side to achieve the desired correction (Video 8.1). However, unless the keystone area is mal-unioned and completely lopsided, it may always be beneficial to place one layer each of AESG on each side of the existing septum.

8.6 Correction of the Bony Axis

It is safe to correct the bony axis after the septal axis has been corrected. This is because it is comfortable to perform the SLEG while the stability of the keystone is secured.

8.6.1 Bone Shaving

The most conservative method of correction is bone shaving for a mild hump on the deviated site. Electric rasping is effective, and a guided electric burr is another option (Video 8.2).

The removal of the hump involves not only eliminating the hump itself but also rasping away the convexity of the lateral nasal side walls. It is possible to correct mild unilateral bony protrusions through extensive rasping and digital pressure. This is particularly true as the nasal lateral walls in Asians tend to be weaker.

8.6.1.1 Medial Osteotomy

During bone shaving, the caudal margin of the nasal bone is carefully dissected to pre-separate the underlying periosteum enough for an osteotome to enter. This pre-determines the path for the osteotome, and in cases where the nasal bone is not large, especially in Asians, a medial oblique osteotomy is preferred. Preserving a substantial bony platform at the radix contributes to the stability of the dorsal graft. In cases of a large nasal bone, avoiding a lengthy medial osteotomy is advisable to prevent a locker deformity. Although paramedial osteotomy is rare, it is sometimes necessary.

8.6.1.2 Lateral Osteotomy

Lateral osteotomy is effective for in-fracturing a convex lateral wall. Although out-fracture of a concave lateral wall is possible, it tends to be less effective than in-fracture, making a complete fracture more efficient. Along with medial oblique osteotomy, a curved high-low-high osteotomy is preferred for lateral osteotomy.

Combining a low-low lateral osteotomy with a transverse osteotomy is effective in cases with a large nasal bone where a paramedian osteotomy is performed.

Osteotomies can be performed internally or percutaneously, but the author prefers the internal continuous method.

8.6.2 Concavity Vs. Convexity of the Side Wall

One aspect that should be considered in correcting the nasal bone's sidewall is the convexity and concavity of the nasal side wall. Although there are methods for intermediate osteotomy for a convex lateral wall, in cases where the overall bone is not large, it may result in small fragments and form a bone defect. Ultimately, to address bony convexity and concavity, the solution may involve segmenting into multiple pieces to achieve flatness. Surprisingly, rasping of the lateral wall can be effective in such cases. Severe convexity might require a double osteotomy or even more segmentation, but most convexities can be flattened with multiple raspings. While the bone thickness may decrease, some areas may remain crushed, contributing to a relatively stable side wall. Electrical rasping can address the convexity of the lateral wall; however, in cases of severe convexity, extensive dissection of the skin's soft tissue envelope might be necessary. For this reason, the author does not perform percutaneous osteotomy on the lateral wall.

The choice between inducing a greenstick fracture and a complete fracture can vary: a complete fracture is preferred for reducing convexity through in-fracture, while a greenstick fracture is favored for resolving concavity through out-fracture.

8.6.2.1 In-Fracture

To correct a broad nasal base that remains unadjusted after rasping the lateral wall to address convexity, an in-fracture of the lateral wall is required. Experience shows that a complete osteotomy through medial and lateral osteotomies has a definitive effect.

In Asian populations, numerous patients undergo lateral wall in-fracture to reduce the width of the bony pyramid. However, it is uncommon for patients to maintain this symmetry long-term. This phenomenon is predominantly attributed to incomplete fractures. To address the convexity and correct an unadjusted broad nasal base following lateral wall rasping, lateral wall in-fracture is deemed necessary. Based on experience, a complete osteotomy, incorporating both medial and lateral osteotomy, is proven effective. Post-osteotomy, excessive packing is discouraged as it may lead to a relapse of convexity. Thus, the use of excessive gauze packing or progressively expanding merocele packing is not preferred. Instead, polyurethane (Nasopore®) is favored for its inability to expand beyond packing pressure, thereby aiding in maintaining the in-fracture's shape. In Asian contexts, while many patients are observed undergoing lateral wall in-fracture to narrow the bony pyramid, the maintenance of symmetry in the long term is exceedingly rare, with most cases believed to be caused by incomplete fractures.

8.6.2.2 Out-Fracture

An attempt is made to create a greenstick fracture to protrude a concave lateral wall outward or to widen a narrow nasal base. After lateral osteotomy, the end of the osteotome is used as a lever to induce an out-fracture. To maintain the out-fracture, ensuring that the previously inserted AESG fits nicely into the medial osteotomy site can be helpful, although technically challenging at times. Excessive open roof creation during hump reduction can render this technique impossible. Thus, as previously mentioned by the author, rasping allows for keeping a portion of the bony platform at the rhinion area, providing more excellent stability. It is crucial to maintain appropriate packing after osteotomy, and if a lateral wall sinking is observed postoperatively, an effort should be made to repack in an outpatient setting.

8.6.3 Packing and Dressing

Proper packing is as crucial as the surgery itself in correcting a deviated nose. Excessive packing should be avoided after an in-fracture. In contrast, appropriate packing following an out-fracture is essential to push the freed lateral wall in the desired direction while simultaneously exerting outward pressure. The dressing for the external part of the nose must also allow for proper compression.

8.7 Turbinoplasty

If one side of the nasal septum is concave, compensatory ipsilateral turbinate hypertrophy occurs. Therefore, it is necessary to reduce the inferior turbinate. There are several types of surgery related to the inferior turbinates, but from a plastic surgery point of view, out-fracture with a simple Freer elevator and packing can expand the nasal cavity easily. A conventional method of reducing turbinate is inferior submucosal turbinectomy (SMT). This method has been used to preserve the function of the nose by minimizing the resection of the mucosa by preserving it and removing mainly the bony part inside. The short-term results are similar in the review of the effects of out-fracture and SMT. Still, in the long term, the Sino-nasal outcome is excellent in SMT compared to radiofrequency-assisted inferior turbinoplasty (RAIT), a minimally invasive technique that can reduce tissue volume. The most powerful effect is achieved with microdebrider-assisted inferior turbinoplasty (MAIT) (Video 8.3). However, the author uses RAIT, which uses high frequency to create lesions within the submucosal tissue of the turbinate to reduce tissue volume. The long-term evaluation revealed reduced resistance and subjective benefits for 2 years after the procedure [8]. The author uses the out-fracture of turbinate with RAIT (Video 8.4).

8.8 Rehabilitation

For bony side wall, deformity found after splint removal more than 10 days after surgery, if the convexity is not corrected or the autograft is placed in the dorsum, it can be corrected by pressing the protruding bone or graft with digital pressing. Especially in green stick fracture, if it is found that the fractured lateral wall is prominent again due to the movement of the transverse nasalis after surgery, it is recommended to teach continuous digital pressing before the bone union so that the convexity can be reduced again by rehabilitation with the patient's manual press.

References

1. Dhong E-S, Na M-W. Secondary septal surgery. In: Dhong E-S, Na M-W, editors. Asian septorhinoplasty: conundrums and solutions. Singapore: Springer Singapore; 2021. p. 147–58.
2. Wang D, Hou K, Zeng N. M-shaped auricular cartilage as modified septal extension graft: a study by three-dimensional anthropometric analysis in Asian rhinoplasty. Aesthetic Plast Surg. 2021;45:2287–94.
3. Boccieri A, Macro C, Pascali M. The use of spreader grafts in primary rhinoplasty. Ann Plast Surg. 2005;55:127–31.
4. Cerkes N. The crooked nose: principles of treatment. Aesthet Surg J. 2011;31:241–57.
5. Rohrich RJ, Gunter JP, Deuber MA, Adams WP Jr. The deviated nose: optimizing results using a simplified classification and algorithmic approach. Plast Reconstr Surg. 2002;110:1509–23; discussion 1524–5.
6. de Oliveira PWB, Pezato R, Gregório LC. Deviated nose correction by using the spreader graft in the convex side. Braz J Otorhinolaryngol. 2006;72:760–3.
7. Guyuron B, Behmand RA. Caudal nasal deviation. Plast Reconstr Surg. 2003;111:2449–57; discussion 2458–9.
8. Garzaro M, Pezzoli M, Landolfo V, Defilippi S, Giordano C, Pecorari G. Radiofrequency inferior turbinate reduction: long-term olfactory and functional outcomes. Otolaryngol Head Neck Surg. 2012;146:146–50.

Reduction-Augmentation Rhinoplasty: Septal L-Strut Extension Graft (SLEG)

9

Pearls

- Asian rhinoplasty often involves both reduction and augmentation due to pseudo-hump noses and a desire for enhanced tip projection.
- In cases where the nasion is very low, it may be necessary to reduce the bony dorsum to improve the overall nasal profile.
- Challenges include avoiding implant use and maintaining structural integrity, especially in secondary surgeries where previous implant complications may necessitate a careful balance between reduction and augmentation.
- Distinguishing between pseudo-hump and mild saddle noses is crucial due to their different septal issues and the common need for tip projection and extension.
- Effective correction often requires careful septal support and consideration of previous septal damage. Techniques like the septal L-strut extension graft (SLEG) are pivotal for maintaining nasal integrity and aesthetics.
- Saddle nose correction in Asian rhinoplasty involves complex grafts to achieve desired tip projection and stability, with SLEG being key for comprehensive reconstruction.
- Autograft resorption can lead to dorsal profile changes, but techniques like anterior extended spreader grafts (AESG) show lower revision rates and minimal post-surgery adjustment needs.
- Long-term, secure AESG integration is crucial for stability, and maintaining tip projection over time may require addressing the membranous septum's role and ensuring strong support from the caudal septum.

Supplementary Information The online version contains supplementary material available at https://doi.org/10.1007/978-981-96-6127-5_9.

9.1 Reduction Vs. Augmentation

One notable characteristic of Asian rhinoplasty is that many patients simultaneously require both reduction and augmentation. Asian rhinoplasty surgeons encounter patients who have a hump nose and complain of inadequate tip projection. The need for reduction decreases as the planned aesthetic line of the dorsum is projected more anteriorly.

In the lateral profile, the areas requiring reduction or augmentation are determined by establishing the positions of the nasion and the subnasale and then by how the nasofacial angle is drawn from the lateral view. One characteristic feature of Asians is the frequent clinical finding of pseudo-hump noses, which means many patients are observed with proper bony dorsum but underprojection of the lower two-thirds of the nose. This occurs frequently with low nasion.

Regardless of the presence or absence of deviation in the frontal view, the development of the bony pyramid may appear normal in the lateral profile. Still, the overall development of the nasal

E. S. Dhong, *Asian Septorhinoplasty*, https://doi.org/10.1007/978-981-96-6127-5_9

bone may be hypoplastic, often resulting in low nasion with proper rhinion area, commonly referred to as having an average profile but a low radix. Asian patients desire a beautifully projected nasal profile. This cohort of reduction-augmentation patients could be another absolute indication for the septal L-strut extension graft (SLEG).

As discussed in later chapters, reduction-augmentation is also applicable in secondary rhinoplasty. Surgeries related to various types of scars and capsules formed by alloplastic implants are subjects for reduction. Asian secondary rhinoplasty, following implant removal, involves the reduction of scars and the augmentation of a new framework, making it a type of reduction-augmentation rhinoplasty.

9.1.1 Error in the Definition of Pseudo-Hump

Many journals define a pseudo-hump as merely a nose with a low radix, a terminology predominantly used in Western society. However, in Asian contexts, one must also consider the underprojection of the tip alongside the radix. The clinical diagnosis between a pseudo-hump and a mild saddle nose can have only subtle differences, depending on where the desired position of the rhinion is placed. A mild saddle nose can be seen as a case where the profile of the radix, rhinion, and tip is average. Still, the cartilaginous dorsum is low, often resulting from trauma or as an acquired condition after septal surgery, such as submucous resection (SMR).

9.1.2 Pitfalls in Correction

In primary rhinoplasty, alloplastic materials are often prioritized when planning surgery to satisfy the patient's desire for an ideal sellion (Si) augmentation and to address the under-projected lower two-thirds of the nose. However, if the diagnosis is a pseudo-hump nose, the insertion of alloplastic material in the dorsum, which does not integrate with the tissue, can lead to excessive pressure at the keystone area and create dead spaces at the nasion and supratip areas. No matter how well an implant is carved, fitting it precisely to the exact curvature is difficult, making it vulnerable to deviation, including see-saw movements. In other words, the original bony dorsum does not require augmentation, but inserting a full-length implant can cause excessive projection in this area.

To overcome this, the efforts are being made to insert multiple layers of alloplastic material at the nasion or supratip area, develop hybrid implants combining Gore-Tex and silicone, or develop 3D-printed implants. However, excessive implantation cannot solve the inherent problems or risks associated with implantation accompanied by septal surgery.

Contrary to the appearances, a pseudo-hump necessitates surgery that preserves the solid keystone area, given that the rhinion area is average height. However, a significant issue arises from enhancing the whole dorsum, which overlooks the problem of weakening the septal framework as a side effect of nose extension, akin to building a castle on sand. These issues are often encountered during submucosal resection and hump reduction. Even if the bony pyramid is not reduced, the L-strut can weaken after SMR, potentially causing problems with the dorsal implant (Fig. 9.1).

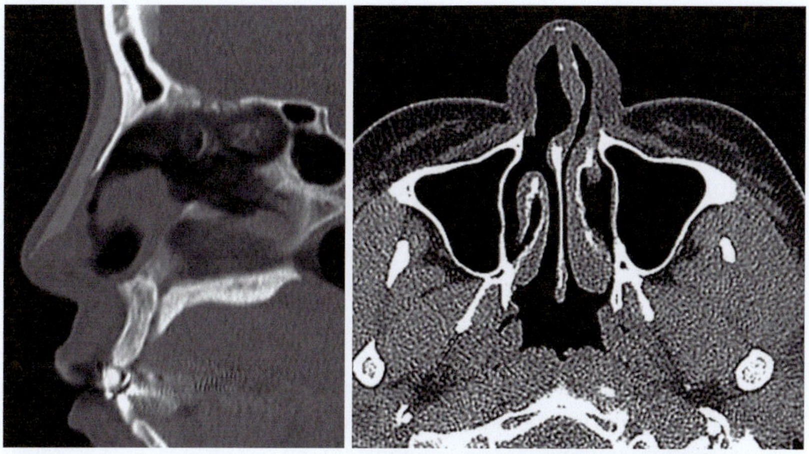

Fig. 9.1 Septal deviation after SMR and dorsal implantation. (Left) Sagittal view of dorsal silicone implant. (Right) Axial view revealed severe septal deviation

9.2 Pseudo-Hump Nose Vs. Mild Saddle Nose

Mild saddle nose and deviation can coexist in patients with a pseudo-hump nose. A more significant characteristic of Asians is the convex profile transitioning into the cartilaginous dorsum and the consequent decrease in tip projection. Therefore, considerations for the tip are mandatory, necessitating planning for both tip projection and extension.

Most author's analyses reveal that the overall upper quarter and the lower two-thirds are underdeveloped, with the hump itself not being significantly pronounced (Fig. 9.2).

It is wise to approach a pseudo-hump nose and mild saddle nose separately, as their septum conditions may differ.

The pseudo-hump nose includes patients with only a low radix area and an overall profile that exhibits a convex profile similar to a small Roman nose. The entire nasal dorsum's aesthetic line is convex, presenting a masculine impression. A straight or slight concave line along the dorsum with tip projection is desired in female patients. Among these patients, those with a trauma history or severe septal deviation upon inspection might have weaker septal support than it appears. It's conceivable that many cases involve simultaneous undergrowth at the radix and overgrowth at the rhinion following unnoticed nasal trauma. Even in cases without a trauma history, it's advisable not to promise surgery solely based on septal cartilage, as it might not be robust and substantial, unlike in generalized hump patients. This is because one might encounter thin and insufficient septal cartilage during surgery.

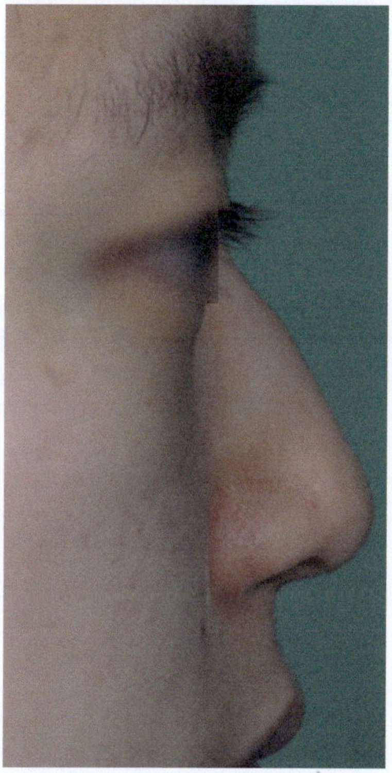

Fig. 9.2 Lateral view of a patient with an underdeveloped nasion and a convex dorsal profile

- Mild saddle nose deformity involves a low cartilaginous dorsum, often accompanied by a significant history of septal trauma and a deviated septum. Septal harvest is likely not enough as you expect it to be.

In both pseudo-hump and mild saddle noses, there's often a history of septal damage, so correction relying solely on dorsal camouflage without proper reinforcement of the caudal septum has limitations. Maintaining the strength of a high dorsum with only anterior spreader grafts without caudal septum support is challenging. Hence, it's difficult to agree that a cantilever type of anterior spreader graft can create a high septum without proper support to an already damaged or weakened nasal base due to SMR, except perhaps in rare cases with undamaged septums. In other words, reinforcing the roof only with an anterior extended spreader graft is likely successful only in cases where the remaining caudal septum is exceptionally sturdy [1].

The author has performed surgeries on pseudo-humps and saddle noses using the SLEG for the past 20 years. It's believed to be a challenging task to maintain the projection of the cartilaginous dorsum only with an anterior extended spreader graft on a weak septum [2–4].

9.3 The Sequence of Reduction–Augmentation

9.3.1 Bone Shaving

Even if the rhinion position in a pseudo-hump nose is minimal, a minor amount of hump may need to be shaved down for the sake of the dorsal aesthetic line. The issue arises from the potential for the rhinion to become flattened after an appropriate shave down and the risk of creating an open roof deformity.

If the base of the bony pyramid has been lowered after bone shaving, it may be necessary to narrow it with bilateral lateral osteotomies. After lateral osteotomy, minimal bone shaving is also required to avoid creating a palpable bony protrusion.

9.3.2 Component Reduction of Dorsal Hump

The rhinion area in a pseudo-hump nose can be composed of a cartilaginous hump and excess cartilage from the upper lateral cartilages (ULC). Therefore, even after bone shaving, it's common to observe protrusion at the lower or lateral parts of the rhinion. Most Asian rhinoplasty surgeons are expected to follow a component hump reduction approach. After bone shaving, an unnoticed septal hump hidden posteriorly may become more prominent. This occurs as the lock at the keystone area is released, making the cartilaginous hump protrude further. Furthermore, the T-shaped roof junction between the ULC and the septum should be adequately separated, ensuring effective reduction of the lateral ULCs.

Excessive resection in this area may necessitate significant augmentation, hence the need for careful component reduction. The inaccurate reduction of the hump is a primary cause of post-surgical hump recurrence, attributable to two main factors. The first involves uncertain management of the cartilaginous hump and the visibility of remnants of the surrounding upper lateral cartilages (ULC) later on. The second issue arises from graft resorption at the dorsum, which leads to the visibility of the convex aesthetic line (Fig. 9.3).

9.3.3 Is it Applicable: Preservation Rhinoplasty in Asians

The recent advancement in rhinoplasty within Western society, termed "preservation rhinoplasty," is heralded as a revolutionary approach. However, the applicability of this technique to Asian populations raises essential questions [5, 6].

Many Western surgeons are enthusiastically exploring this new field with a mix of anticipation and concern. However, the author remains skeptical about its applicability to Asian patients due to anatomical challenges. The concept of achieving hump reduction through posterior reduction, as is often done in preservation rhinoplasty, is chal-

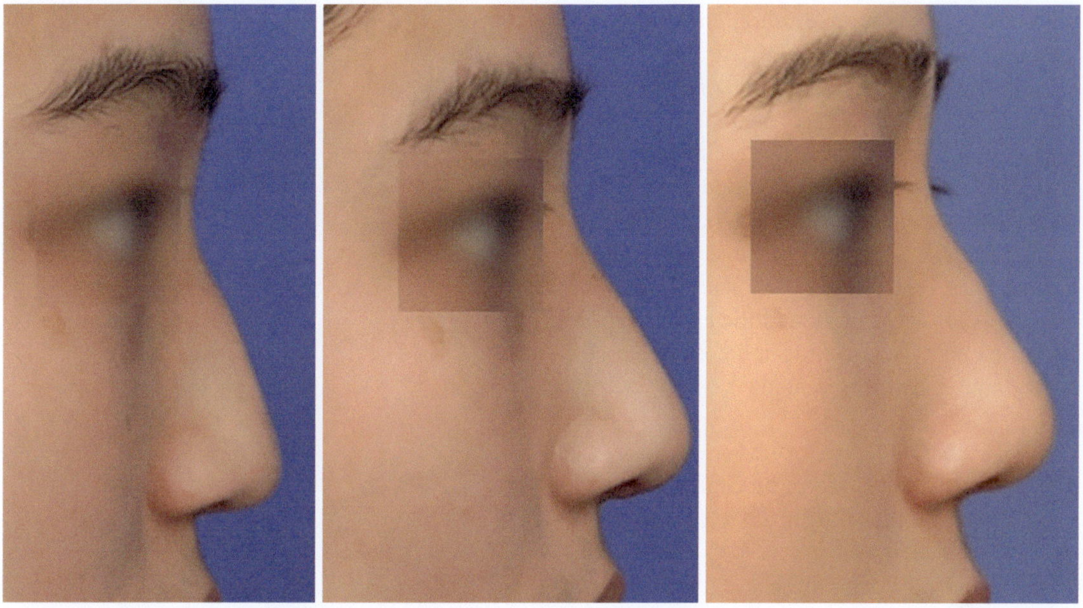

Fig. 9.3 Dorsal graft resorption of superficial mastoid fascia (SMF). (Left) Preoperative lateral view. (Middle) Postoperative 3 months. (Right) Postoperative 18 months: Dorsal soft-tissue graft resorption required minor revision

lenging to apply in Asians who typically do not possess the anatomical structure suitable for such a procedure. While it might apply to a few patients with significantly big noses, such cases are expected to be exceedingly rare.

9.3.4 Septal L-Strut Extension Graft (SLEG): Caudal Septal Extension Graft (CSEG) + Anterior Extended Spreader Graft (AESG)

After appropriate reduction, SLEG is necessary to augment the lower two-thirds. This method is similar to the deviated nose correction discussed in Chap. 8.

Therefore, in Asian patients undergoing septorhinoplasty with submucous resection, there is a distinctive need for extra cartilage harvest almost universally. The primary choice for graft material is the cymba concha, followed by the cavum concha as the second preferred donor site. Rib cartilage is considered in cases where severe septal deformity is observed upon preoperative inspection, in patients where ossification of the septum is anticipated, or in the presence of septal perforations. Below, we discuss methods previously introduced for addressing the lower two-thirds.

9.4 Augmentation of the Lower 2/3

The traditional saddle nose correction uses alloplastic material in the dorsum.

Different reconstructive methods are required depending on the condition of the lower 2/3 of the nose and the degree of underprojection of the cartilaginous dorsum.

The severity of a saddle nose can range from mild middle vault depression due to the extent of trauma to the cartilaginous dorsum to more severe cases presenting as L-strut depression and, in the most extreme instances, manifesting as nasal shortening. The desired state of the tip position varies among patients, but most aim for a higher tip projection than what they had preoperatively.

Consequently, cases where anterior spreader grafts alone provide satisfactory results are exceedingly rare, often leading to issues with stability.

Severe saddle nose requires more grafting, and several methods have been introduced as composite reconstruction. The composite meaning here is that the anterior and caudal septum are reconstructed simultaneously [7–9].

The anterior septum is divided according to whether it is a solid rib in the form of a spreader graft or a cantilever graft, and the caudal septum is divided into a septal strut or a columellar strut depending on how it is treated.

9.4.1 Bilateral Spreader Graft with Columellar Strut: Tongue and Groove

This technique employs bilateral spreader grafts combined with a caudal columellar strut graft (Fig. 9.4). It is particularly effective in addressing mild cases of saddle nose deformity or pseudohump nasal configurations.

As reported earlier, while increasing nasal length can be effective, the impact on tip projection is relatively limited. Achieving the same level of projection force with a columellar strut as with a septal extension graft (SEG) is challenging.

For an effective tongue-and-groove technique, shaping solely with septal cartilage can be difficult, making using costal cartilage more advantageous when harvested [10].

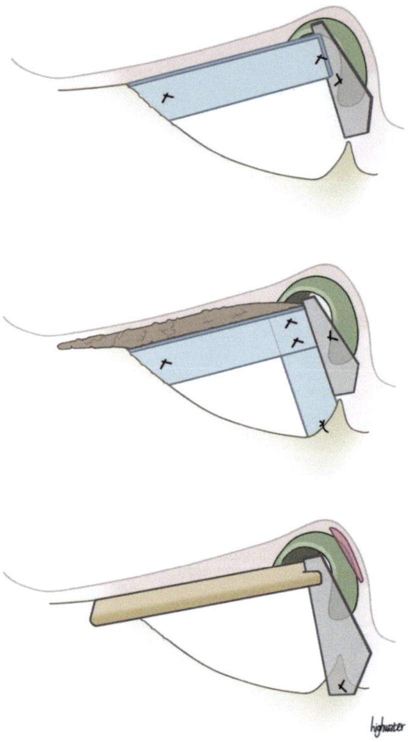

Fig. 9.4 Various types of framework reconstruction. (Above) Bilateral spreader graft with columellar strut. (Middle) Pistol: extended spreader graft + septal end-to-end strut. (Low) Solid rib + columellar strut (redrawn the figure from Ref. [9])

9.4.2 Pistol: Extended Spreader Graft + Septal End-to-End Strut

9.4.2.1 Solid Rib + Columellar Strut

In addition to the columellar strut method above, a septal strut is added to the caudal septum (Fig. 9.4). This approach is utilized when a more stable caudal septum is desired. The difference lies in extending the dorsum using spreader grafts or incorporating solid rib material [8].

The distinction may seem complex and convoluted, but it can be simplified into deciding whether to employ a columellar strut, a septal strut, or a combination of both. Additionally, it involves choosing between using a spreader-type graft for the high septum or creating the dorsal profile with a solid rib.

9.4.2.2 Caudal Septal Replacement Graft: L-Shape Strut

Reconstructing the anterior and caudal septum simultaneously is theoretically feasible, but there are significant constraints in Asian patients (Fig. 9.5). These include the technical challenge of harvesting a suitably sized piece of cartilage in an L-shape. Harvesting costal cartilage in this specific shape is also tricky. In reality, procuring entire septal cartilage is essential for application in primary rhinoplasty.

9.4.2.3 SLEG: AESG + CSEG

This method is distinct in that the extension of the caudal septum involves a batten-type bilateral

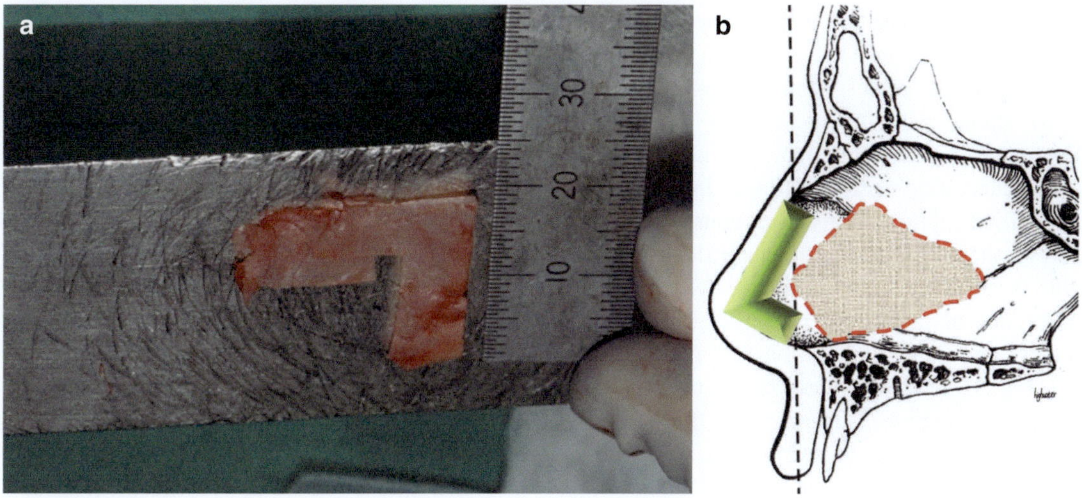

Fig. 9.5 Caudal septal replacement graft (**a**) L-shape strut. (**b**) Schematic of L-shape strut

graft. Additionally, it subtly differs by directly enhancing and expressing the anterior extension through the lower 2/3 of the nose. This technique was developed due to the unique characteristics of Asian noses, which require different surgical approaches than Western noses.

In Asian primary rhinoplasty, patients often prefer not to harvest rib cartilage when correcting pseudo-hump noses and mild saddle noses. However, in most secondary cases, rib cartilage is necessary. The resistance is encountered with the hard nasal tip, followed by concerns regarding scars, anesthesia, and cost issues.

The alternative approach, therefore, is to maximize the stable projection of the lower two-thirds of the nose using available septal and ear cartilage. Employing an AESG can reduce the burden on the dorsal onlay, while a CSEG can simultaneously reinforce, extend, and project the caudal septum. This strategy applies to both primary and secondary rhinoplasty (Fig. 9.6).

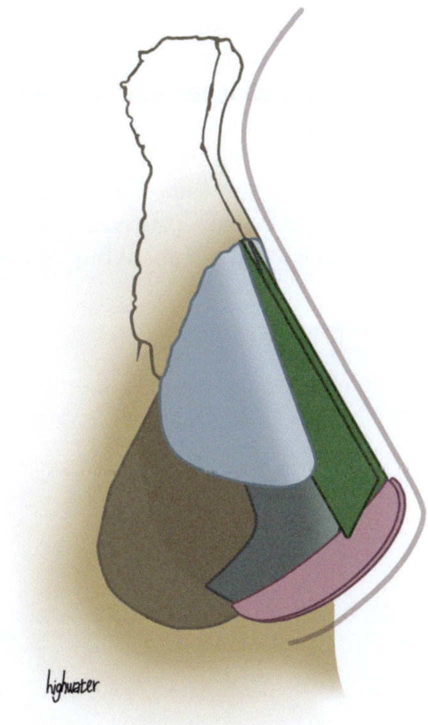

Fig. 9.6 Schematic of SLEG: AESG + CSEG (illustration from Ref. [4])

9.5 Strategy for Very Low Nasion

When patients reject alloplastic materials, the most stable radix graft requires a solid rib. However, young Asian females may prefer to avoid harvesting costal cartilage. In such cases, alternative options must be considered. The author, therefore, favors diced cartilage wrapped with fascia (DCF) in this scenario. Although various types of fascia can be utilized, the author mainly prefers superficial mastoid fascia (Video 9.1; Fig. 9.7) Many patients refuse to leave scars even at the temple. Depending on the necessity, fine dicing may not be carried out, and alternatives, such as crushed bone fragments from SMR or EPP corrections or even from the maxillary crest during convexity corrections, can be helpful. If septal cartilage remains available, preserving its flat surface by wrapping it with SMF rather than dicing can yield a higher layer of grafts.

Due to the decreased absolute requirement of dorsal onlay grafts for the lower 2/3 using AESG, achieving the desired nasion graft approximation can be accomplished with SMF and small amounts of cartilage alone. Patients must be adequately informed about the possibility of resorption, and consent must be obtained regarding the potential need for retouch procedures.

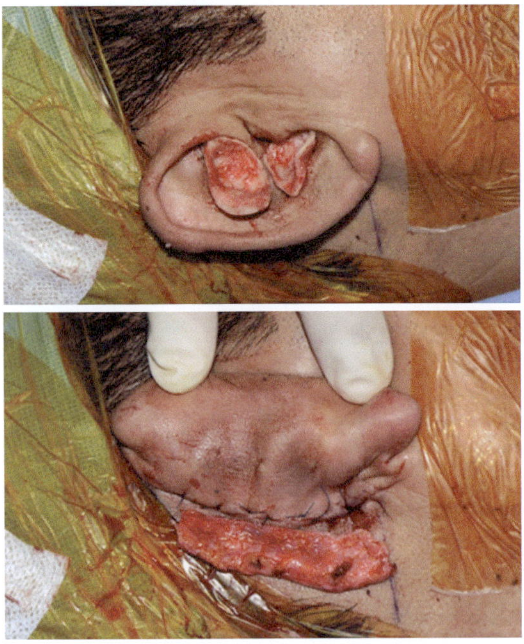

Fig. 9.7 Materials for nasion graft. (Above) Cavum and cymba concha. (Low) Superficial mastoid fascia

9.6 Pseudo-Hump Nose Mixed with Deviated Nose

As mentioned in Chap. 8, the usefulness of SLEG in correcting a deviated nose has already been explained. However, pseudo-humps are frequently present during preoperative analysis of patients with deviation. This increases the likelihood of weakening the rhinion during surgery, making applying SLEG more difficult.

When lateral osteotomy is required, it is safer to reconstruct it using shaving and in-fracture techniques whenever possible.

9.7 Long-Term Problems

9.7.1 Dorsal Profile Change: Resorption

If the limited longevity of alloplastic implants is a disadvantage, then the downside of autografts is the unexpected resorption rate. When only soft tissue is used for a dorsal graft, one must anticipate a resorption rate of more than 30–50%. Since resorption can continue for more than 18 months post-surgery, it is advisable to use grafts made from harvested cartilage and bone whenever possible. However, when comparing cases where dorsal grafts were performed from the nasion to the tip without AESG to cases where AESG was performed together, the latter showed a relatively lower revision rate. Even if a revision is needed, the volume to be augmented is minimal.

While filling the entire nose with filler may not be feasible, retouching with filler or fat grafts in the small area is relatively less burdensome.

9.7.2 Sinking Tendency of AESG

Rarely does saddle nose deformity recur due to instability in the rhinion area after AESG. Some suggest that the hump may regrow, but in the author's experience, there haven't been instances of hump regrowth in patients operated on outside of their growth period.

It's important to differentiate between the visibility of an undercorrected bony dorsum and a separate issue caused by the resorption of the soft tissue.

There have been no experiences of AESG grafts becoming fractured due to trauma.

Reports exist of discovering unnoticed saddling of the septal cartilage after the removal of implants in secondary cases. Often, this is attributed to cartilage erosion due to alloplastic implants or physical depression rather than gravitational tilting, which may occur due to the weak physical properties of the cartilaginous dorsum.

The author emphasizes the importance of a secure union of AESG connected to the high septum for achieving a stable dorsal aesthetic line. In most primary reduction-augmentation procedures, using a TCC suture is unnecessary [11]. The need for this suture indicates a loss of stability in the rhinion during surgery. To adequately anticipate the posterior displacement of AESG, a small wedge at the caudal end or conservatively dissecting at least one side of the high mucosal pocket should be considered. Suturing between the high septum and AESG should be done multiple times with various types of sutures, and the number of attempts may vary depending on the patient's condition. However, trying at least five different ties is essential to ensure security.

9.7.3 Decrease in Tip Projection

As time passes, tip projection may decrease. Among the sutures related to projection, such as interdomal suture, lateral crural spanning suture, medial crural approximation, and columella-septal suture, are associated with the long-term position of the tip [12]. The decrease in tip height in patients who attempted tip projection with SLEG is primarily attributed to the resorption of the soft-tissue tip graft. Strong support can be maintained through multiple sutures between the LLC and the high septum. LLCs can catch up with the projection using subdomal grafts or mid-crural extension grafts fixed to the CSEG.

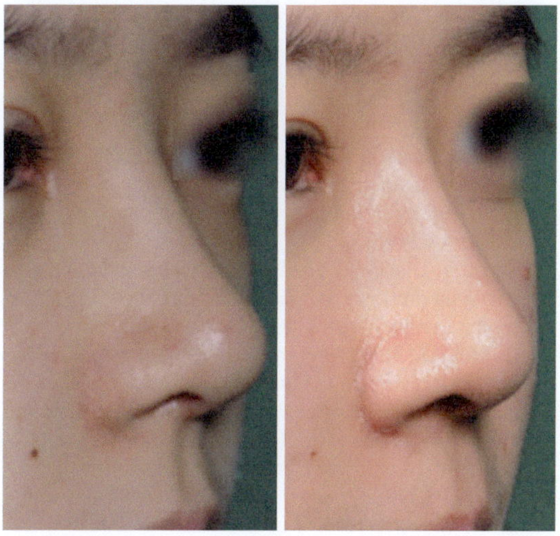

Fig. 9.8 Decrease in tip position after SLEG: In the long term, the reduction in tip projection is caused by the resorption of the soft-tissue graft. (Left) Postoperative 3 months. (Right) Postoperative 18 months

However, the essential factor in the correlation between the LLC complex and the caudal septum is the membranous septum, which acts as a buffer zone between the tip and the membranous septum, where natural factors cause a decrease in tip projection. If the force of the tip tripod is weak, the loosening will be more severe. If the LLC complex is not projected due to a high septum, for example, as in the case of a columellar strut, the degree of decrease in tip projection will be more severe [13]. Even if a practical tip projecting onlay graft is multilayered, if it does not provide direct support from the caudal septum, a decrease in tip projection can be expected due to pressure from the soft-tissue envelope, gravity, edema reduction, and tissue repositioning during the healing process. In SLEG, the decrease in tip projection is minimal due to the possibility of septum-dependent tip positioning in long-term observations (Fig. 9.8).

References

1. Kim B-K, Han J. Use of an augmentation spreader graft for management of nasofacial angle in patients with pseudo-hump. Ann Plast Surg. 2019;82:369–74.
2. Namgoong S, Kim S, Kim H-R, Jeong S-H, Han S-K, Dhong E-S. Folded cymba concha: is it large and sta-

ble enough for caudal septal extension graft in Asian rhinoplasty? Aesthet Surg J. 2021;41:NP737–47.
3. Hwang N-H, Dhong E-S. Septal extension graft in Asian rhinoplasty. Facial Plast Surg Clin North Am. 2018;26:331–41.
4. Kim SB, Baik SH, Lee KI, Dhong ES, Jeong SH,Han SK. Functional evaluation of septal L-strut extension graft in East Asians. J Plast Reconstr Aesthet Surg. 2024;94:178–186.
5. Saban Y, Daniel RK, Polselli R, Trapasso M, Palhazi P. Dorsal preservation: the push down technique reassessed. Aesthet Surg J. 2018;38:117–31.
6. Daniel RK. The preservation rhinoplasty: a new rhinoplasty revolution. Aesthet Surg J. 2018;38:228–9.
7. Romo T 3rd, Sclafani AP, Sabini P. Reconstruction of the major saddle nose deformity using composite allo-implants. Facial Plast Surg. 1998;14:151–7.
8. Daniel RK. Rhinoplasty: septal saddle nose deformity and composite reconstruction. Plast Reconstr Surg. 2007;119:1029–43.
9. Daniel RK, Brenner KA. Saddle nose deformity: a new classification and treatment. Facial Plast Surg Clin North Am. 2006;14:301–12, vi.
10. Guyuron B, Varghai A. Lengthening the nose with a tongue-and-groove technique. Plast Reconstr Surg. 2003;111:1533–9; discussion 1540–1
11. Haack S, Hacker S, Mann S, Gubisch W. Bony fixation of the nasal framework. Facial Plast Surg. 2019;35:23–30.
12. Petroff MA, McCollough EG, Hom D, Anderson JR. Nasal tip projection. Quantitative changes following rhinoplasty. Arch Otolaryngol Head Neck Surg. 1991;117:783–8.
13. Akkus AM, Eryilmaz E, Guneren E. Comparison of the effects of columellar strut and septal extension grafts for tip support in rhinoplasty. Aesthetic Plast Surg. 2013;37:666–73.

Part III

Secondary Nose

10 Blind Faiths in Asian Rhinoplasty

Pearls

- In Asian rhinoplasty, people often try new methods and materials before there is enough evidence to prove they are safe and effective. Without strict regulations, this can harm patients. This shows why it's important for doctors to be careful and base their practices on solid evidence, focusing on the long-term safety of their patients rather than seeking quick results or peer acclaim.
- In Asian rhinoplasty, there's misplaced confidence in the safety and efficacy of alloplastic implants, even on osteotomized nasal bones, despite varying complication rates and potential severe outcomes, including irreversible damage.
- Additionally, the belief that septorhinoplasty is inherently a clean surgery underestimates the complexities and risks involved, especially when using empirical antibiotics, highlighting the need for more evidence-based approaches and caution.
- In secondary Asian rhinoplasty, there are absolute indications for exclusively using autologous grafts, particularly when addressing complications related to the soft tissue envelope, nasal framework, and functional issues.
- While innovative, the advent of 3D manufactured materials in rhinoplasty often overlooks the complexity of nasal anatomy and surgical nuances, leading to misplaced trust in their ability to precisely match the desired outcome.
- Reconstructing the septal L-strut and minimizing the need for additional grafting or alloplastic implants by utilizing autografts, particularly in secondary surgeries, offers a comprehensive solution to many challenges in Asian rhinoplasty, focusing on preserving nasal integrity and functionality.

Asian Rhinoplasty: The "Myth"

In Asian cultures, aesthetic surgery saw significant development starting in the 1970s. It is characterized by a unique perspective, often summarized by the belief that "my way is the only way." This has led to a notable acceptance of surgeries that incorporate alloplastic materials.

Viewing the situation impartially, when a patient seeks exceedingly sophisticated cosmetic results driven by the desire for perfection, it often stems from vanity. It is essential for both the patient and the medical professional to ensure that vanity does not dictate their decisions. Here, mutual disengagement or the expectation of a satisfactory outcome diminishes concerns about the procedures. The long-term viability of implanted alloplastic materials remains uncertain for medical professionals. Although there is no universally recognized "guarantee period for the safety"

Supplementary Information The online version contains supplementary material available at https://doi.org/10.1007/978-981-96-6127-5_10.

E. S. Dhong, *Asian Septorhinoplasty*, https://doi.org/10.1007/978-981-96-6127-5_10

of these materials, this lack of certainty is not typically communicated between doctors and patients.

Breast augmentation procedures use relatively large alloplastic materials, and modern implants often include bags equipped with barcode tracers for identification and tracking. However, the materials used in Asian rhinoplasty procedures are subject to fewer regulations, and there is often a lack of consistency in the documentation and tracking of the source materials across medical facilities.

Surgeons should be aware of the potential for underestimating the overall complication rates of using materials such as silicone or Gore-Tex in surgical procedures. This underestimation is often due to a reliance on literature that may not fully account for the potential complications. Compared to the simple rhinoplasty of the past, the surgery in the recent decade has become very complex, especially when the septum is involved.

- A highly respected American rhinoplasty surgeon I hold in high esteem once remarked to himself after watching one presentation on Asian rhinoplasty at a Korean Society meeting, "It's not a good idea to use so many grafts." It seemed that even such a distinguished doctor might not fully grasp the methodological necessities unique to Asian rhinoplasty.
- In this specific surgical context, the extensive use of grafts is often required.

10.1 Blind Faiths in Asian Rhinoplasty

All doctors become independent research institutions, each operating based on their morality and an Individual Review Board (IRB)-based research system. This underscores the necessity for extensive medical education, which facilitates the development of innovative medical practices that adhere to bioethical standards. Given the diverse and unpredictable nature of situations encountered in the operating room, such education is critical to equip medical professionals with the ability to make nuanced judgments. While universally valid methods exist, adventurous surgical actions within the legal framework are legal and medical. However, the outcomes can often be adverse if non-standard methods are used. This is particularly true in Asian rhinoplasty, which requires a significant amount of material and where new substances are constantly being tested and sometimes fail. The issue arises because applying new methods is not illegal per se, but the burden of any adverse outcomes falls entirely on the patient. If a technique introduced as the best practice is abandoned within 3–4 years, it raises questions about the patients who underwent surgery using that method.

Self-regulation within medical societies has limits, and the severity of these issues is widespread since cosmetic surgery is not performed in all specialties. In Asian rhinoplasty, which frequently uses alloplastic materials, many new substances have been introduced, failing later, even though the KFDA initially approved them. It's particularly concerning that the use of such materials gets published in SCI journals and gains scientific impact, with the patients bearing the brunt of the damage 4–5 years later, and the task of rectifying such harm falls to conscientious doctors. A notable example of this is the absorbable mesh plate.

The typical issues are as follows:

- "I might be using a new material or method without perfect evidence, but it should be fine.
- I've tried this method on several patients over a few months, and although one or two experienced complications, the overall outcomes were satisfactory.
- I don't know the causes of these complications, but they should be manageable.
- I've been a successful doctor so far. Why wouldn't I continue to do well?
- I need to present this content quickly at a conference or seminar."

When a paper is published, it undergoes peer review. However, presentations at seminars, especially to young doctors, significantly impact the next day's surgery. Doctors might adopt methods with scant evidence after hearing about them at conferences or symposia or following information from developers of new materials. This is particularly common among young doctors when the method is simple or involves ready-made materials. Asian septorhinoplasty often requires significant material to achieve the desired appearance.

Even peer-reviewed papers can be problematic for direct clinical application to patients due to the novelty of the content, which might be valued for its rarity rather than its clinical relevance. Moreover, rhinoplasty surgeons who primarily operate on other ethnicities may be largely unaware of new Asian techniques and their consequences. It's wise for doctors to be conservative and approach new methods cautiously.

A clinic that caused a significant issue in Korean society years ago due to complications from nasal surgeries still practices and advertises alloplastic materials for extension grafts in the septum to create long, high tips. Patients continue to suffer. Beyond disputes between plastic surgery and otolaryngology, doctors must adopt a self-regulating approach to quality control.

- Intraseptal surgical site infections can leave unimaginable deformities.

Because the person performing the final surgery assumes all responsibility once legal and financial issues are resolved, the patient and the last doctor ultimately suffer the consequences.

Faith is based on collective scientific evidence from multiple doctors, while blind faith is the hope that good things will happen. A 1% devastating outcome can overshadow 99% good outcomes. Anyone can be the victim of that 1–5% of bad results.

When a new technique gains blind faith, the damage from a bad outcome can be unimaginable.

Additionally, there is a "false hope" that problems caused by alloplastic implants can be resolved with more alloplastic materials. This is entirely a false hope. While believing what one wishes is a matter of personal freedom, such an approach is unacceptable regarding patient care.

A rational doctor should aim for long-lasting surgical outcomes and, ideally, be the last surgeon to operate on the patient. However, it's even more crucial to ensure that if another surgeon must operate on the patient later, the patient's condition should be such that further surgery is feasible. The prevalence of cases where revision is nearly impossible is often due to ignorance or a selfish form of blind faith.

Ultimately, the message is to avoid new techniques or methods that could lead to severe complications due to a lack of evidence. There's a need for a broader perspective on Asian operations or a more conservative approach. Even though a method is published in a journal, it still needs to be validated or widely accepted by most doctors. If complications arise from the authors' techniques, it's important to publicize these issues and reflect on and share their methods. The author strongly opposes using materials like Medpor and absorbable mesh in the intraseptal area, as dealing with the complications caused by these materials has been mentally and emotionally taxing.

10.2 Typical Blind Faiths of Asian Rhinoplasty

10.2.1 Alloplastic Implants Have Healthy Longevity Even over Osteotomized Nasal Bone

The use of alloplastic implants in Asian rhinoplasty is common, and the reported complication rate varies between 4 and 15%, depending on the source [1]. However, this should be distinguished from the current situation, which involves more complex surgeries and more aggressive use of materials. This book does not discuss the use of dorsal implants with minimal manipulation and without septal surgery; instead, it addresses the issue of devastating complications that leave no possibility for reoperation due to deviation or cosmetic dissatisfaction. My intention is not to be confrontational but to acknowledge the problems associated with implants placed on osteotomized bone or the severe deformities resulting from implants used in conjunction with septal surgery.

- Silicone implants can cause bone resorption of the undersurface due to pressure, gravity, and the constant physical force exerted by the soft tissue pocket.
- Alloplastic material on osteotomized bone can lead to malunion of the lower bony pyramid.
- Lower bony irregularities may be anticipated in cases of reoperation following implant removal, and a CT scan is necessary for diagnosis.

Apart from the problem of nonunion or malunion of the osteotomy itself, the problem of the dorsum implant pushing down on the underlying bony base can cause unwanted lateral nasal wall deviation (Fig. 10.1).

A nasal mucosal tear that can occur after medial osteotomy and the wound problem that arises here can lead to capsule formation of the alloplastic implant located in the dorsum and subsequent fibrous granuloma or mucosal invagination [2].

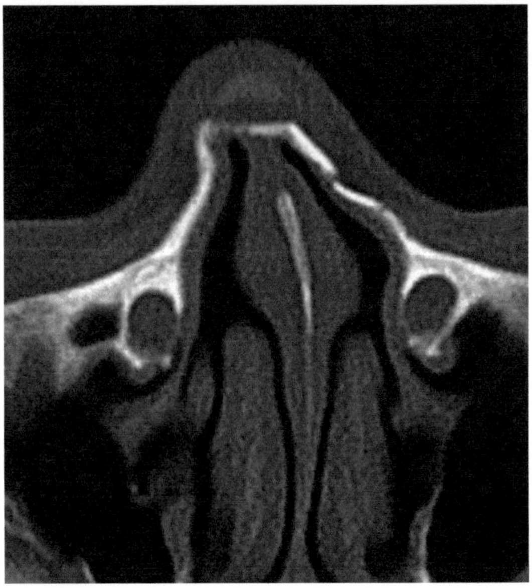

Fig. 10.1 Malunion of both nasal walls: silicone over the osteotomized bony pyramid

10.2.2 Asian Septorhinoplasty Is a Clean Surgery; Empirical Antibiotics Generally Provide Adequate Coverage

- When accompanied by septal surgery, or following an ear cartilage harvest with grafting, and finally during implantation, Asian septorhinoplasty becomes a clean-contaminated surgery.
- Preoperative, intraoperative, and postoperative antibiotic therapy is essential.

It is highly unscientific to treat postoperative infections (acute surgical site infections) with empirical antibiotics, even with continuous postoperative antibiotics.

It is essential to use appropriate antibiotics based on the potentially infectious normal flora (PINF) and the physiology of the patient's nasal cavity [3].

If the burden of PINF in the preoperative nasal swab is high, it is helpful to prepare the patient for surgery by cleaning the nose with a nose bidet using normal saline.

Dorsal implantation should be successful over a cartilaginous platform that has been resected, such as a septum that has undergone submucosal resection

- If an implant is placed on a platform weakened by SMR, the underlying platform will not be able to withstand the load (Fig. 10.2).
- Problems with septal deviation can occur after surgery.

No author has reported the long-term effects of using a spreader graft beneath an implant. The effectiveness of combining an implant with a subimplant spreader graft in Asian rhinoplasty has not yet been documented. The functionality of a spreader graft under the implant warrants careful consideration. The author believes that functional improvement will not occur unless the cross-sectional area of the nasal cavity is increased or the angle between the upper lateral cartilage (ULC) and the septum is widened. The opposite phenomenon will adversely affect the function of the nose, i.e., the platform of the ULC depressed by the implant will cause nasal narrowing.

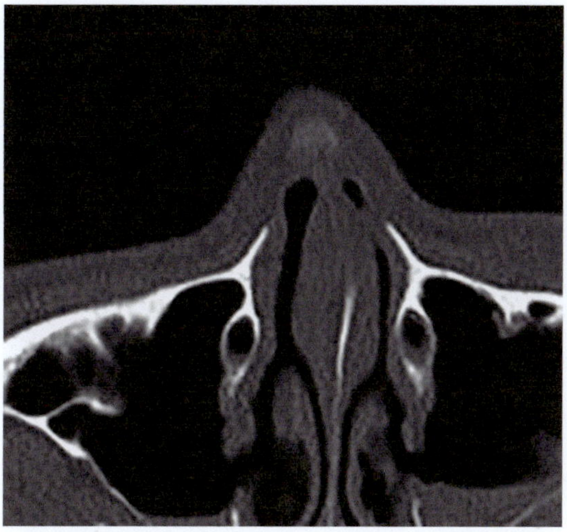

Fig. 10.2 Silicone over the septum after submucosal resection

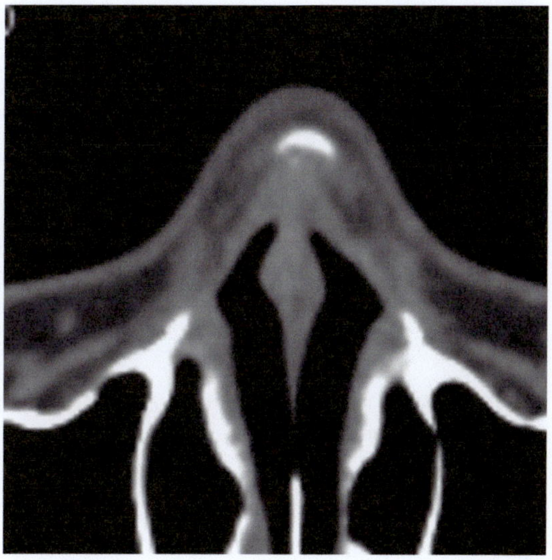

Fig. 10.3 Low internal nasal valve: low valvular roof just at the junction of LLCs and ULCs

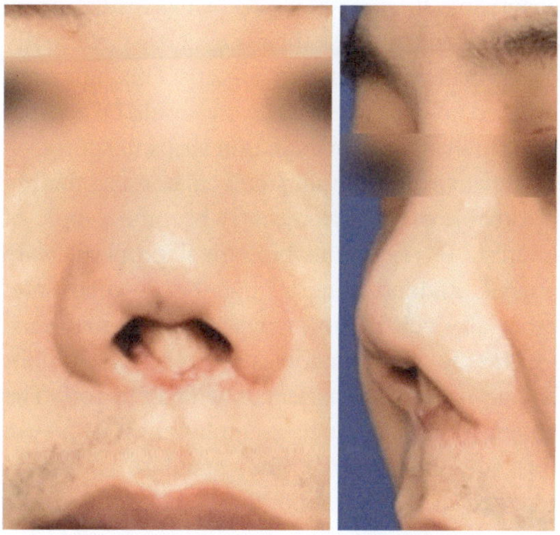

Fig. 10.4 A victim of intraseptal PCL mesh use

10.2.3 Massive Tip Projection and Tip Rotation Will Be Fine Functionally

- Any tip projection that fails to consider function does not accurately describe the functional deterioration after surgery.
- There is no evidence that using an onlay on the supratip or a spacer graft on the derotation or lateral genu improves nasal function.
- The projected tip complex results in a more acute internal nasal valve angle.

Any implant, suture, or graft that causes an abrupt INV depression will worsen the function of the nose. This nasal obstruction comes from an imbalance between the ULC and LLC (Fig. 10.3).

This functional derangement cannot be improved without a procedure to lift the upper lateral cartilage (ULC) with high septal support. Excessive tip projection can result from the lateral genu of the lower lateral cartilage (LLC) not being supported by the high septum after gathering in the center. This is problematic because these two procedures are the most common in Asian rhinoplasty. Ultimately, an over-projected tip and a heavy dorsal implant with insufficient high septal support are the causes of the problem.

10.2.4 Intraseptal Alloplastic Materials Will Be Fine as a Septal Framework

- PCL mesh, representative of new materials, is risky and necessitates further evidence due to potential inflammation and destruction following absorption (Fig. 10.4).

Using alloplastic materials in the septum may seem unthinkable in Western rhinoplasty. Of

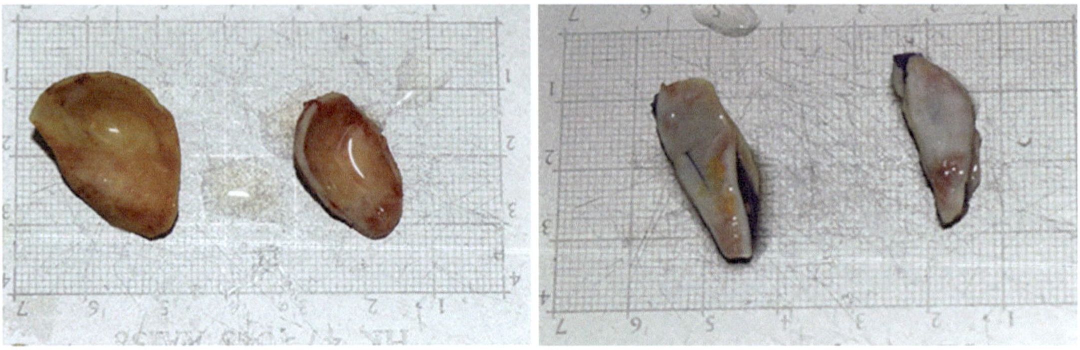

Fig. 10.5 Folded PDS foil used in the middle of conchas. (left) Cymba and cavum conchas. (right) Folded PDS foil is used for straightening the conchas

course, a few years ago, we saw the development of an absorbable support or support thread that widens the internal nasal valve of the nose (LATERA® absorbable nasal implant system, Stryker, MI, USA). It's still early days, but if absorbable threads show promising results, there is no reason to oppose their use, at least externally on the nose, in functional surgery. This judgment is based on current evidence and could be comparable to using nasal ventilation strips in sports.

However, developing new materials, mainly resorbable plates, has recently become a topic of interest. Physical and biological properties are crucial, and no material can be deemed safe, especially considering that absorption may lead to chronic inflammatory reactions. The author has no negative experiences with PDS foil. The author minimizes its use, employing it as a strut for strength. Unlike the standard practices reported in the literature, the author folds it and places it in the cartilage or the folded cymba concha to achieve straightness (Fig. 10.5).

However, this approach is not immune to long-term complications, necessitating the evaluation of potential inflammation and other issues [4].

10.3 Absolute Indications of Autogenous Graft only Rhinoplasty

All surgeries should utilize an appropriate graft, but there are instances when autologous tissue must be employed. This is particularly characteristic of secondary Asian rhinoplasty. Below are some examples:

- Problems with the soft tissue envelope
- Issues with the nasal framework
- Complications about functional issues

These three problems are characteristic of secondary rhinoplasty, which is not found in primary rhinoplasty and is characteristic of Asian rhinoplasty. Most autograft reoperations are due to the incorrect use of alloplastic material. When surgery is not feasible due to complications with alloplastic materials, patients usually present with very severe deformities. When addressing issues with alloplastic materials, simply reinserting the alloplastic material in the same field is misguided.

10.4 Problems with the Soft Tissue Envelope

It is not uncommon for the thickness of the soft tissue envelope to decrease after a secondary operation. While the scar may become thicker, its removal during revision surgery can result in a thinner envelope than before the original surgery. This issue arises after proper scar removal during surgery and is influenced by the decision to remove the anterior capsule and the thickened scar.

10.4.1 Scar: The Management of Anterior Capsule

In a sense, silicone implants can generate a new soft tissue called a capsule. Consequently, scarring of the soft tissue may generate new soft tissue without an inflammatory response. However, a notable characteristic of silicone implants is the variability in individual capsule formation, which can lead to bone erosion and resorption beneath the surface.

Implant capsules can be classified as unhealthy with contracture and healthy without contracture. The author, however, holds a nuanced view: a capsule is considered healthy if it is pliable and thin and unhealthy if it fails to be so.

No matter how thick the capsule is, if an avascular layer outside the implant does not bleed well when dissected, the scar tissue should not be used again as a substitute for soft tissue.

The severity of the implant's demarcation can be attributed to its initial placement depth; if inserted too superficially, the implant's outline may become pronounced.

The anterior capsule should be preserved without skin demarcation or severe contracture. Removing it risks the skin flap's circulation, as the anterior capsule is in direct contact with the dorsal skin. Excision of this capsule would result in an excessively thin skin flap (Fig. 10.6). Furthermore, if the inflammation of the anterior capsule is severe, removing it is essential to address the sequelae. Thinning of the overlying skin flap is also observed following removing granulomas or paraffinomas.

The issue of a thinned skin flap following scar removal cannot be remedied without soft tissue supplements. In cases of poor circulation within the skin envelope, high-tension oxygen therapy (hyperbaric oxygen therapy: HBOT) proves beneficial. The author advises two daily sessions of oxygen tank therapy. HBOT therapy has also been reported to be effective in controlling inflammation.

- A scar that is not inflamed and has good circulation can be repurposed for flap thickness augmentation or cartilage support without requiring complete removal.
- Inflammation, capsules with a mucous membrane-like surface, and hard avascular scars should be removed.
- Contracture is typically attributed to scar tissue surrounding the capsule, and its orientation is invariably longitudinal, mirroring the implant's shape. Furthermore, inflammation often stems from the implant's surface within the capsule. Therefore, complete removal is recommended if there is suspicion of synovial metaplasia or mucous-like drainage (Fig. 10.7).

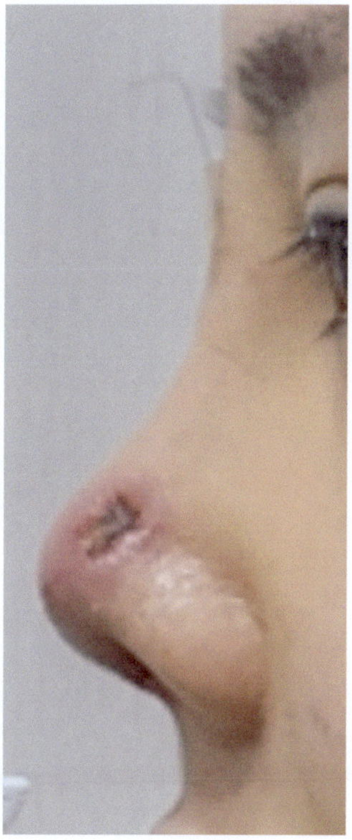

Fig. 10.6 Referred due to the tip skin necrosis: on palpation, the skin of the tip was very thin

A dermis graft is crucial for reinforcing thinned dorsal skin. Direct application of a rib graft to thin skin, mainly if the onlay rib is solid, may lead to rib demarcation upon long-term observation. Additionally, demarcation may occur with capillary hyperplasia due to inadequate circulation. A soft tissue cover is essential for layered

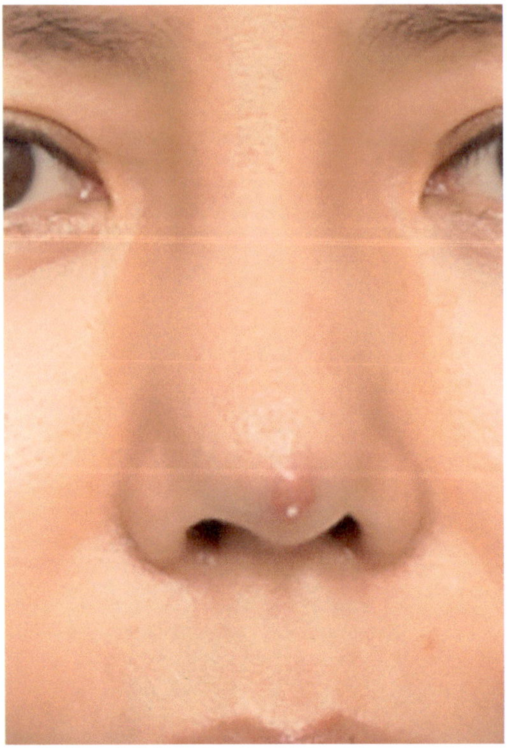

Fig. 10.7 Skin puncture with drainage: pustule-like skin lesion

coverage, even in small quantities. When using a solid rib, a layered cover consisting of a perichondrial graft, rectus fascia, or Scarpa's fascia, harvested during the rib harvest, is necessary beneath the thin skin.

10.4.2 Pus Drainage and Puncture of the Tip Skin Following Late-Onset Inflammation (LOI)

In the advanced stage of late-onset inflammation, the implant may protrude from inside the nostril, the columella, or directly through the lower part of the tip skin. The mucocele-like texture is easily found in the capsule (Fig. 10.8, Video 10.1).

Below are the typical disease courses. Postoperatively, the wound initially heals completely before unexplained recurrent swelling occurs. Subsequently, the nose progressively swells, leading to puncture of the skin or mucosa and drainage of pus. In scenarios where the unidentified edema responds to over-the-counter medications, it is fortunate as it indicates the infection is fluctuating between active and subdued states. The progression to an uncontrollable infection characterized by pus drainage is attributed to resistant strains unresponsive to empirical antibiotics. These strains may include pseudomonas, MRSA (Methicillin-resistant Staphylococcus aureus), MRSE (Methicillin-resistant Staphylococcus epidermidis), enterobacter, etc. [3].

The primary determinant in such cases is the severity of the overall nasal soft tissue, mainly whether there is significant cellulitis enveloping the area.

- Even when an antibiotic-susceptible strain is identified and a perfectly matched antibiotic is administered, severe cellulitis may necessitate the removal of the implant or graft, postponing reconstruction.
- If the cellulitis is mild, the dorsum and caudal parts are relatively unaffected with no widespread inflammation, or if pus within the septum can be drained, reconstructive surgery may not need to be delayed.
- Removing the infection focus and proceeding with autograft reconstruction is often feasible in cases with septal mucus drainage.
- Postoperative management should include administering the identified susceptible antibiotics following extensive irrigation, which is beneficial for the patient's recovery.

When encountering a patient with such a condition in an outpatient clinic, it's crucial to follow a specific procedure to determine the appropriate timing for surgery. This involves assessing the strain, the extent of the infection, the patient's response to antibiotics, and the overall health of the surrounding tissues (Table 10.1).

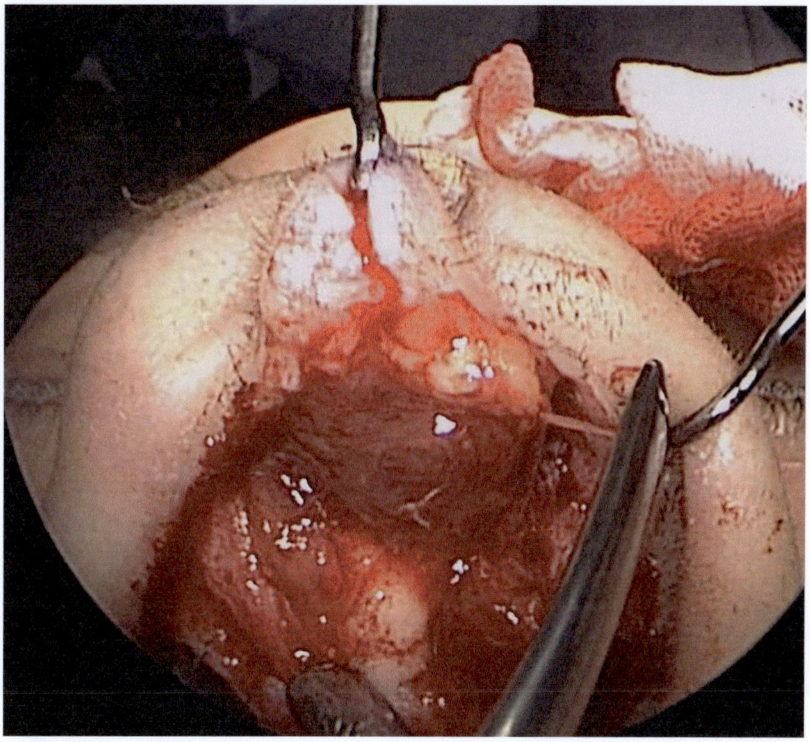

Fig. 10.8 Mucocele under the tip area

Table 10.1 Comparison between Medpor and PCL mesh

	Medpor	PCL mesh
Septal inflammation	+/−	+++
Pain when pressing	+++	+
Intraseptal dead space formation	+/−	+++
Intraseptal dissectibility	+/−	−

10.5 Problems of 3D Manufactured Materials

Here are a few examples of blind faith that 3D has brought to the forefront.

A simple X-ray is the most accessible modality for determining the implant's position and relationship to the current lesion.

Recently, a manufacturer introduced a novel technology by producing a silicone implant designed to adhere to the nasal bone and cartilaginous dorsum, utilizing 3D CT imaging for precision. However, this approach outlines a basic technique and overlooks the intricate intraoperative manipulations of bone and septum. Rhinoplasty surgeons are not mere painters or plasterers; they are akin to artistic sculptors, adept at altering the structural anatomy.

- Unwanted scar tissue forms between the undersurface platform and the implant, more easily found in the cartilaginous dorsum, the area from the rhinion to the supratip.
- It is blind faith that the manufactured implant will sit exactly where you want it to.
- Most cartilaginous dorsum is subject to modification, including spreader grafts, so considering this intraoperative change, 3D manufacturing makes little sense.

10.6 Alloplastic Implantation Is Mostly Found Regardless of SEG or Derotation Graft

In addition to the SEG extending to the caudal septum, a derotation graft was introduced to achieve a lateral crural spanning extension to fulfill Asian rhinoplasty without touching the septum [5]. Neither the SEG nor the derotation graft can adequately delineate the lower two-thirds of the dorsum and the bony dorsum. In secondary surgeries, it is common for many surgeons to revert to alloplastic materials on the dorsum after extending its length.

Almost all cartilage is used to extend the length of the nose, and the dorsum is expected to be addressed by implanting alloplastic material. Even when laminated ribs are used for nose extension, many doctors often use silicone for reliable dorsum augmentation. It's by no means a reliable method. Therefore, one should be prepared for this scenario.

10.7 Solving the Myths: Septal L-Strut Extension Graft (SLEG)

A way to solve many of the problems mentioned above is to reconstruct the L-strut and represent most of the nose as a septum. Since it uses autograft, it solves most of the secondary surgery.

The septal structure can essentially characterize the nasal profile, particularly the cartilaginous dorsum of the lower two-thirds of the nose. This allows for a reduction in the extent of augmentation required. Consideration should primarily be given to augmenting the bony dorsum from the nasion to the rhinion, which also permits a decrease in the volume of the graft utilized. An extended spreader graft can elevate the ULC and the LLC concurrently, enhancing the nasal minimal cross-sectional area.

– Unlike the onlay graft, the spreader graft functions as an orthotopic graft, enveloped by the nasal mucosal barrier, rendering it physiologically compatible.

Using spreader or derotation grafts is key to invisible grafting techniques. These standard methods focus on keeping the nose's length and rebuilding its function but cannot reshape the nose independently. Because of this limitation, additional grafts or alloplastic implants along the dorsum are often needed. In this context, the authors have creatively used the spreader graft as a visible element, calling it the "septal L-strut extension graft."

This technique involves extending the L-strut forward and downward, combining the roles of a visible spreader graft and a caudal extension graft. This approach significantly reduces the need for extensive grafting for the dorsum, allowing the septum to shape most of the lower two-thirds of the nose.

References

1. Kim YK, Shin S, Kang NH, Kim JH. Contracted nose after silicone implantation: a new classification system and treatment algorithm. Arch Plast Surg. 2017;44:59–64.
2. Moon K-C, Lee K-I, Lee J-S, Kim A-R, Dhong E-S, Kim D-W, et al. Late-onset inflammation in Asian rhinoplasty using alloplastic implants. Aesth Plast Surg. 2021;45:670–8.
3. Moon K-C, Jung J-E, Dhong E-S, Jeong S-H, Han S-K. Preoperative nasal swab culture: is it beneficial in preventing postoperative infection in complicated Septorhinoplasty? Plast Reconstr Surg. 2020;146:27e–34e.
4. Wang LL, Frankel AS, Friedman O. Complications of polydioxanone foil use in nasal surgery: a case series. Facial Plast Surg. 2018;34:312–7.
5. Paik MH, Chu LS. Correction of the short nose using derotation graft. Arch Aesthetic Plast Surg. 2012;18:35–44.

Secondary Septal Surgery: Dissectable Septum vs. No Man's Land

11

Pearls

- In secondary septal surgery, the balance between means and ends is crucial. Secondary septal dissection requires careful consideration of mucosal damage and the potential for long-term complications like inflammation and mucosal contraction.
- A preoperative review of previous surgeries and the condition of septal materials is essential for planning corrective measures.
- Using a donated rib in the septum poses challenges, including the risk of inflammation and the need for careful graft viability assessment.
- In revision rhinoplasty, it's critical to determine if the septal deviation is residual or developed after previous surgery, with a focus on the impact of dorsal implants on the nasal structure and function.
- Post-rhinoplasty nasal obstruction often stems from changes to the internal nasal valve or graft complications, requiring precise evaluation and septal revision. Detecting nasal obstruction caused by iatrogenic complications is crucial to tailor effective treatment strategies.
- When septal mucosa becomes a single layer, dissection becomes challenging, often leading to perforation. Materials like PCL mesh and Medpor® can cause severe inflammation or mucosal synechia, complicating revision surgery.
- Mucoceles, potentially linked to alloplastic materials and surgical trauma, can further complicate septal reconstruction, underscoring the importance of cautious surgical planning and material choice.

There is a trend toward increasingly complex secondary septal surgeries in Asian patients, which tend to become more severe. This is likely due to the rising number of surgeries among all patients. Another issue is the influx of young surgeons taking on challenging cases to sustain their practices. Despite educational efforts like conferences and publications, adventurous techniques continue to be explored, possibly driven by practitioners' desires for convenience or cost efficiency.

There are a few cases that may require secondary septal surgery, including the following:

- Persistent symptoms: If nasal obstruction continues after the initial surgery, a secondary surgery may be necessary to correct the septal deviation further.Incomplete correction leads to worsening of symptoms over time.
- Accumulated destruction: Destruction of the septal framework caused by previous surgery, among other factors, can reduce nasal length and deformity, necessitating secondary septal surgery.
- Ongoing inflammation due to intraseptal materials implanted: Perforation or inflammation after mechanical stress from Medpor® remains

E. S. Dhong, *Asian Septorhinoplasty*, https://doi.org/10.1007/978-981-96-6127-5_11

a problem, and the use of PCL mesh and donated IHCC is the most serious problem encountered in the author's outpatient practice.

Secondary septorhinoplasty often necessitates more autograft material than initially expected. Frequently, a substantial amount of cartilage from rib donations or previous surgeries using alloplastic materials is needed to reinforce this weakened septal support. A significant challenge in secondary Asian septorhinoplasty is addressing alloplastic materials previously applied to the quadrangular cartilage.

If the aim is to correct nasal obstruction or deviation, reconsideration of re-dissecting the septum is crucial. Despite the tendency in many Asian cases to use submucosal resection for cartilage in primary rhinoplasty, even for small noses and under-projected dorsum, this approach paradoxically weakens septal support while aiming to lengthen the nose. The viewpoint presented here might not align with the majority in the medical community and could be seen as unconventional. Surgeons, despite their expertise and intentions, may face significant challenges with unexpected infections or delayed inflammation, where the condition of the septal cartilage significantly influences the outcome. A compromised septum can lead to severe complications, mainly if the inflammation originates there.

Asian rhinoplasty surgeons often describe the method as a "rhinoplasty that takes less than an hour." It is a simple endonasal approach in which a silicone implant is placed, and autologous tissue, such as ear cartilage, is placed on the tip of the nose for projection.

It is better to emphasize that it takes a surgeon's experience to make such a prediction. It may be better for the patient to be underdone than overdone, as we have seen with patients suffering from serious complications.

It is a straightforward premise.

- The septal cartilage should be preserved if it is small and pliable.
- Due to lacking evidence, direct application of alloplastic material to quadrangular cartilage is not a safe option.

11.1 Multifactoral Considerations in Secondary Septal Surgery

A phrase says, "Putting the cart before the horse." This is another way of saying that the end and the means are out of proportion. The means are so excessive that they cause an adverse effect before achieving the end.

It should not be done if harvesting the septum does not improve nasal shape and function. This perspective is even more crucial in secondary operations.

Even if septal dissection is feasible, it's important to anticipate potential circulatory problems and limitations in the tissue's ability to stretch back to its original size.

When releasing a contracted nose, the part stretched by septal dissection is mostly the membranous septum.

- The mucoperichondrium in the center must be preserved, and the author has heard a speaker say to do a supraperichondrial dissection of this part, which is a method that should never be done. Supraperichondrial dissection of the septum is not feasible and should be avoided.

11.1.1 Is Secondary Septal Surgery Essential?

The distinction between surgeries involving septal mucosal dissection isn't merely about time but also the necessity for antibiotics due to a transient bacteremia state during the dissection [1]. The approach to the entire surgery differs significantly, whether it's a secondary procedure or not.

- When a septal dissection is included in a secondary rhinoplasty, the type of surgery changes to clean contaminated surgery [2, 3].
- An anterior septoplasty or caudal septoplasty is necessary to resolve deformity or obstruction caused by the septal extension graft.

If you're dealing with localized septal deviation without issues in the structural support, it's fortunate that it can be addressed locally without needing total septal surgery. Septoplasty with a batten-type graft or an additional layer of spreader grafts could be a viable solution for deviations in the anterior or caudal septum. It's advised to interact with the caudal septum minimally or to graft the anterior septum instead of performing extensive dissection. Yet, most contracted nose cases necessitate dissecting the entire septum.

11.1.2 How Was the Previous Septal Surgery Performed?

It's essential to review all medical records for any type of primary surgery, as relying solely on the patient's memory might not be accurate. First, the surgical record, obtainable from the hospital or the doctor's notes, must be reviewed to understand the materials used on the septum and the surgical approach taken. This information is crucial for planning corrective measures. In many secondary surgeries, the structural framework may be compromised or weakened due to prior submucosal resection (SMR), necessitating cartilage grafts from other areas for reinforcement. Specifically with Medpor®, expect cartilage destruction in the high or caudal septum [4].

This is the primary reason Western rhinoplasty differs from Asian secondary rhinoplasty. A more significant reconstructive challenge has recently emerged with the use of absorbable PCL mesh to extend the septum, which has led to more severe complications.

- PCL absorbable mesh can cause severe septum destruction in cases of prolonged inflammation, complicating reconstruction efforts.
- Chronic inflammation may lead to significant adhesion of the surrounding mucoperichondrium, rendering dissection challenging.

It is challenging to distinguish this by palpation. It can only be estimated by the degree of stiffness, which, together with imaging, should be used to assess the extent and size of the alloplastic material used. Most importantly, we need to see how much of the membranous septum remains.

11.1.3 Donated Rib (IHCC) in the Septum

Here, we only discuss irradiated homologous costal cartilage (IHCC). A sliced section of donated rib applied to the septum can also be found to be inflamed. The author has never seen a case of bleeding from a donated rib. The author believes that the donated rib is a dead graft. In some cases, it is found stacked in thin capsules (Fig. 11.1). The original condition of the donated rib is unknown, so it is not possible to compare. Still, most of the time, its physical properties are weakened, and it breaks easily. I have never seen a case where it can be repaired enough to be used again. In principle, the authors remove the donated rib if it is found.

In Asian rhinoplasty, perforation of the membranous septum or foreign body protrusion is accompanied by a wider mucosal defect than seen because of asymmetrical coaptation of mucosal flaps.

If the central septum retains only a thin layer of mucosa, surgeons should be cautious of dissection for any septal perforation, regardless of size. For minor perforations, septal reconstruction might coincide with external rhinoplasty.

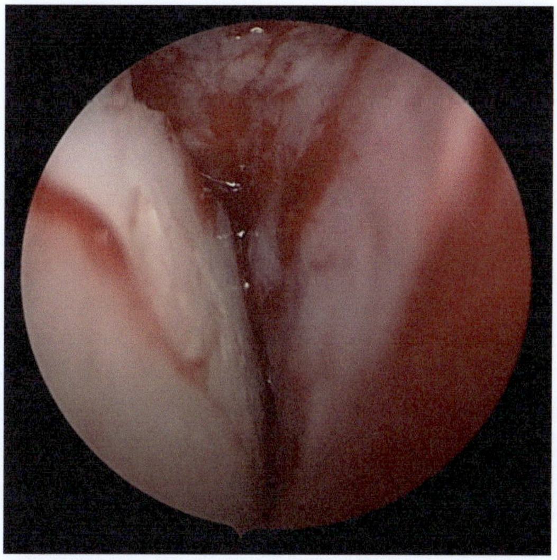

Fig. 11.1 Thin capsule around the IHCC: dissected at the membranous septum where the donated rib was used as a septal extension graft

However, separating the surgeries into stages may increase the likelihood of success for significant defects in the high or central septum.

If there is cellulitis at presentation or ongoing purulent drainage, it's highly likely that donated rib or absorbable plates were used.

- Cultures should be taken for ongoing bacterial identification, and suitable antibiotics must be administered.
- Operating on the structural framework concurrently with abscess drainage is not advisable. Planning for septal surgery should follow once a manageable bacterial strain is identified.
- The extent of cellulitis in the flap is a critical factor in deciding on the feasibility of surgery.

11.1.4 Is the Current Infection or Inflammation Controlled?

Cultures are often negative due to the prevalent use of oral antibiotics. However, identifying the strain through multiple bacteriologic tests is crucial, especially in external nasal and membranous septum drainage cases. In the presence of fluctuation in the membranous septum or septal infection with columella redness, initial incision and drainage to remove fluid and assess the septal flap's integrity are vital. The first treatment step combines systemic antibiotics with incision and drainage. Definitive surgery involves removing all grafts and alloplastic materials. Skin survival takes precedence, especially if the dorsal skin is thin; even localized skin defects can be critical. Empiric antibiotics may not always target the correct strain. Therefore, using a strain-specific and susceptible antibiotic in preoperative preparation is crucial. After I&D, systemic antibiotics are used to reduce the bacterial burden and monitor the extent of cellulitis in the nasal cavity or cellulitis of the dorsum and tip skin to determine the timing of surgery.

- In acute surgical site infection with severe cellulitis, removing all alloplastic implants from the dorsum and septum to irrigate and salvage the area is crucial. Reoperation at the same time is not advised.

In cases of late-onset inflammation, the treatment approach, including the possibility of two-stage surgeries, varies by surgeon and depends on the type of pus drained. The author opts for simultaneous secondary septorhinoplasty if the infection is deemed controllable, not resistant to antibiotics, or caused by a mucocele. Uncontrolled infection pockets, characterized by continuous pus drainage despite systemic antibiotics and irrigation, suggest ongoing internal graft destruction and are unsuitable for immediate reconstruction. Definitive surgery is recommended once pus drainage decreases or stops and the septal mucosal flap's cellulitis stabilizes. The operation should be decided on the extent of cellulitis, not just the presence of pus drainage.

11.1.5 Was the Intranasal Inspection Appropriately Done?

In secondary septorhinoplasty, conducting an anterior rhinoscopic or endoscopic examination is crucial. Initially, the primary objective is to assess the septal condition relative to the patient's symptoms, including identifying perforations in unexpected areas. Symptoms reported by patients during the examination may exacerbate post-surgery, and subjective symptoms vary so greatly that surgery reconsideration may be necessary if patients expect these symptoms to be resolved surgically. The subjective symptoms in secondary septorhinoplasty are complex and challenging to address, often leading to surgeon frustration when patients seek reoperation for cosmetic rather than functional concerns.

11.1.6 Unexplained Nasal Pain

A small number of patients report pain immediately post-surgery, often improving within days, but some experience persistent pain beyond a year, necessitating evaluation alongside nasal obstruction symptoms. Asian rhinoplasty may involve a pulling sensation or unexplained pain, particularly after multiple surgeries, potentially due to sensory nerve damage. Persistent sensations post-implant removal, especially without total capsulectomy, may require treatments akin to those for neuropathic pain. Medpor® implants in the nasal tip can cause pain due to restricted tissue movement. Pain in the membranous septum may arise from excessive nasal tip projection or irritation from non-dissolvable sutures. Functional issues like empty nose syndrome or airway vortices might contribute to symptoms, necessitating thorough patient questioning and possibly long-term topical steroid treatment for relief. Direct pain from alloplastic implants suggests the need for implant removal.

Neuropathic pain following septorhinoplasty will be thoroughly examined in Chap. 14.

11.2 Septal Deviation: Is It Persistent or Newly Developed?

The author notes that many patients present with cosmetic concerns and nasal obstruction. The deviation of the caudal septum was observed to be a more frequent cause of tip asymmetry. The caudal septal deviation was prevalent among patients seeking functional improvement for nasal obstruction. Most patients had previously undergone septoplasty or submucosal resection. The issue is that even after correcting a deviated nasal septum, many cases still experience obstruction due to the failure to correct the bony deviation at the inferior part. An even bigger problem is the occurrence of newly-onset nasal obstruction caused by a weakened L-strut after submucous resection (SMR).

- During an evaluation, it is essential to determine whether the patient's nasal deviation has not been adequately corrected or if it was initially satisfactory but deteriorated postoperatively.
- Insights should be derived from visual inspections, computed tomography (CT) scans, and endoscopic evaluations.

A heavy implant on the dorsum can destabilize an already weak lower septum. The discovery of an unforeseen saddle deformity upon removal of a dorsal implant during secondary rhinoplasty often stems from overlooking the interaction between a weakened septum and the implant's weight. Such heavy implants may distort the caudal septum, leading to nasal obstruction complaints. In revision rhinoplasty, where patients are typically dissatisfied cosmetically or functionally, it's essential to proceed with caution without preoperative photos or CT scans, as cosmetic concerns may mask the actual cause of nasal obstruction. A detailed preoperative nasal exam is crucial to assess previous grafts and the state of the septum. The last surgeon performing the secondary septorhinoplasty bears the responsibility for the outcome, with strategies like bilateral ANS reinforcement with batten grafts for the caudal septum and possibly unilateral spreader grafts for high septum deviation in fortunate cases while addressing the LLC's position for internal nasal valve collapse. After a proper swing door procedure, the caudal septum is resolved by reinforcing both sides of the ANS with a batten graft (Fig. 11.2).

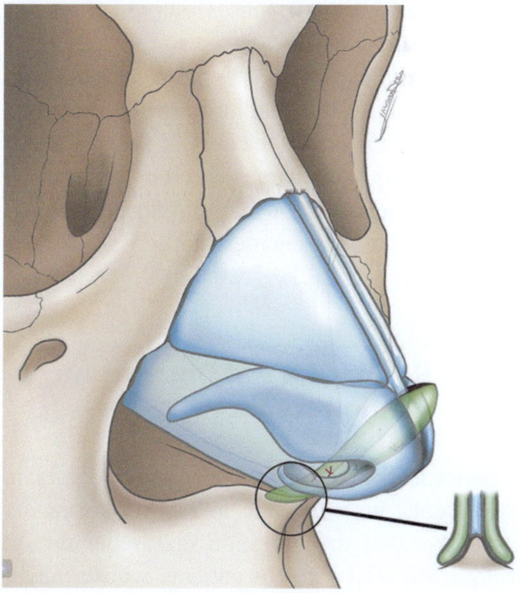

Fig. 11.2 Bilateral batten graft at ANS: folded cymba concha as a caudal septal extension g graft: CSEG (Aesthetic Surgery Journal, Volume 41, Issue 7, July 2021, Pages NP737–NP747)

11.2.1 Anterior Extended Spreader Graft (AESG) and Caudal Septal Extension Graft (CSEG)

Secondary septal surgery is mainly resolved with a batten-type graft. It is rare for simple sutures and excisions to resolve the problem. In cases where correction of the total nasal framework is necessary, the rib cartilage is usually utilized, which requires reconstruction of the total nasal framework with total mucosal flap elevation. However, if dissection is not possible, only a localized anterior or caudal batten graft may be possible.

If the caudal septal tilt is the primary cause, the external manifestations can range from tip asymmetry to nostril asymmetry to loss of tip projection.

Correction of caudal septal tilt is best accomplished by re-dividing and swinging the ANS and PSA, re-suturing, and placing batten grafts. This is the revisional CSEG.

If the nasal dorsum deviates after a spreader graft using rib cartilage, suture failure or cartilage warping should be suspected. The extended spreader profile of the dorsum is represented as a direct dorsal aesthetic line. However, there are not many surgeries in Asia where the direct aesthetic line of the dorsum is expressed by the high septum alone, so the alloplastic material applied to the dorsum is often the cause of the deviation.

This is why secondary Asian septorhinoplasty is more complex, and using alloplastic material in the dorsum adds another hurdle to diagnosis and surgery.

11.3 Recurred Nasal Obstruction in Adolescents

It is not advisable to perform septal surgery in adolescents, including the insertion of spreader grafts, because the deviation may recur due to overgrowth afterward. In patients whose maxillofacial growth has not yet been completed, attempting hump nose correction, even due to psychosocial issues, may result in regrowth problems, potentially leading to the recurrence of the deviated nose. Patients should be informed preoperatively that septal overgrowth can reoccur during growth, potentially necessitating revision surgery [5].

Even without harvesting a large amount of septal cartilage, septal dissection can affect growth, potentially leading to deviation. Inadequate release of the internal tension in the quadrangular cartilage may cause the septal tilt to relapse, presenting both cosmetic and functional issues.

In such cases, the surgical options include excising the deviated portion or using a caudal batten graft. In the author's experience, a batten graft is often preferred for most patients with cosmetic concerns. This preference is because correcting tip deviation and enhancing tip projection frequently necessitate reinforcing the anterior septum, including the caudal septum. Since patients are often already in an SMR state at this time, planning must consider the extent of detachment and potential surgery.

11.3.1 Excision vs. Batten Graft

If convexity is observed in the quadrangular cartilage, excising this area, if dissection is feasible, may offer a solution while providing the necessary cartilage for grafting.

The bony spur on the maxillary crest can sometimes pose a challenge, but if the area is accessible without causing a mucosal tear. Performing a chondrotomy through the maxillary crest and dislocating the ANS is often essential for correcting the tilt of the caudal septum. The outcome of the caudal septal tilt depends on whether this area acts as a "swinging door." To avoid excessive thickening of the columella area, opt for a batten graft only when necessary. A thickened columella is expected due to excessive grafting in secondary septal surgery. The over-insertion of donated rib cartilage and scar tissue, often used as a columellar strut, frequently causes this condition (Fig. 11.3).

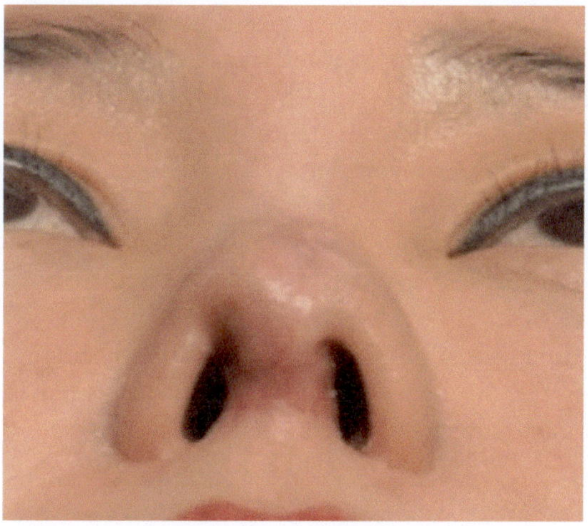

Fig. 11.3 Thick columella containing a donated rib strut

11.4 Newly-Onset Nasal Obstruction

Patients visiting our clinic with complaints of new-onset nasal obstruction, which did not exist before their surgery, often have already undergone complex grafting. In Korea, numerous surgeries aim to alleviate nasal obstruction, including rhinitis, while enhancing the nasal profile. Depending on the insurance system, this can appear as a sales tactic to secure coverage from insurance companies, for instance, by performing more septal surgeries than necessary to harvest cartilage for tip plasty. From an advertising perspective, the dual benefit of improved nasal function and achieving the desired appearance is overly produced. However, it is crucial to acknowledge that the repercussions of excessive surgery are on the rise. Furthermore, if the use of alloplastic materials in the nasal septum is the cause, this represents a severe example of an iatrogenic complication.

The causes of newly-onset obstruction can be categorized into two main groups: those who have undergone septal surgery in their initial or previous surgeries and those who have not. Most newly-onset nasal obstruction cases are due to the narrowing of the internal nasal valve area, including the external nares, often resulting from the surgical techniques used in Asian rhinoplasty to increase tip projection. This narrowing leads patients to experience a sensation of obstruction. The characteristic features of these cases are described below.

11.4.1 Post-septal Surgery

If septal surgery was performed in the previous surgery, some cases complaining of new nasal obstruction can be divided into the following categories.

- Septal collapse after too much harvest of the quadrangular cartilage
- Septal tilt after improper SEG
- Deviation after the spreader graft
- Septal tilt after dorsal onlay implanting: weak L-strut
- Any type of septal collapse after septal surgical site infection
- Thick caudal septal graft using costal cartilage
- Thick caudal septal graft using donated rib cartilage
- Resorption or breakage of the prior septal graft using donated rib cartilage

When quadrangular cartilage is harvested, the issue arises of the entire load being placed on the rhinion and caudal septum. Should the caudal septum be weak, the unilateral septal extension graft (SEG) may easily tilt to one side, and the presence of an alloplastic implant in the dorsum could further weaken the lower L-strut due to gravity and pocket pressure.

Reinforcing the caudal septum with thick donor costal cartilage increases the overall thickness of the membranous septum and reduces the external nares' size, leading to complaints of nasal obstruction. With IHCC or Tutoplast, lamination options are limited. From the author's experience, achieving thin lamination is not always feasible in IHCC and tends to break easily. In recent years, there has been a significant increase in the number of patients requiring secondary septal surgery due to complications associated with the use of donated ribs (Fig. 11.4).

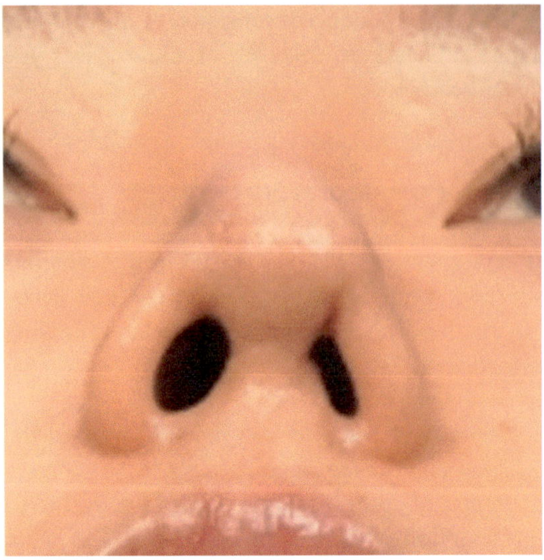

Fig. 11.4 Destructed nose after complicated septorhinoplasty using IHCC

Due to the nature of the donated rib, if it is double-layered, it shows a thickness of more than 3 mm, leaving a relatively thicker caudal septum than before surgery. This is a direct cause of nasal obstruction if warping or tilting occurs. The same applies to older patients whose rib autografts have failed to make thin laminated pieces.

The donated rib is characterized by a thick, hard, implant-like texture on preoperative physical examination, easy separation from the surgical field of view, and little bleeding. At the time of surgery, it can be found to be easily broken, and in some cases, it is encapsulated in a thin layer.

The author published many years ago that IHCC is an unproblematic and beneficial material for tip surgery [6]. At the time of publication, the author had attempted thin lamination within 2 mm but later encountered limitations and stopped using IHCC due to unsatisfactory results. Furthermore, there have been complaints of severe nasal obstruction in instances where the nasal cavity has narrowed due to the previously mentioned high septum issue, as well as in cases of breakage. One meta-analysis examining the use of donated rib in dorsal augmentation showed no significant differences in outcomes between autologous and homologous costal cartilage grafts, including aspects such as warping, resorption, infection, contour irregularity, or the need for revisions. En bloc dorsal onlay grafts are frequently utilized in this type of rhinoplasty to enhance the contour and structure of the nasal dorsum [7]. However, donated ribs have limited utility in septal reconstruction as laminated thin rib cartilages.

11.4.2 Tip-Related Nasal Obstruction

The types of nasal obstruction caused by postoperative tip changes that are frequently seen in Asians are as follows:

- Excessive alar base reduction
- Excessive grafting in the supratip area, including tip grafts
- Septal extension graft involving approximating the lateral genu
- Overly projected tip extension: change in the steepness of the internal nasal valve (INV) angle following tip projection
- Tip tilting

If you examine patients from past rhinoplasties where only silicone was inserted and the tip surgery was conducted with a simple suture, the function of the internal nasal valve is rarely compromised. However, if the dome angle of the lower lateral cartilage (LLC) becomes acute with recent septal extension grafts (SEG) or the lateral crura are brought together by cephalic rotation for tip projection and approximated to the supratip again, an acute tip complex in the internal valve area can be observed (Fig. 11.5).

In addition to various types of grafts, cases are often observed where, due to excessive tip projection during surgery combined with SEG of the caudal septum, when the INV angle is diminished. Patients commonly report symptoms of nasal obstruction, describing insufficient airflow during inhalation. These symptoms improve when the lateral crus is manually elevated with an instrument. The external nares may appear too oval, deviating from the typically round shape characteristic of Asians, leading some patients to complain of nasal obstruction. It is hypothesized that the transition from the external nares to the LLC might obstruct or cause vortexing of the airflow due to a sharp decline in the lateral genu.

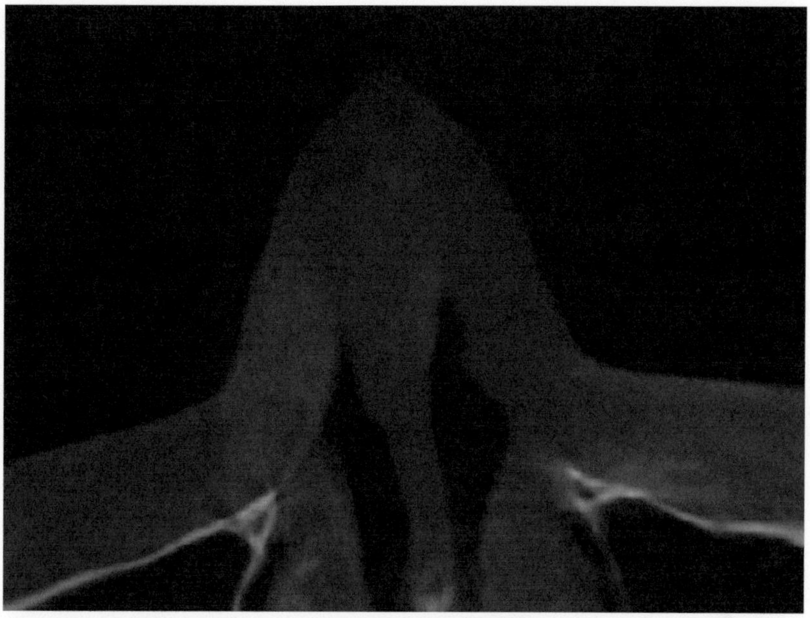

Fig. 11.5 Internal nasal airway problem: low and narrow nasal cavity

This phenomenon is also noted in cases of derotation, where extra cartilage is added to the supratip, pushing the lateral genu downward. Excessive grafting in the supratip area reduces space in the internal valve area, leading to decreased nasal airflow for the patient.

Thus, the question arises: How is it possible to preserve the shape of the supratip while supporting the entire LLC with the force of the lateral genu?

If the position of the ULC does not catch up with the projected tip, a sharp space reduction into the transition to INV can lead to step ladder deformity in the cross-section. Sometimes, the roof of the INV is directly observed on nasoscopy, and it is caused by a low roof regardless of whether the INV angle (the angle formed by the genu and septum) is acute or obtuse.

11.4.3 Other Iatrogenic Problems

- Intranasal synechia after improper nasal packing (Fig. 11.6)
- Sinking problems of prior implanted dorsal alloplastic materials (Fig. 11.7)

After the nasal packing removal, wounds on the mucous membrane can adhere to each other, leading to synechia and causing nasal narrowing as they heal. This is primarily due to the convex parts of the septum and the inferior turbinate coming into contact. While this is not an issue during surgery and can be easily addressed during a secondary procedure, it is crucial to monitor packing methods and check the location of any bleeding that occurs during packing removal to prevent synechia.

Bleeding observed during packing removal can be effectively managed by temporarily placing a silicone sheet and maintaining it for 1 week.

In rare instances, a silicone implant placed in the dorsum may be displaced into the nasal cavity due to gravity and pocket tension. In such cases, it is essential to recognize and preoperatively address whether the implant is deviating from the tip or descending in the rhinion area.

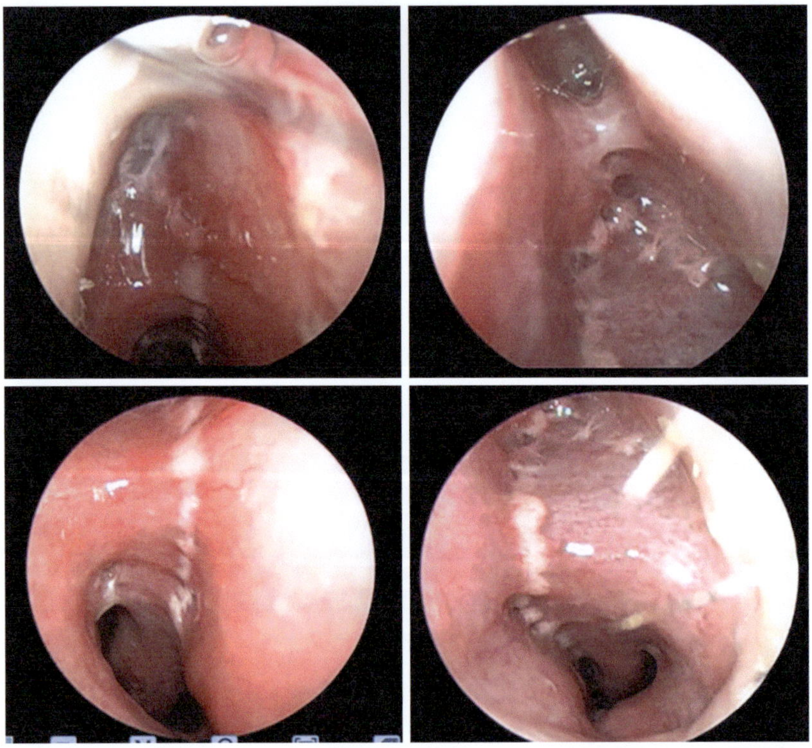

Fig. 11.6 Bilateral nasal mucosal synechia due to the traumatic nasal gauze packing removal

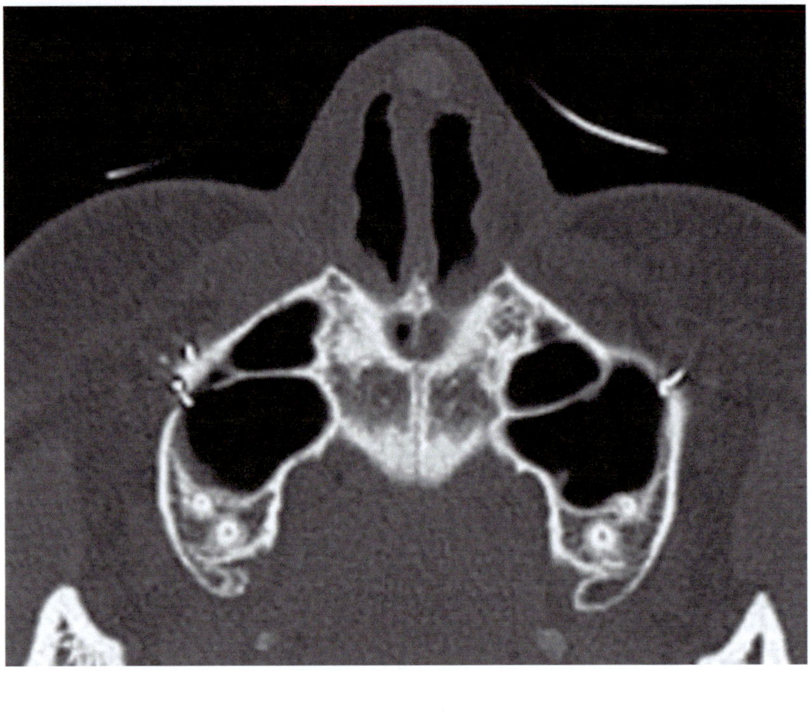

Fig. 11.7 Sinking of implanted dorsal silicone

11.5 Single Septal Mucosal Flap: No Man's Land

The issue arises when the mucosa of the septum becomes a single plane. In such cases, dissection is not feasible, and usually, a perforation is found (Fig. 11.8).

Most surgeons aim to re-debulk the mucoperichondrium from the reconstruction field of view, but I have encountered numerous cases where this is not achievable. This is likely due to two reasons: the previous surgeon failed to preserve the perichondrium and dissected it, the inflammation destroyed this plane, or possibly both occurred. The final feature is severe contracture of the central compartment, with severe nasal retraction.

11.5.1 Single Mucosal Plane Due to Inflammation

PCL (polycaprolactone) mesh plates are associated with the most severe inflammation.

Adhering to scientific ethics would involve conducting and publishing long-term follow-ups until 2–3 years after the PCL has completely resorbed and vanished. The potential harm to young surgeons who rely on anecdotal reports from journals, and more importantly, the potential damage to patients, even if it involves only one or two cases of total practice, is so severe that it should be prohibited. It is valid to challenge the positive outcomes reported in published papers [8, 9]. But the author is entitled to argue against the good results of a paper that has already been published. There is enough clinical experience and evidence to criticize PCL mesh.

Medpor® may lead to persistent thinning of the septal mucosa due to its physical properties. This thinning can also result from constant nasal irritation. The nature of Medpor® allows soft tissue to grow into its pores, creating a strong attachment that differs in strength from the surrounding area. Therefore, when Medpor® is applied to the septum, it can cause persistent irritation and pain due to its firmness. The report suggesting that dissection was relatively easy in 2 of the 29 patients who experienced extrusion is speculative, but it may indicate cases where the perichondrium was well preserved [10]. In patients without preserved perichondrium, adhesions are so severe that dissection often leads to perforation, making reconstruction more challenging. It's essential to be cautious of the pitfalls of meta-analyses using small-sized clinical report series. This is because the surgical methods and the application areas are different. Should we accept that Medpor® is a superior material just because its complication rate is below 6% and the revision rate for autogenous costal cartilage is 10%? [11]. Is it worth following the many papers that claim Medpor® can be safely used as a spreader graft? However, if Medpor® leaves a

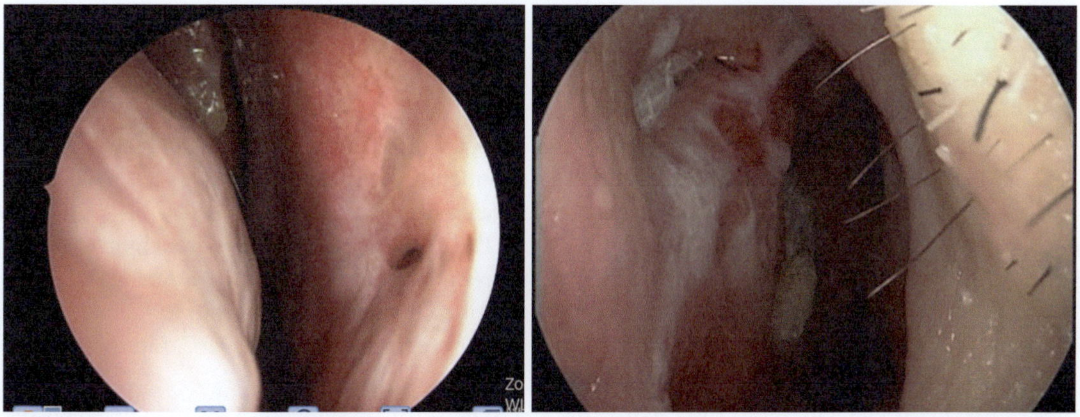

Fig. 11.8 Various types of septal no man's land. (Left) Tiny perforation but coapted septal mucosa. (Right) Multiple septal perforations revealed by contralateral gauze packing

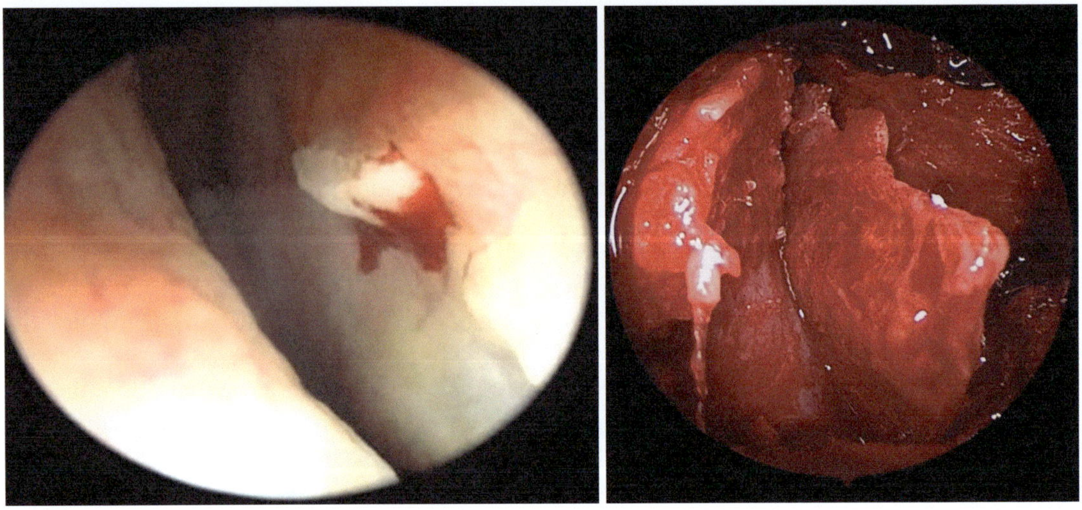

Fig. 11.9 Various types of Medpor complications. (Left) Removing scabs showed Medpor extrusion. (Right) High septal destruction after Medpor removal

septal defect in the high septum in referred cases, as shown in the photo, one must doubt whether it is medically acceptable (Fig. 11.9). The more significant issue is that the dorsum is predominantly augmented with a silicone implant. The quality of the meta-analysis on the complication rate of Medpor® use, or the number of papers it references, does not alter the fact that outcomes can vary greatly depending on whether it is used in conjunction with an alloplastic implant in the dorsum and whether or not an osteotomy is performed on the nasal bone. Additionally, the authors advise against sequelae in intraseptal use due to its potential for significant destruction [4].

11.6 Mucocele Invading into Septum

Several potential causes for mucoceles exist. Pathologically, a pseudocyst containing mucin deposits resembles a typical mucocele. It is believed that mucin from the mucosal membrane has extravasated and accumulated inside the capsule surrounding the silicone. In some instances, the mucosal membrane may be intact or disrupted, making it challenging to fully assess the pathology due to the difficulty of en bloc extirpation. This difficulty arises because the capsule's thickness varies among patients, and removing the anterior portion of the capsule during surgery is often challenging.

It is hypothesized that invagination of the nasal cavity mucosa due to trauma may occur, but mucoceles are frequently found even in the absence of a trauma history. If the swelling fluctuates, with periods of improvement and worsening, it may suggest an association with chronic inflammation. This could be due to synovial metaplasia, endothelial ingrowth, or mucocele formation within the capsule. Over time, the patient's nose may appear progressively shorter due to ongoing contracture.

Contracture around the capsule occurs when the capsule remains after silicone removal. This contracture is more severe in thick and avascularized capsules than in thin ones, and the degree of contracture is exacerbated when accompanied by inflammation.

The role of endothelial-mesenchymal transition (EndoMT) in the eventual contraction around the silicone and its relationship to mucocele formation represents an area for future research [12].

The most problematic cases occur when the dorsum and septal pockets are connected. However, in rare instances, the pockets contain-

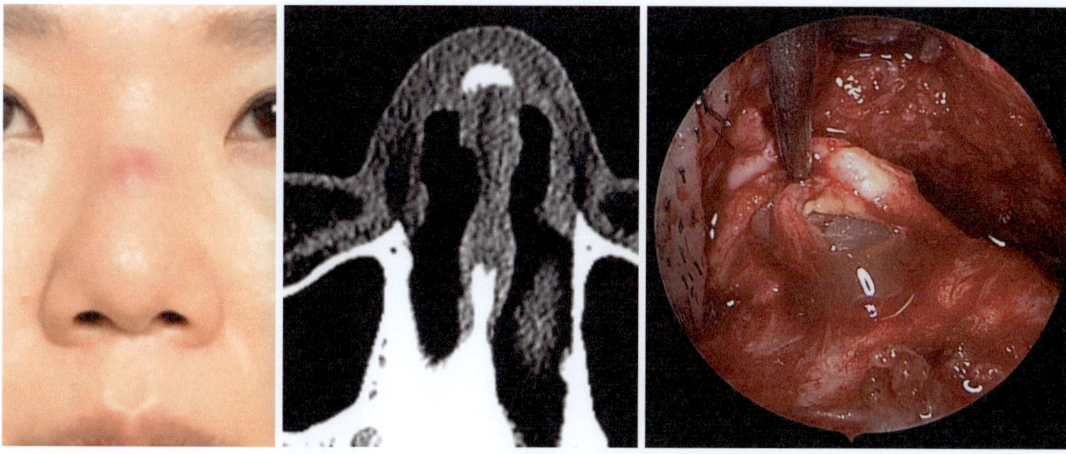

Fig. 11.10 Clinical features of late-onset inflammation (LOI) after silicone and septal Medpor use. (Left) Dorsal skin lesion. (Middle) CT scan showed T-shaped silicone with double-layered Medpor used. (Right) Mucocele connected dorsum and tip

ing alloplastic material in the columella or caudal septum may also be interconnected. Late-onset inflammation resulting from a pocket created by the use of Medpor® in the columella can be connected with a Medpor® pocket in the high septum, leading to a huge mucocele-like pocket. In some cases, the caudal septum pocket is connected to the silicone pocket on the dorsum, and the sequence of events depends on where the issue first arose. Patients with a history of lateral osteotomy or humpectomy, combined with silicone implants in the dorsum, often develop a mucocele-like pocket originating around the silicone implant [13].

Late-onset inflammation primarily occurs due to exposure accompanied by mucosal invagination. Rarely a large mucocele-like pocket extending from the tip and columella to the dorsum is observed using L-type silicone implants (Fig. 11.10).

This will be discussed in more detail in Chap. 15.

References

1. Okur E, Yildirim I, Aral M, Ciragil P, Kiliç MA, Gul M. Bacteremia during open septorhinoplasty. Am J Rhinol. 2006;20:36–9.
2. Ricci G, D'Ascanio L. Antibiotics in septoplasty: evidence or habit? Am J Rhinol Allergy. 2012;26:194–6.
3. Mäkitie A, Aaltonen LM, Hytönen M, Malmberg H. Postoperative infection following nasal septoplasty. Acta Otolaryngol Suppl. 2000;543:165–6.
4. Moon K-C, Jung J-E, Dhong E-S, Jeong S-H, Han S-K. Septorhinoplasty for destructed septal L-strut in patients with previously applied porous high-density polyethylene implants (Medpor®). Aesth Plast Surg. 2019;43:1286–94.
5. Dhong E-S, Na M-W. Secondary septal surgery. In: Dhong E-S, Na M-W, editors. Asian septorhinoplasty: conundrums and solutions. Singapore: Springer Singapore; 2021. p. 147–58.
6. Suh M-K, Ahn E-S, Kim H-R, Dhong E-S. A 2-year follow-up of irradiated homologous costal cartilage used as a septal extension graft for the correction of contracted nose in Asians. Ann Plast Surg. 2013;71:45–9.
7. Vila PM, Jeanpierre LM, Rizzi CJ, Yaeger LH, Chi JJ. Comparison of autologous vs homologous costal cartilage grafts in dorsal augmentation rhinoplasty: a systematic review and meta-analysis. JAMA Otolaryngol Head Neck Surg. 2020;146:347–54.
8. Park YJ, Cha JH, Bang SI, Kim SY. Clinical application of three-dimensionally printed biomaterial Polycaprolactone (PCL) in augmentation rhinoplasty. Aesth Plast Surg. 2019;43:437–46.
9. Ahn TH, Heo CY, Ahn KC. A compound osteocartilaginous graft with polycaprolactone (PCL) mesh in Asian rhinoplasty. J Plast Reconstr Aesthet Surg. 2020;73:e6–7.
10. Kim YH, Kim BJ, Jang TY. Use of porous high-density polyethylene (Medpor) for spreader or extended septal graft in rhinoplasty: aesthetics, functional outcomes, and long-term complications. Ann Plast Surg. 2011;67:464–8.
11. Liang X, Wang K, Malay S, Chung KC, Ma J. A systematic review and meta-analysis of comparison between autologous costal cartilage and alloplastic

materials in rhinoplasty. J Plast Reconstr Aesthet Surg. 2018;71:1164–73.

12. Piera-Velazquez S, Li Z, Jimenez SA. Role of endothelial-mesenchymal transition (EndoMT) in the pathogenesis of fibrotic disorders. Am J Pathol. 2011;179:1074–80.
13. Moon K-C, Lee K-I, Lee J-S, Kim A-R, Dhong E-S, Kim D-W, et al. Late-onset inflammation in Asian rhinoplasty using alloplastic implants. Aesth Plast Surg. 2020;45:670. https://doi.org/10.1007/s00266-020-01648-8.

12 Septal L-Strut Extension Graft (SLEG) Using Laminated Rib: Salvaging the High Septum

Pearls

- In secondary septorhinoplasty, the septal L-strut extension graft is preferred for reconstructing the framework when significant perforations or infections are present.
- The cantilever grafts are, presumptively, more susceptible to infections and complications due to their non-physiological nature and lack of integration within a few weeks.
- The septal L-strut extension graft offers a more robust solution against late-onset inflammation and complications, particularly in complex revisions where the extension of the mucosal layer is critical.
- Securing the anterior nasal spine (ANS) and rhinion is crucial in septal L-strut extension graft (SLEG) procedures to ensure stability and prevent deviations.
- If the ANS is compromised, the rhinion becomes an alternative fixation point, though achieving stability can be challenging without both secure anchors. Techniques vary based on the presence of residual cartilage and bone, with options ranging from suturing to drilling for anchor placement.
- The donated rib cartilage presents alternatives where rib cartilage calcification or patient-specific concerns necessitate their use, albeit with careful consideration of their respective challenges and limitations.
- Repairing high septal perforations is crucial in secondary septal surgery to maintain the integrity of the nasal framework and avoid complications. Various techniques, including surgical closure, local and regional flap techniques, and perichondrial grafts, can be employed based on the specific clinical scenario.
- The perichondrium plays a vital role in wound healing, with its rich-cell layers contributing to the repair process. This highlights the importance of careful surgical planning and the selection of appropriate repair methods to ensure successful outcomes.

12.1 Anatomic Considerations Selecting the Costal Cartilage: The Sixth vs. Seventh Rib

12.1.1 Preferred Rib for Laminated Costal Cartilage

The seventh rib is often straighter and narrower than the sixth rib, which is generally wider but more curved. For the author's SLEG technique, a straight laminated rib measuring at least 20–25 mm in length and 10 mm in width is required (Fig. 12.1). Therefore, the seventh rib is often more favorable than the sixth rib [1, 2].

In secondary surgeries, many patients present with more than one rib already harvested, making it challenging to obtain the desired amount of costal cartilage. Due to previous incisions, harvesting the seventh rib in the preferred location is often not feasible. If central or marginal ossifica-

E. S. Dhong, *Asian Septorhinoplasty*, https://doi.org/10.1007/978-981-96-6127-5_12

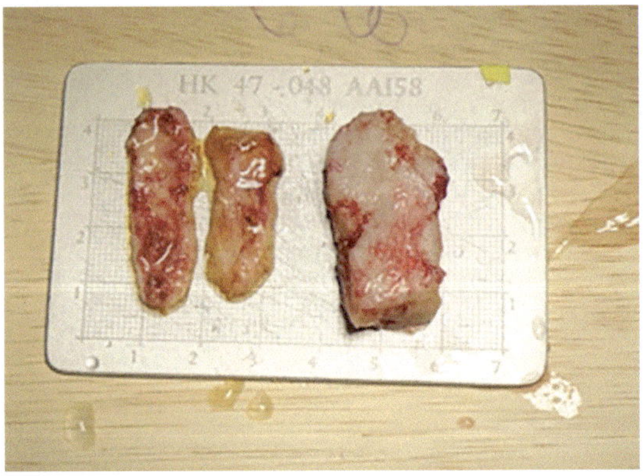

Fig. 12.1 Seventh rib, perichondrium, and Scarpa's fascia

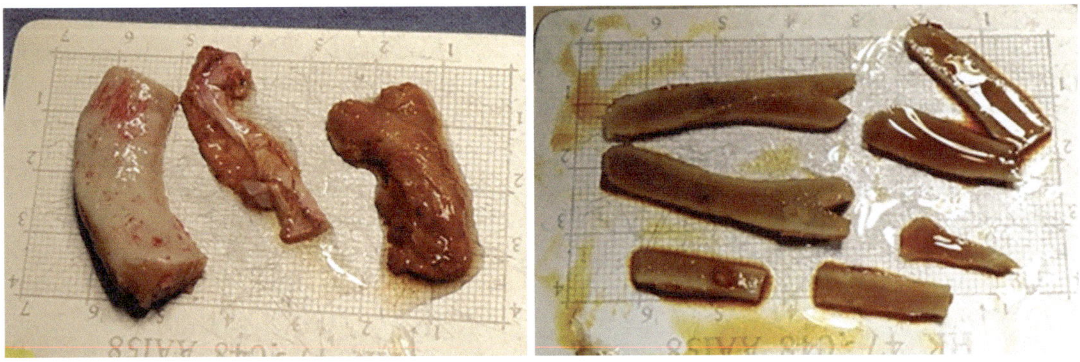

Fig. 12.2 Seventh rib of a 50-year-old female. (Left) Rib, perichondrium, and rectus fascia. (Right) Yellowish trabeculae with central ossifications, thin laminated rib pieces for two AESGs; wedge cut included, two CSEG, columellar strut, and shied graft, etc.

tion is present, rib lamination may not be achievable. Therefore, patients over 45 should be considered for the presence of a central trabecular core within the hyaline cartilage, which can reduce suture stability during repair (Fig. 12.2).

Males were prone to peripheral calcification, and females to central costal cartilage calcification (CCC). Diffuse CCC was observed as an age-independent sign for high CCC levels. This study has reported that calcification of the seventh rib costal cartilage is independent of gender. Contrary to previous beliefs that it does not occur before age 40, calcification has been observed in 6.3% of the population under 40 [3].

Although the authors sometimes opt for a rib cage view, performing surgery based on a chest CT is rare. If calcification is detected and a sufficient length of the seventh rib is not obtainable, an adjacent level of rib or ear cartilage harvesting may be considered an alternative. For patients over 40, a direct physical examination using needle pricking during local anesthesia can be conducted.

12.1.2 Encountering Unexpected Bleeding

Surgeons performing rhinoplasty with costal cartilage rarely encounter issues with the internal mammary artery. Plastic surgeons, especially those experienced in breast reconstruction, are well-acquainted with the anatomy of the internal mammary artery, including its location and thickness, particularly around the third to fourth rib. They understand the associated risks, although complications are more likely with less experienced surgeons or due to patient-specific factors. Additionally, the significant size of the internal mammary vein should not be overlooked. In female patients, the fifth to sixth rib is sometimes chosen for harvesting to align the scar with the inframammary fold. Compared to the seventh rib, harvesting from the upper five ribs poses a greater risk of damaging the internal mammary pedicle.

When a patient lies down, the diaphragm elevates, with the right side higher than the left. Direct hemostasis can be challenging if arterial bleeding occurs on the underside of the costal cartilage. Severe bleeding may occur at the moment of vessel severance, and partial severance can be particularly hazardous. Applying pressure with a gauze or a fingertip to the lower part of the harvested rib can temporarily halt the bleeding. It's crucial to remain calm and, if necessary, extend the skin incision to expedite the rib cartilage harvest. Attempting to stop the bleeding without rib harvesting is only a temporary solution and risks causing pneumothorax by damaging the visceral pleura underneath.

The seventh rib, above the abdominal cavity and with the internal mammary artery more medially located, presents a lower risk during cartilage harvesting. The intercostal artery, easier to manage, is cauterized with caution. The intercostal arteries from the first to the sixth rib originate from the internal thoracic (mammary) artery. At the same time, those of the seventh, eighth, and ninth spaces come from the musculophrenic artery. Thus, severing the internal mammary artery during the seventh rib harvest is highly unlikely unless there is significant dissection medially.

The seventh rib, favored in the author's SLEG technique, is harvested away from the medial costal border, minimizing the risk of pedicle injury.

12.2 L-Strut vs. L-Cantilever: Which Should Be Applied in Secondary Septorhinoplasty?

In cases where a patient has an acute surgical site infection that has spread to the septum, secondary dissection of the septum may be infeasible if there is a large perforation or damaged perichondrium. Under such circumstances, septal reconstruction becomes impossible, leaving a cantilever graft as a secondary option. If severe septal perforation is present due to previously used alloplastic materials and the perforation cannot be closed, septal reconstruction is unfeasible as exposed laminated rib grafts are susceptible to acute surgical site infections.

The author does not prefer cantilever grafts over L-strut reconstruction. Extending the foreshortened soft tissue septum may be necessary in many secondary rhinoplasty cases. Although releasing the soft tissue envelope sufficiently can enhance the appearance through a cantilever graft, skin repair becomes unachievable without releasing the mucosal layer, including the hinge area. Releasing the mucoperichondrium is more intricate and challenging than releasing the soft tissue envelope.

12.3 L-Strut vs. L-Cantilever: Which Is more Robust Against Infection?

The authors have not experienced late-onset inflammation in patients with septal L-strut extension graft in secondary septorhinoplasty. The most challenging aspect of secondary septorhinoplasty is the risk of surgical site infections (SSI). The biofilms may only be partially removed in some cases. This situation can be divided into two types: cases where the biofilm from previous surgeries was not completely eliminated and cases where new inflammation occurs. However, in our experience, the primary concern is residual biofilm.

Therefore, the quick integration of autologous cartilage is crucial for overall healing. The authors believe that SLEG heals faster than L-cantilever grafts.

Cartilage lacks a main vascular pedicle and relies on plasma imbibition for survival, leading to survival with resorption. Regeneration of cartilage is not typically expected. However, the use of perichondrium significantly impacts its survival.

A rib used as a cantilever graft does not receive blood supply from the septal mucosa on both sides, unlike the laminated costal cartilage in the septum, and therefore must endure prolonged ischemia. Even with the imbibition of surrounding plasma, it is impossible to completely prevent resorption during healing. Specifically, costal cartilage placed on exposed bone or within a skin envelope where the capsule remains will suffer from poor blood supply.

L-cantilever grafts are not biological and are believed to be more susceptible to late-onset inflammation due to their prolonged healing time. Conversely, SLEGs are supposed to heal faster and be more resistant to late-onset inflammation, as most of the cartilage is embedded within the mucoperichondrium of the septal mucosal layer.

Cantilever grafts are non-physiological and purely aesthetic, focusing solely on the external features of the nose. Employing an appropriate perichondrium, either below or above the graft, can be advantageous.

12.4 Preparation of Laminated Costal Cartilage: Proper Use of Perichondrium

The success or failure of frame rebuilding hinges on the preparation for rib lamination. To mitigate warping, the balanced technique, introduced six decades ago and now widely endorsed by doctors, plays a crucial role. Since the outer layer of costal cartilage, akin to skin, is primarily responsible for warping, utilizing only the central portion's cartilage from the entire cartilage's cross sections is advised [4]. Reports indicate that harvesting concentric costal cartilage yields better long-term results due to reduced warping compared to eccentric harvesting. This method requires essential symmetric perichondrial shaving and systematically removing the perichondrial ring with a scalpel. For implant-type rib dorsal grafts, ensuring the convex curve faces dorsally is crucial [5]. Concentrically carved cartilage grafts have been the gold standard for preventing warp in nasal reconstruction.

Reports indicate no significant difference in warping between the anteroposterior and cephalocaudal axes in the balanced harvesting technique of the central portion [6].

Other reports suggest including the outer cortex in the laminated rib method. Good outcomes have been noted with transverse cuts along the axis of the sixth and seventh rib junction. This technique reportedly results in less warping compared to concentric or eccentric carving [7]. However, there are reports that oblique cutting is better for long axes [8, 9]. Warping, to some degree, is an unsolvable issue. The author employs anteroposterior lamination by slicing along the long axis of the harvested seventh costal cartilage. The resultant laminated rib is then immersed in a betadine double antibiotic solution containing 50 mL of povidone-iodine, 1 g of cephazolin, and 80 mg of gentamicin in 500 mL of normal saline for over an hour to monitor warping (Fig. 12.3). Although this solution is contentious due to concerns about resistance or lack of evidence, the author has opted for it for over 20 years, especially after discontinuing widely used broad-spectrum polypeptide antibiotics like bacitracin. The literature on breast surgery has acknowledged the efficacy of such irrigation methods [10].

Direct contact between the costal cartilage and the dorsal skin envelope may result in a small amount of fibrotic tissue encapsulation, potentially leading to the demarcation of the costal cartilage. This phenomenon has been observed in animal

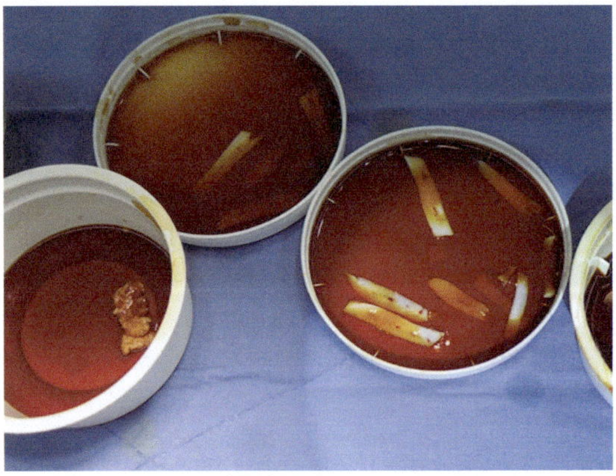

Fig. 12.3 Preparation of laminated rib in modified Adam's solution

studies conducted for other purposes [11]. Occasionally, increased vascularity can be observed in the dorsal skin above the demarcated costal cartilage [12]. This issue is often encountered when there is poor blood supply, especially when a carved graft from a costal cartilage block is utilized for dorsal augmentation following the removal of a silicone implant. Demarcation of the costal cartilage is more likely if the dorsal skin envelope or the patient's dermis is thin. To prevent this, soft tissue can be placed between the dorsal skin envelope and the costal cartilage, or the perichondrium can be grafted. However, in many patients, hypervascularity spontaneously resolves over a long-term follow-up of more than 2 years. However, evidence is needed to support how the soft tissue facilitates the integration of the costal cartilage. Furthermore, using a laminated rib for dorsal augmentation might need the interposition of perichondrium or soft tissue between the graft and the dorsal skin.

12.5 Securing the ANS and Rhinion in SLEG

The fixation at the anterior nasal spine and the rhinion is essential for ensuring the stability of the septal L-strut extension graft (SLEG). Securing these two areas before considering any deviation to the left or right is crucial. The author recommends securing the ANS area by first adjusting the tip height and then the rhinion area. However, fixating the rhinion first becomes an alternative if the ANS is compromised or destroyed by previous surgery. Placing bilateral AESGs secured with high septal cartilage can lead to significant stability. However, achieving adequate support is challenging if the rhinion is unstable. Stabilizing these two anchors is vital for controlling further deviations.

12.5.1 Securing Caudal Septal Extension Graft at ANS

Surgery is easier if there is even a tiny amount of residual cartilage on the ANS. The attachment of the bone and cartilage junction around the ANS is very tight and usually consists of several layers of thickening as the attachment of the perichondrium transitions to the periosteum, and the periosteum is located in a deeper layer, so it is often well damaged from previous surgery and scar formation is frequently found.

12.5.2 When the Remaining Cartilage, Bone, and Soft Tissue Are Repairable

If residual cartilage exists, a bilateral CSEG can be easily placed starting on either the left or right side to complete the caudal support. The priority is dissecting the posterior septal angle over the anterior nasal spine. Subsequently, a decision should be made regarding the width and length that offer better support or stability. Given the laminated rib's thickness, a bilateral graft is preferred if the bilateral application is feasible. It consistently provides more stability than a unilateral graft.

For stable repair, a small portion of periosteum and soft tissue may be attached to ANS rather than completely detaching from ANS to repair the batten graft. One or two non-absorbable sutures and several absorbable ones will be placed. Careful attention must be given to avoid suture exposure during the mucoperichondrial repair around the anterior nasal spine.

Suppose no soft tissue remains around the nasal spine prominence or if substantial fixation of the posterior septal angle is required. In that case, drilling through the prominence can complete the fixation anchor. Use the smallest diameter drill and carefully orient the drill through the prominence to allow the suture to pass through.

12.5.3 When the Remaining Cartilage, Bone, and Soft Tissue Are Absent?

In patients where the ANS area has been destroyed for some reason, anchoring the CSEG to the midline becomes a challenging attempt. Drilling or suturing the protruding bony portion is easier than fixation on the depressed portion.

In cases of ANS loss, if the AESG has firm cephalocaudal support, anchor the CSEG to the caudal end of the AESG. Limiting the amount of caudal mucosal dissection is essential to create a tight dissection pocket. However, it should be noted that the smaller the dissection amount, the less the overall length will be extended. If stability cannot be achieved with the above method, the ANS area should be anchored with a GII® Anchor/Mitek (DePuy Synthes) suture anchor and sutured.

In Asian patients, the alveolar bone of the maxilla is protruding, and the midface is relatively concave, so it is difficult to perform a transcutaneous suture with bilateral perialar to transverse tunneling.

12.5.4 Securing SLEG at Rhinion

Among the factors determining the stability of the entire septal L-strut graft, the stability at the keystone area is crucial for defining the dorsal profile. Even with thorough bilateral mucosal dissection, stability may be challenging if the rhinion's bony caudal portion is not secured. Suppose the caudal ends of the bony dorsum on both sides are well preserved. In that case, the stability can be easily achieved by creating *"a wedge section"* in the anterior extended spreader graft (AESG) and interlocking it (Fig. 12.4). After inserting the wedge into the bone's end, it is repaired with the upper lateral cartilage to achieve stability, and the dorsal margin around the rhinion can be sculpted to minimize irregularities for a smooth dorsal line. The stability of the AESG in the rhinion area may be compromised by a significant open roof deformity after humpectomy or bony imprinting of previous overlying silicone implant. In such cases, the decisive factor for stability is the height of the remaining nasal sidewall bone. If the nasal bony height is sufficient, transcutaneous transosseous cerclage suture is a viable option [13].

However, if the nasal bone height is insufficient, making transverse bony tunneling challenging, the only option may be ULC repair. In Asian secondary rhinoplasty, the dorsal soft tissue is often thickly scarred, the ULC is weak, and finding the ULC in dorsum areas treated with alloderm, making rhinion fixation unstable, may be impossible. Increasing pocket stability with limited septal pocket dissection or obtaining stability from CSEG should be considered in such cases. However, instability in the rhinion area can lead to a recurrence of saddle nose deformity, necessitating a switch to a cantilever graft approach.

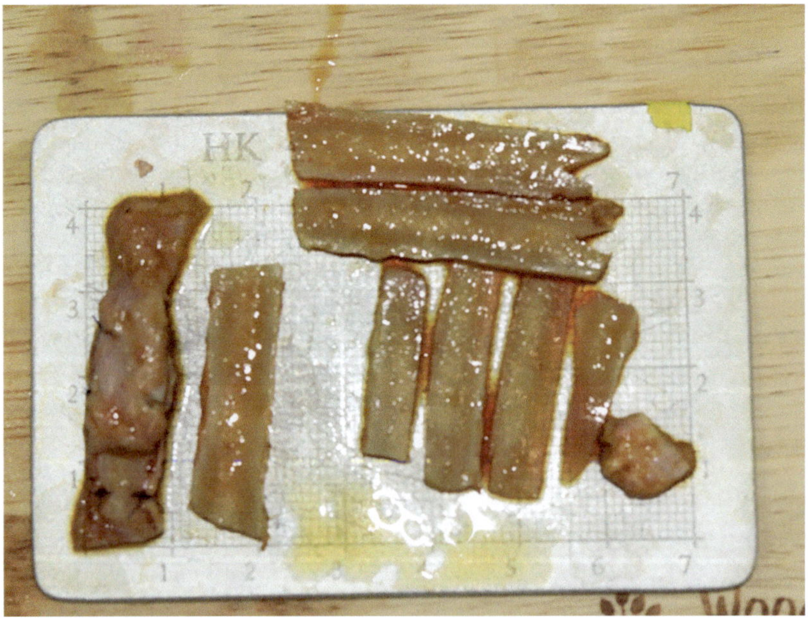

Fig. 12.4 Preparations for SLEG: two laminated rib cartilage show wedge section for AESG (above)

Even with stable rhinion fixation, extending the anterior dorsal line requires a higher spreader graft than the existing dorsal height. The method limits unilateral mucosal dissection to increase support from the rhinion to the new tip. The author aims to increase pocket support by dissecting only the necessary portion of the right mucoperichondrium to accommodate the AESG. For instance, if the dorsal height projection is 3 mm and the width of the rib slice for the AESG is 7 mm, the author limits the dissection to no more than 4 mm deep to maintain pocket stability.

The transcutaneous transosseous cerclage suture (TTC suture) method is worth considering if the midface is convex, making the maxilla below the anterior nasal spine (ANS) palpable. However, this technique is challenging in patients with thick cheeks and often requires significant effort, particularly in many Asian individuals.

12.6 Simultaneous Soft Tissue Harvest from the Chest

Soft tissue is necessary for the radix graft, which includes the bony dorsum and the smoothing of the dorsal line. Adequate soft tissue coverage is also essential to prevent the demarcation of the costal cartilage at the tip. Despite the thicker dermis in Asians, secondary rhinoplasty often involves scar removal and the removal of previously applied alloderm, which can leave a very thin soft tissue envelope.

12.6.1 Scarpa's Fascia

In secondary cases, or when a significant amount of soft tissue is needed, preparing Scarpa's fascia before approaching the rectus fascia is helpful. After passing through the superficial fatty layer, a very thin lamellar layer will be encountered.

12.6.2 Previous Operative Scar

Some patients rarely wish to remove a previously unsightly chest scar. The undersurface scar tissue can be utilized as soft tissue while excising the desired amount of scar. Complete deepithelialization is essential.

12.6.3 Rectus Fascia

Before harvesting ribs, ensuring adequate preharvesting of the fascia before encountering the rectus muscle is helpful. More than 4 × 4 cm of fascia is required for wrapping, and a Colorado microdissection electrocautery tip allows for less bloody harvesting (Fig. 12.5).

Rectus fascia can be used for wrapping diced cartilage (DCF), but the author primarily uses it for soft tissue coverage of the dorsal margin of laminated rib (Fig. 12.6).

12.6.4 Perichondrial Graft

The perichondrium contains blood vessels, which can nourish the transplanted tissue and promote healing, potentially leading to better outcomes in tissue viability and longevity. Although the layer's thickness or volume is small, it is the most effective healing soft tissue. It is often used with a cartilage graft or to facilitate contact healing with the nasal bone (Fig. 12.7).

In patients with significant open roof deformity, a laminated rib graft is necessary to contour the dorsum even after SLEG. In this case, a large piece of perichondrium covers the high septal defect and simultaneously covers the undersurface of the laminated rib, promoting rapid healing (Fig. 12.8).

12.6.5 Fat Injection

You can use the multiple folding method to achieve the volume of a soft tissue graft. However, there is a limit to the amount of fascia that can be harvested. Fat injection can be performed within the perichondrium to obtain a larger volume of perichondrial graft and achieve the desired volume [14]. The author considers fat grafting a beneficial procedure following the release of contracture in the foreshortened nose. The author has experience with multiple injections of

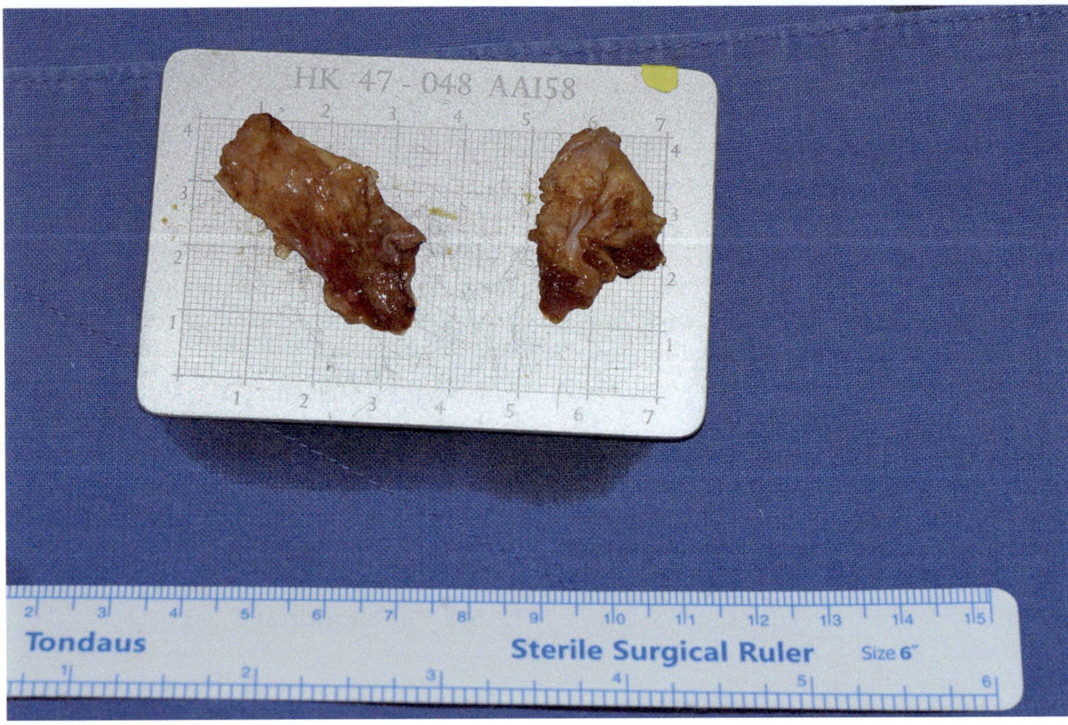

Fig. 12.5 Rectus fascia strips

Fig. 12.6 Rectus fascia covering laminated rib

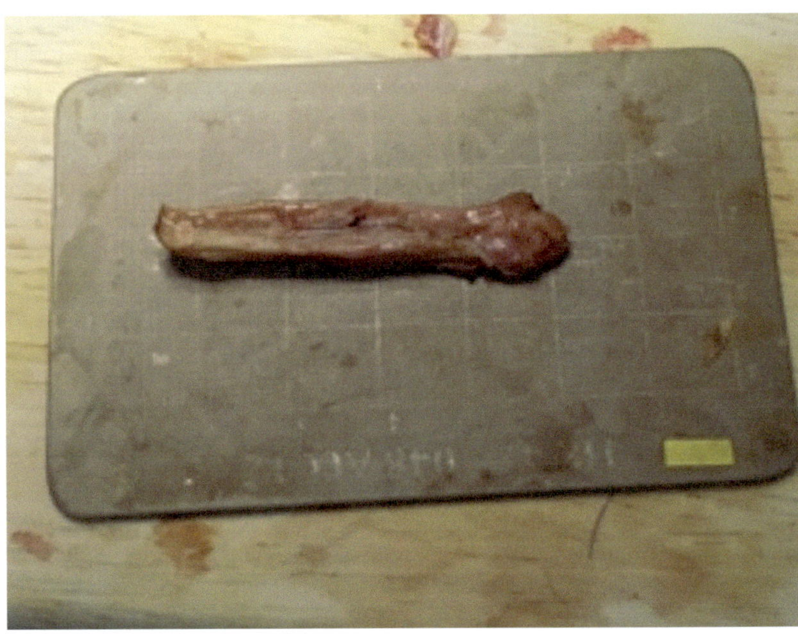

adipose-derived stromal/stem cells (ADSCs) in patients with contracted noses but believes they have no effect. The author notes that, during the inflammatory phase, ADSCs can differentiate into fibroblasts or myofibroblasts, potentially worsening the contracture. This observation is based on findings that ADSCs exhibit behavior similar to fibroblasts when treated with traditional inflam-

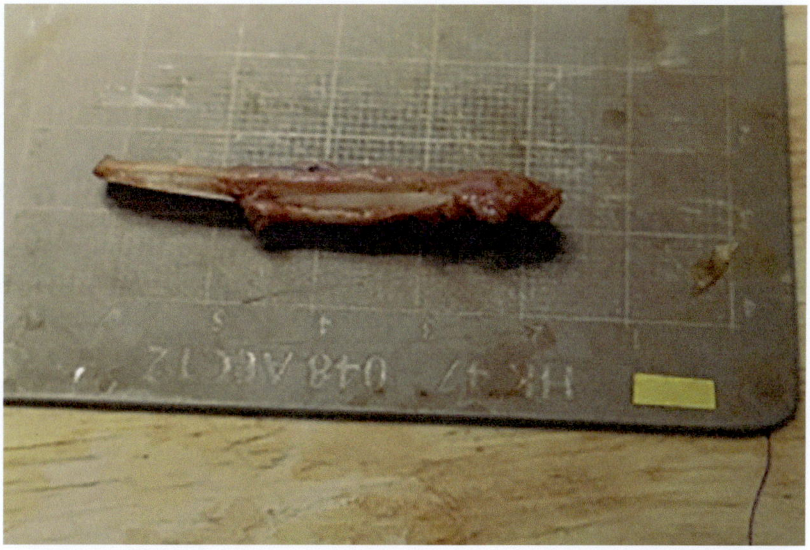

Fig. 12.7 Attaching perichondrium to the undersurface of the laminated rib for a dorsal onlay graft; lateral view

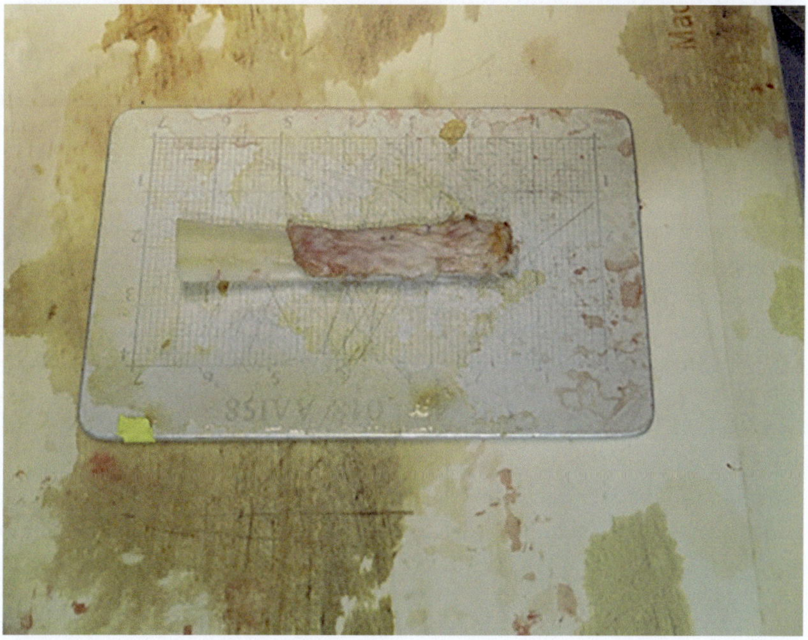

Fig. 12.8 A massive open roof deformity requires perichondrial coverage under the laminated rib

mation-related cytokines [15]. However, fat injection or fat grafting involves fatty tissue containing oil, which relieves contracture.

12.7 DCF vs. Laminated Rib Graft

Neither the cantilever graft nor the SLEG with laminated rib is completely free from warping.

The author prefers the diced cartilage wrapped in the fascia (DCF) method for augmentation from the radix to the supratip, utilizing SLEG to shape the lower two-thirds of the dorsum as a pronounced septum. However, the issue of resorption presents a limitation, necessitating overcorrection. For a young female patient seeking a high-quality result, it raises the question: how many would be willing to undergo surgery knowing they must overcorrect by 20–30% to account for future resorption and monitor for resorption for over 12 months? Additionally, the use of laminated ribs is constrained by the necessity of employing soft tissue on the dorsum for edge smoothing. Septorhinoplasty using autografts is fundamentally a struggle against resorption. While DCF is challenged by resorption, laminated rib faces warping issues, highlighting the advantages and disadvantages of both methods.

Consequently, what are the implications of inserting silicone for dorsal augmentation after SLEG? There are two primary concerns with placing a silicone implant atop a well-constructed SLEG base. It is not safe to insert silicone into the dorsum after complex septal surgery.

- The implant may also pose risks for minor mucosal defects in the septum or an open roof.
- In the case of secondary surgery, excessive thinning of the skin envelope may occur due to the removal of the previous capsule.

A multilayer laminated rib can be sutured in place, but I do not believe using non-absorbable suture material will prevent warping. The cartilage prone to warping will eventually overcome the force of the suture, leading to warping. When augmentation is achieved using only soft tissue, the graft must be prepared to account for more significant resorption [16].

Diced rib cartilage can be inserted using a syringe without being wrapped in fascia. Surgeons who have conducted secondary surgeries on such patients understand this approach's challenges for secondary dissection and recognize that it should be avoided. Unwrapped diced rib cartilage can lead to significant scar tissue formation, complicate dissection in subsequent surgeries, and result in an irregular soft tissue envelope. All surgeries should be performed in a way that considers the surgeon who will come after you. This is because you might not be the last surgeon for this patient.

Currently, the author prefers using a graft combining laminated rib, perichondrium, and rectus fascia for cases where minor dorsal augmentation is needed after SLEG.

12.8 Donated Rib Cartilage Use: Irradiated Homologous Costal Cartilage (IHCC) and Tutoplast

In older patients or when calcification of the rib cartilage is discovered, opting for ear cartilage is prudent. Both central and peripheral calcification can hinder lamination and obstruct the acquisition of the intended rib piece. Presently, surgeries employing donated ribs are prevalent in private clinics. Two or three varieties of donated ribs are used in Korea, yet new companies continue to emerge. One study reported that low-dose gamma irradiation ensures a sterility assurance level A SAL of 10−6 (SAL6) for the final packaged graft. No differences were noted in outcomes between autologous and homologous costal cartilage grafts, including rates of warping, resorption, infection, contour irregularity, or revisions, in patients undergoing dorsal augmentation rhinoplasty [17].

Irradiated homologous costal cartilage (IHCC) constitutes the majority of the usage. Regarding IHCC, the authors have previously published papers asserting that it poses no problems. More recent studies have provided additional data, yet even with a complication rate of less than 2–4%, there exists a population bias. The application of IHCC differs significantly between primary and secondary rhinoplasty or septorhinoplasty. Its use in extension grafts under tension is not recommended nor advised for contracted noses with inflammation. The indications for IHCC are deemed to be very limited.

Utilizing IHCC as bilateral spreaders for anterior septal extension grafts (AESG) of the entire L-strut can yield unpredictable outcomes. The authors observed that a capsule formed around the donated rib, leading to inadequate blood supply. Finding IHCC integrated with the patient's septum during secondary operations was rare. The material often exhibited a breakage and scar formation pattern, with most margins showing signs of fragmentation. Therefore, it is considered an unsafe material for long-term use for the septal framework.

Tutoplast® (RTI Surgical Holdings Inc.) tissue sterilization process, initially developed as a chemical sterilization methodology, involves osmotic, oxidative, and alkaline treatments (if indicated) to break down cell walls, inactivate pathogens, and remove bacteria. Solvent dehydration permits room-temperature storage of tissue without damaging its native structure. The author has no experience with Tutoplast and cannot comment on it.

12.9 SLEG for High Septal Defect Repair

Repairing a high septal perforation in the nose is a challenging task that requires careful consideration of healing, re-perforation, and a disaster.

While some surgeries focus solely on repairing perforations, in Asian secondary septal surgery, repairing high septal perforations is essential in reconstructing the framework. Without repairing the high septum, the integrity of the exposed laminated costal cartilage cannot be ensured. These situations include:

- Removing a large granuloma (late-onset inflammation) that has invaded the septum
- Dissecting a very low upper lateral cartilage (ULC) that requires anterior projection
- Tearing during extensive capsular release
- Perforation caused by chronic inflammation due to PCL mesh
- Exposure of Medpor

Depending on the specific circumstances, various methods can be used, individually or in combination [18].

- Surgical closure: This is the most direct approach when encountering a very small laceration between the septal dorsum and ULC junction
- Local flaps: Utilize the surrounding septal mucosa to create flaps to close the perforation. Flaps can be based on the mucoperichondrium or mucoperiosteum and may include the rotation flap or bilateral advancement flaps. However, repairing a high septal defect without a posterior or inferior backcut is complex, and the author does not favor it.
- Regional flaps: In cases where local tissue is insufficient or compromised, tissue may be brought in from adjacent regions, such as an anterior ethmoidal artery (AEA) flap and greater palatine artery (GPA) flap. However, although theoretically possible, repairing a high septal defect is challenging using these flaps.
- Button technique: This involves placing a custom-made "button" made of silicone or other biocompatible material, sized to cover the perforation and secured in place. This method is less commonly used due to potential complications and the non-biological nature of the repair.
- Connective tissue grafts: These involve using fascia or cartilage to provide a scaffold for tissue growth across the perforation. The author's favorite is the perichondrial graft.

12.9.1 Why Is the Perichondrium Essential for Wound Healing?

The perichondrium is crucial in cartilage growth, maintenance, and repair. It consists of two distinct layers:

- Outer fibrous layer: This is the more superficial layer of the perichondrium. It consists mainly of dense, irregular connective tissue and is rich in fibroblasts (Fig. 12.9).
- Inner cambium layer: Located just beneath the fibrous layer, the cambium layer is more cellular and contains progenitor cells that have the potential to differentiate into chondrocytes (cartilage cells).

There was a report on the healing capacity of cartilage structures focusing on the role of the perichondrium's inner (cambium) and outer (fibrous) layers of rabbits in cartilage wound healing in vitro. It examines the healing process under three conditions using rabbit ear cartilage explants: both perichondrium layers intact, only the outer layer removed, and both layers removed. There was fibrous cell growth over the wound edges starting from day three from the outer layer. New cartilage formation was noted around the entire

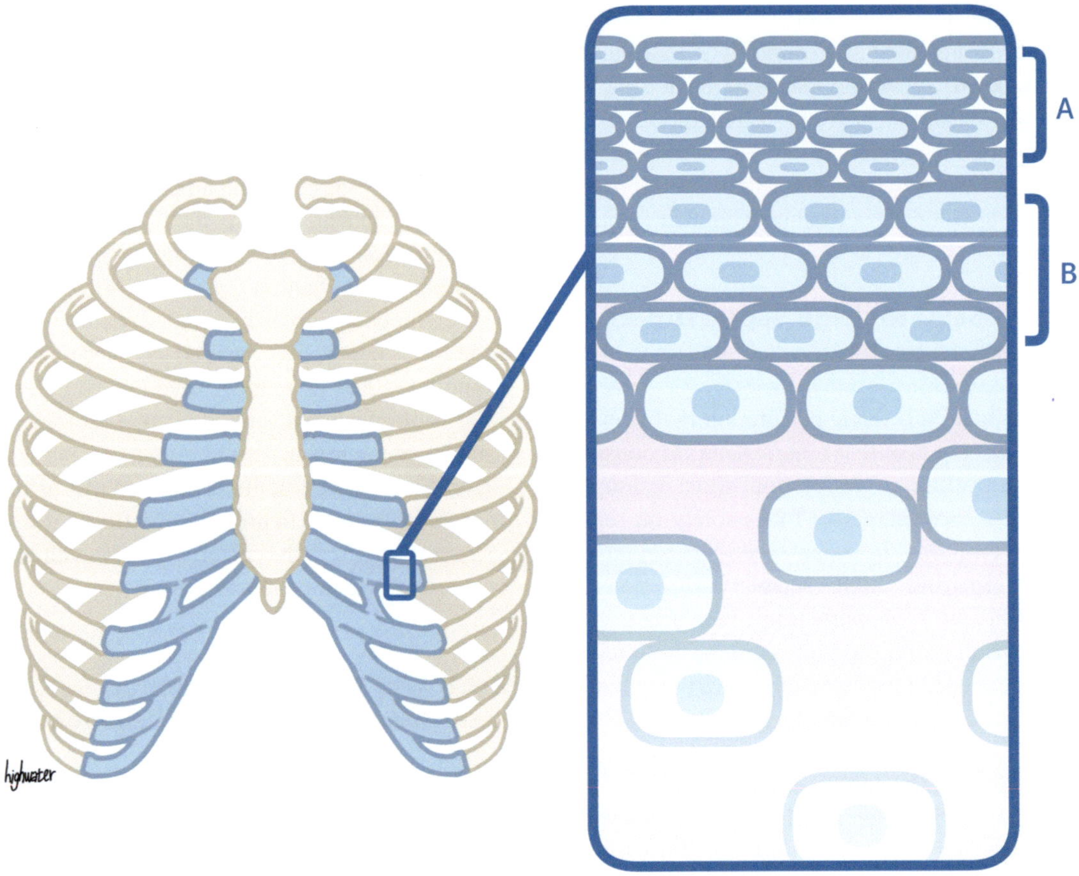

Fig. 12.9 Perichondrium composed of inner and outer packed cells

explant by day 21, suggesting the inner layer plays a crucial role in generating new cartilage cells.

Notably, TGFβ1 levels remained high in the outer perichondrium layer and the fibrous cell layer growing over the explant, hinting at its involvement in promoting fibrous tissue growth during healing [19].

- Therefore, even laminated costal cartilage exposed in the high septum can be highly beneficial to future healing and wound repair if the exposed area can be covered with proper perichondrial wrapping.

References

1. Jung D-H, Choi S-H, Moon H-J, Chung I-H, Im J-H, Lam SM. A cadaveric analysis of the ideal costal cartilage graft for Asian rhinoplasty. Plast Reconstr Surg. 2004;114:545–50.
2. Yi. Preoperative considerations, operative preparation, and postoperative care for rib cartilage use in rhinoplasty. Plast Aesthet Res. https://parjournal.net/article/view/3017
3. Hawellek T, Beil FT, Hischke S, Saul D, Hoffmann DB, Kleiss S, et al. Costal cartilage calcification: prevalence, amount, and structural pattern in the general population and its association with age: a cadaveric

study. Facial Plast Surg Aesthet Med. 2021;26:481. https://doi.org/10.1089/fpsam.2021.0063.
4. Gibson T, Davis WB. The distortion of autogenous cartilage grafts: its cause and prevention. Br J Plast Surg. 1957;10:257–74.
5. Kim DW, Shah AR, Toriumi DM. Concentric and eccentric carved costal cartilage: a comparison of warping. Arch Facial Plast Surg. 2006;8:42–6.
6. Farkas JP, Lee MR, Lakianhi C, Rohrich RJ. Effects of carving plane, level of harvest, and oppositional suturing techniques on costal cartilage warping. Plast Reconstr Surg. 2013;132:319–25.
7. Teshima TL, Cheng H, Pakdel A, Kiss A, Fialkov JA. Transverse slicing of the sixth–seventh costal cartilaginous junction: a novel technique to prevent warping in nasal surgery. J Craniofac Surg. 2016;27:e50.
8. Taştan E, Yücel ÖT, Aydin E, Aydoğan F, Beriat K, Ulusoy MG. The oblique split method: a novel technique for carving costal cartilage grafts. JAMA Facial Plast Surg. 2013;15:198–203.
9. Adams WP Jr, Rios JL, Smith SJ. Enhancing patient outcomes in aesthetic and reconstructive breast surgery using triple antibiotic breast irrigation: six-year prospective clinical study. Plast Reconstr Surg. 2006;118:46S–52S.
10. Adams WP Jr. Commentary on: surgical site irrigation in plastic surgery: what is essential? Aesthetic Surgery J. 2018:276–8.
11. Fukuda N, Asato H, Umekawa K, Takada G, Kan T, Sasaki S. Costal cartilage graft with perichondrium, a possible anti-adhesive material. J Plast Surg Hand Surg. 2017;51:247–53.
12. Robotti E, Leone F. The SPF-SPLF graft: building the ideal dorsum in revision rhinoplasty. Plast Reconstr Surg. 2020;145:1420–4.
13. Haack S, Hacker S, Mann S, Gubisch W. Bony fixation of the nasal framework. Facial Plast Surg. 2019;35:23–30.
14. Toriumi DM. Dorsal augmentation using autologous costal cartilage or microfat-infused soft tissue augmentation. Facial Plast Surg. 2017;33:162–78.
15. Lee J-S, Tae S-S, Kim D-Y, Han S-K, Kim W-K, Dhong E-S. Do IL-3/GM-CSF effect on the myofibroblastic differentiation of human adipose derived stromal cells? Exp Cell Res. 2017;355:67–82.
16. Lee T-Y, Lee K-I, Dhong E-S, Jeong S-H, Kim D-W, Han S-K. Long-term resorption rate of autogenous Onlay graft in east Asian rhinoplasty: a retrospective study. Plast Reconstr Surg. 2022;149:360–71.
17. Vila PM, Jeanpierre LM, Rizzi CJ, Yaeger LH, Chi JJ. Comparison of autologous vs homologous costal cartilage grafts in dorsal augmentation rhinoplasty: a systematic review and meta-analysis. JAMA Otolaryngol Head Neck Surg. 2020;146:347–54.
18. Santamaría-Gadea A, Mariño-Sánchez F, Arana-Fernández B, Mullol J, Alobid I. Innovative surgical techniques for nasal septal perforations: management and treatment. Curr Allergy Asthma Rep. 2021;21:17.
19. Duynstee MLG, Verwoerd-Verhoef HL, Verwoerd CDA, Van Osch GJVM. The dual role of perichondrium in cartilage wound healing. Plast Reconstr Surg. 2002;110:1073–9.

13 Composite Graft Revisited: Creating a De Novo Soft Triangle

Pearls

- Composite grafts are generally reserved for complex cases such as severe alar retraction, often in revision surgeries to expand the nasal framework and internal lining or for columellar defects.
- The choice and success of composite grafts hinge on detailed surgical planning and an understanding of nasal anatomy, particularly in addressing the limitations of the internal nasal lining and achieving the desired elongation and contour of the nasal tip and alar regions.
- For more significant defects, bilobed flaps are preferred because it can conform to the nose's curved surfaces. Techniques such as the nasolabial perforator flap are chosen for their aesthetic match and minimal scarring, especially in cases of alar reconstruction.
- Composite grafts, frequently harvested from the posterior aspect of the ear for aesthetic reasons, offer a direct solution for nasal tip defects but come with varied success rates.
- Understanding the mechanisms of revascularization is key to enhancing graft survival. Strategies such as hyperbaric oxygen therapy promise to improve outcomes by promoting revascularization and reducing tissue edema.
- A clean recipient bed with well-defined margins and sharp debridement is crucial for successful composite grafting, particularly at the skin's edge, where revascularization is most likely.
- Incorporating more cartilage than skin in the graft not only provides structural support but also enhances the potential for revascularization, especially when preserving the perichondrium, highlighting the technique's importance in ensuring graft survival and addressing defects in areas like the columella, alar, lobule, and soft triangle.
- Correcting soft triangle deformities in secondary rhinoplasty is challenging due to its lack of cartilaginous support and vulnerability to scarring from repeated surgeries.
- Innovative grafting techniques to restore structural support and suture techniques to maintain the natural contour and fullness of the soft triangle, ensuring a harmonious nasal aesthetic, are crucial for reconstructing the soft triangle.

13.1 Composite Graft in Asian Rhinoplasty

In East Asian rhinoplasty, composite grafts are generally considered a last resort. The reluctance to use composite grafts is particularly evident in cosmetic surgery involving alloplastic implants for dorsal augmentation due to the potential complications associated with wound healing. Indeed, wound complications are tantamount to surgical failure.

Primarily, composite grafts are utilized to address alar retraction by augmenting the caudal

E. S. Dhong, *Asian Septorhinoplasty*, https://doi.org/10.1007/978-981-96-6127-5_13

portion of the lower lateral cartilages and the internal nasal lining. In revision surgeries, the indication shifts toward expanding the nasal framework and internal nasal lining as part of contracture release measures rather than solely correcting alar retraction. This expansion is necessary to accommodate the increased soft tissue envelope of the dorsal nasal region, which is achieved through extensive dissection and scar excision. However, the limited release achievable in the nasal mucosa necessitates further enlargement of the internal nasal lining to align with the expanded dorsal skin-soft tissue envelope (SSTE).

Applying alloplastic implants in the nasal dorsum carries inherent risks, mainly when extensive modification necessitates composite grafts due to insufficient internal nasal lining during redraping. The choice of a composite graft becomes particularly challenging if delayed wound healing occurs, given the concurrent risk to the dorsal implant.

Consequently, composite grafts are predominantly reserved for initial rhinoplasty procedures without implants, as an independent intervention in multi-stage surgeries, or in conjunction with rib grafts during autologous tissue reconstruction in revision surgeries.

Due to the lack of tissue, a composite graft may be used for congenital anomalies. Correction of cleft lip and nose deformities may require a definite rhinoplasty.

- The most common need for a composite graft in Asian rhinoplasty is in cases of severe alar retraction, where no redraping method can compensate for the lack of inner alar lining (Fig. 13.1).

Addressing the elongation of a contracted nasal tip in secondary rhinoplasty necessitates a nuanced approach. Successful elongation hinges on adequately releasing the outer nasal envelope: the skin-soft tissue envelope (SSTE). The author calls it a sleeve-down technique. This involves extensive dissection to detach the surrounding skin, allowing for its lengthening. Such a procedure ensures that the SSTE can expand, facilitating a multidirectional peel-off of the skin to achieve the desired elongation. This approach is critical for attaining an optimal aesthetic outcome while preserving the integrity of the nasal

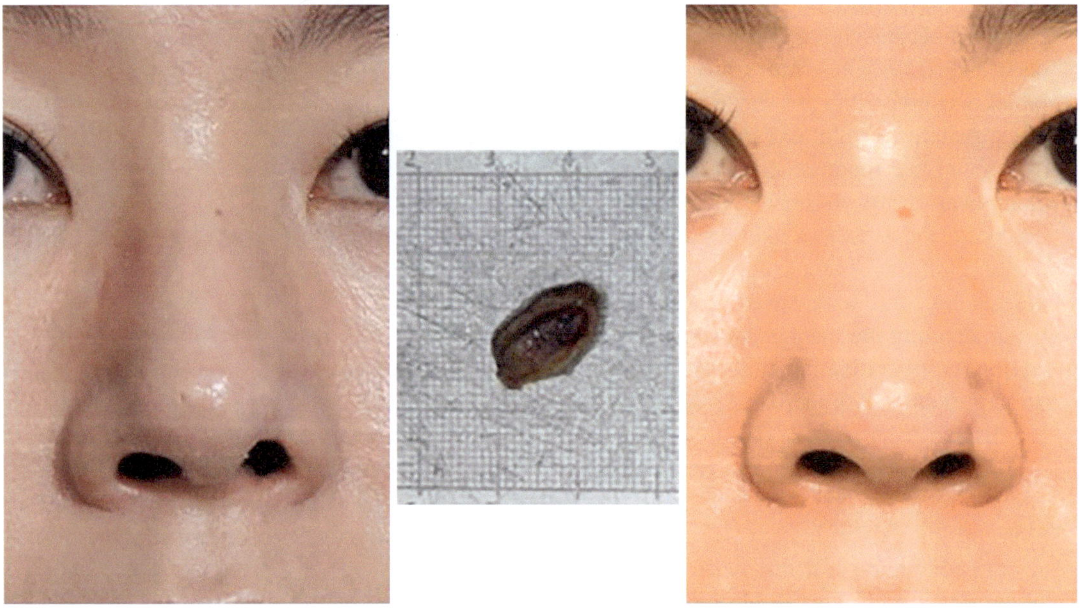

Fig. 13.1 Composite graft for left alar retraction. (Left) Preoperative view. (Middle) Cavum concha donor. (Right) Long-term postoperative view

structure. The skin flap can be cross-hatched with scar excision of the undersurface of the skin flap. However, there is a limit to the extension of the internal nasal lining. A composite graft is applied if the internal nasal lining cannot be lengthened to the desired framework by dissecting the hinge and scroll areas between the ULC and LLC (Fig. 13.2). The defect is mainly along the incision line and below the lateral marginal incision. No matter how well the outer skin envelope is stretched, the effectiveness of the extension is reduced if the inner lining cannot catch up (Fig. 13.3).

Technically, the decision is to place the composite graft on the caudal margin of the internal nasal lining or between the upper lateral cartilage and the lower lateral cartilage for alar extension. The composite graft applied to the margin is close to the nostril, which can cause nostril thickening and visible scarring, and the composite graft between the ULC and LLC often does not provide sufficient extension. The position of the composite graft should be determined according to the alar shape and the resilience of the alar skin. Still, to create a beautiful soft triangle, the author believes the composite graft should be positioned more cephalically, and the soft triangle should be made with the full "sleeve-down" of the nostril margin.

13.1.1 Nasal Lining—Composite Graft

Suppose the desired elongation of the nasal lining is not achieved when tip projection is performed or the lower lateral cartilage is extended. In that case, an extra SSTE cover is required to fill the gap between the stretched soft tissue envelope and the caudal margin of the internal nasal lining. The most commonly used part of this is a composite graft directed down the concave surface of the concha to which the skin is attached (internal nasal lining).

This means that the skin on the inner surface of the cymba or cavum must be used.

In some cases, it may be necessary to harvest skin more than 3–5 mm wide from the anterior side of the concha.

If the cartilage width and skin width are too much, harvesting the skin behind the ear may also be considered, but the convex skin may be directed to the internal lining.

The anterior skin attachment of the concha cartilage is much thinner, and the subcutaneous tissue on the posterior side is thicker. However, because the incision in front of the ear leaves a visible scar, the author prefers the back of the ear. You should choose a method that leaves a minimal scar.

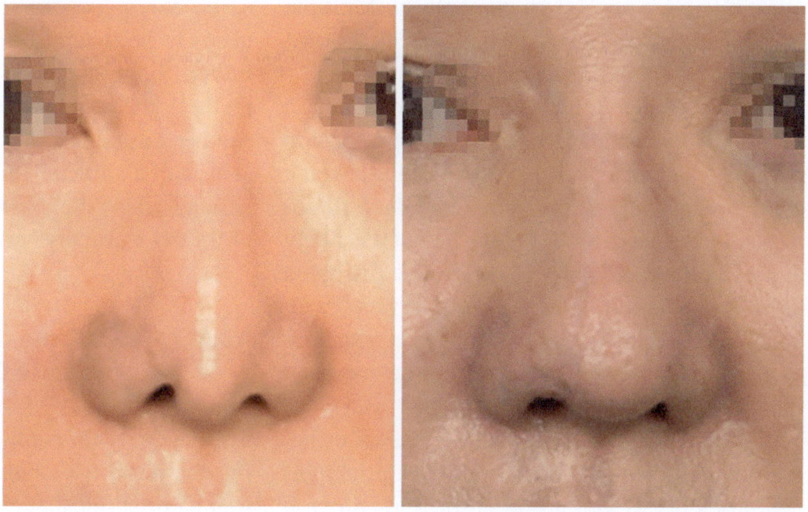

Fig. 13.2 Sleeve down of soft triangle. (Left) Preoperative view. (Right) Long-term postoperative view

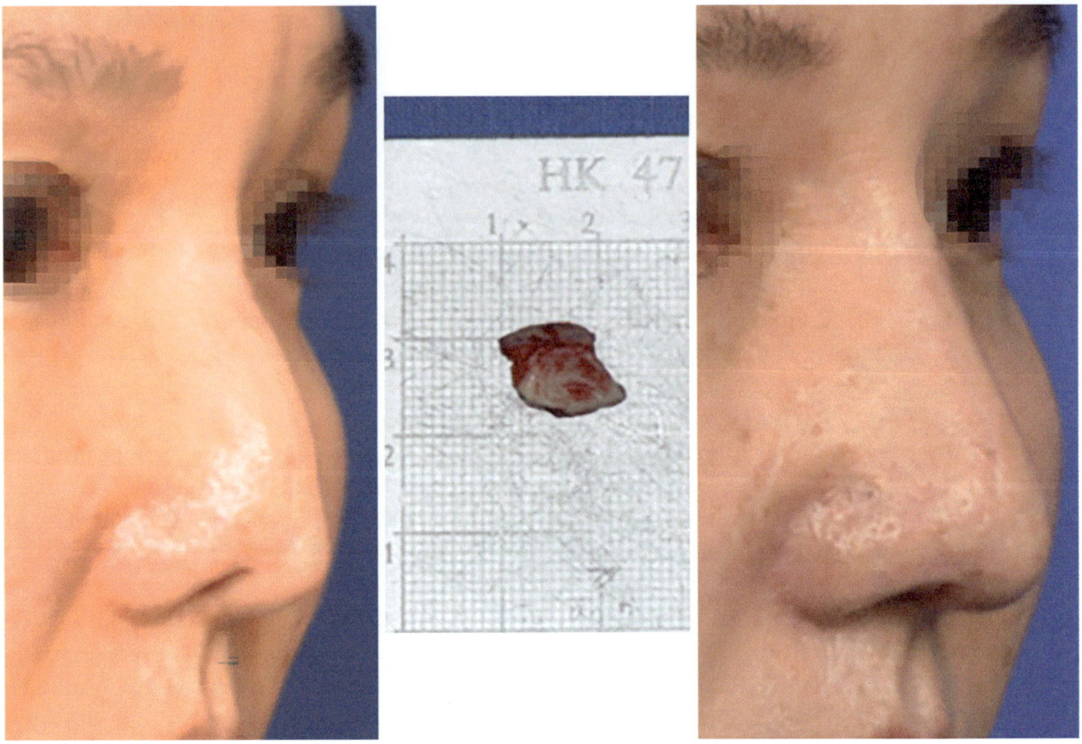

Fig. 13.3 Sleeve down of soft triangle. (Left) Preoperative quarter view. (Middle) Composite graft from cavum concha. (Right) Long-term postoperative view

13.1.2 Columella-Composite Graft

The need for a composite graft of the columella is often due to necrosis caused by iatrogenic complications from secondary rhinoplasty. Multiple operations usually result in surgical errors that impair skin circulation to the columella.

It is speculated that failure to maintain a proper dissection plane or excessive tip tension may have caused circulatory disturbances, which are frequently seen in Asian secondary rhinoplasty. The exact cause is unknown, but it is likely due to columellar flap elevation that disrupted dermal circulation. When a patient visits with columellar necrosis, they are usually in a state of despair and have a fear of a midline forehead flap, seeking alternative methods (Fig. 13.4).

It is essential to consider the flap's tension, but it is not possible to define it in terms of principles and protocols. If you are a plastic surgeon, you will have been trained in flap monitoring during your training, so that you will need experience with this. The most important thing is to draw the template accurately behind the ear before harvesting. It is crucial to harvest more cartilage and perichondrium than skin (Fig. 13.5).

As noted with the columellar defect, the graft needs to be much thicker than the internal nasal lining. Since the open rhinoplasty of the columella skin is accompanied by the loss of the anterior layer as thick as the vestibule incision, surface skin with a sufficient amount of concha cartilage is required, so the donor site in the posterior part of the ear is usually sufficient (Fig. 13.6).

13.1.3 Tip Lobule, Alar Margin-Composite Graft

The necessity for composite grafts in reconstructing the nasal tip lobule often arises from direct trauma or surgical excision, particularly in cases involving carcinoma removal. Traumatic defects typically result from bite injuries or lacerations

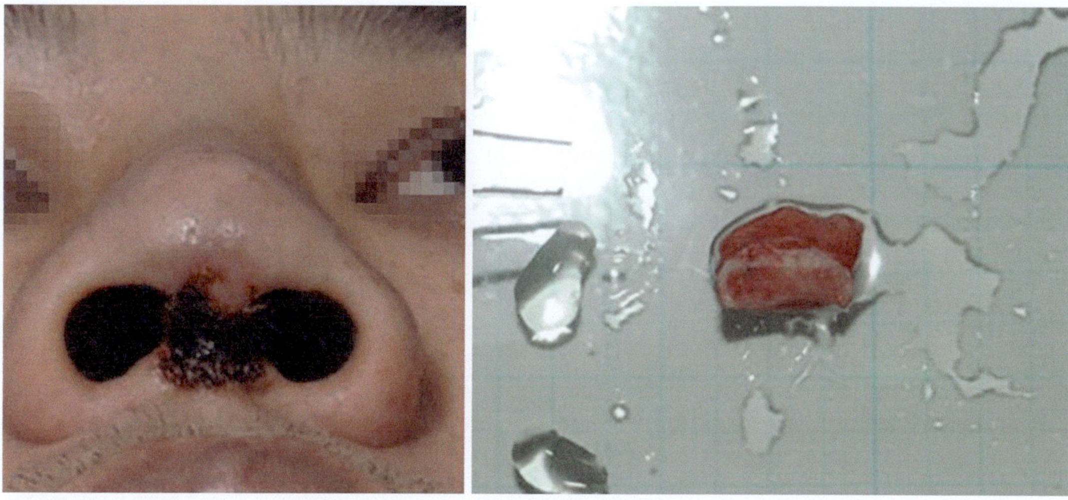

Fig. 13.4 Columella necrosis. (Left) Basal view when transferred. (Right) Donors from cavum concha

Fig. 13.5 Template for the columellar defect. (Left) Paper template. (Right) Posterior left ear donor

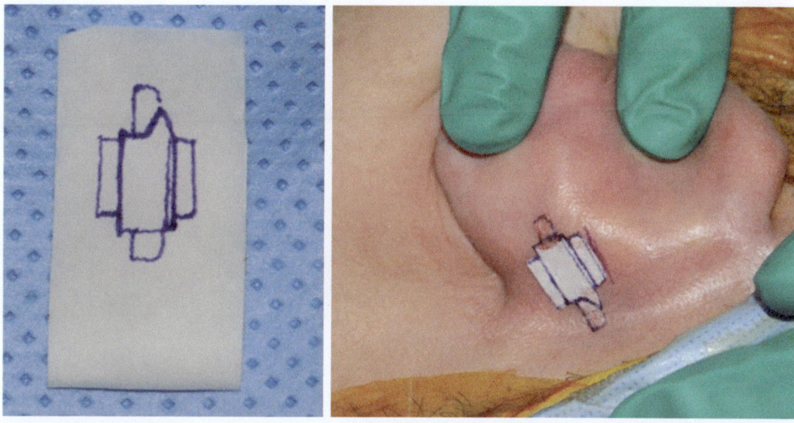

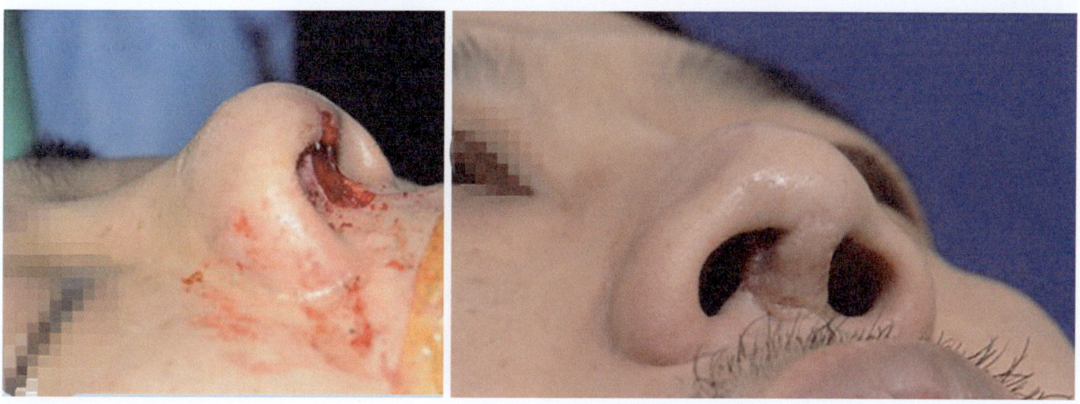

Fig. 13.6 Columellar defect reconstruction. (Left) Preoperative full-depth defect. (Right) Long-term postoperative view

inflicted by sharp objects. Similarly, surgical resections for carcinoma are characterized by well-defined margins. For defects involving the alar margin, which may extend to the tip lobule or soft triangle, reconstruction is commonly achieved using a dorsal nasal flap or a bilobed flap. However, composite grafting is a specialized solution when margin defects result in full-thickness deficits (Figs. 13.7 and 13.8).

Addressing full-thickness defects necessitates a strategic approach, often involving manipulating the upper lateral cartilage (ULC) or lower lateral cartilage (LLC) to convert a full-thickness defect into a partial-thickness one. For example, transposing the LLC toward the margin reduces the full-thickness defect at the caudal margin.

Given the complexity of replicating the intricate contours of the alar margin with local flaps, applying a composite graft to the external surface becomes crucial. Although such defects are rare, their reconstruction is uncommon, and using composite grafts, selected for their volume and robustness, remains a viable option for managing marginal defects. The author prefers to use posterior skin with cartilage in the longitudinal direction of the cavum and cymba concha (Fig. 13.9).

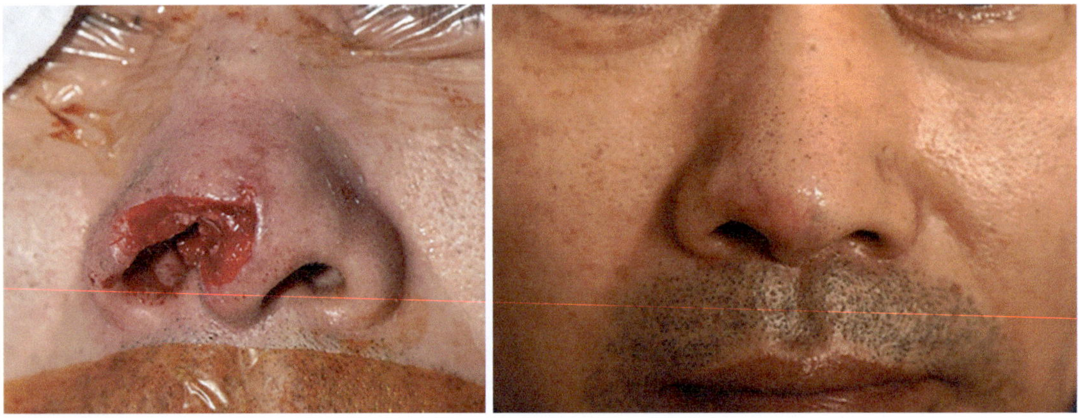

Fig. 13.7 Traumatic right alar defect. (Left) Preoperative view. (Right) Long-term postoperative view

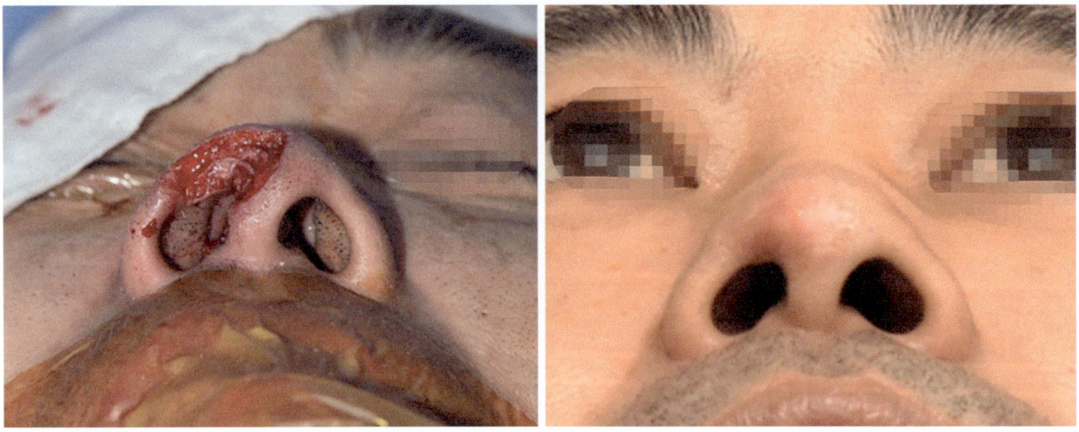

Fig. 13.8 Traumatic right alar defect. (Left) Preoperative basal view. (Right) Long-term postoperative view

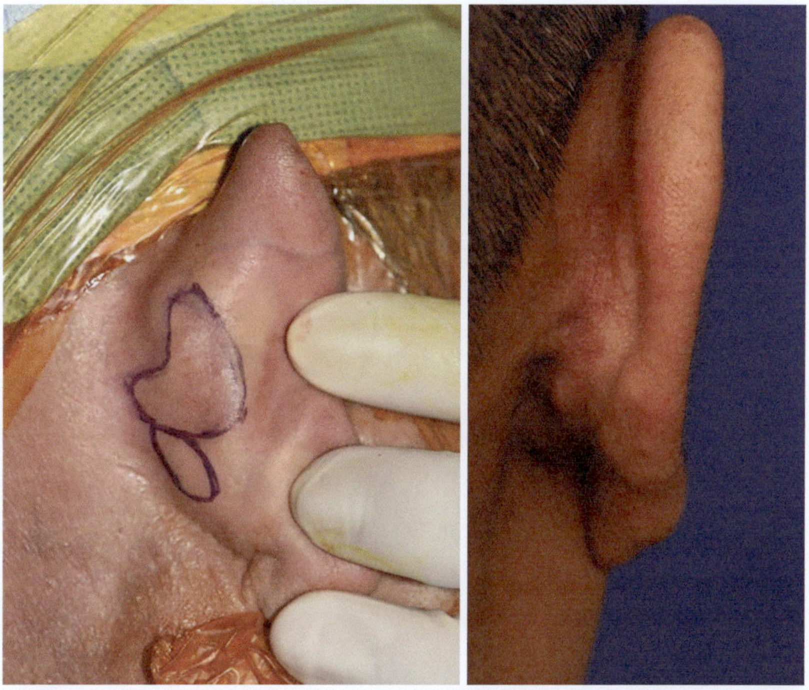

Fig. 13.9 Donor site for two different composite grafts. (Left) Design. (Right) Long-term postoperative scar

13.2 Larger Defect, Including Tip Complex-Beyond the Composite Graft

Although this reconstruction falls under the category of aesthetic rhinoplasty, from a broader perspective, there is no boundary between aesthetics and reconstruction. Local flaps or transposition flaps are preferred for sizes beyond the range that a composite graft can cover.

A bilobed flap is a local flap suitable for covering curved surfaces. It is used to reconstruct the nose's spherical shape.

A heavily tensioned dorsal skin flap can cause deformation of the lower nasal framework in the direction of the long axis of skin tension. As a result, it can cause problems such as tip shortening. For this purpose, absorbable plates introduced in craniofacial surgery can play a role in overcoming this longitudinal tension if adequately utilized. To overcome the longitudinal tension of the soft tissue envelope, the absorbable plate is anchored to the upper lateral cartilage and lower lateral cartilage in the form of an onlay, which maintains its length during adequate soft tissue creeping substitution (Figs. 13.10 and 13.11).

Full-through defects in the alar area are among the most difficult to reconstruct, and the author prefers the nasolabial perforator flap for reconstructing the outer and inner lining. A thin and long flap is required to cover a total alar defect, and a nasolabial flap with a perforator is practical. Midline forehead flap or paramedian forehead flap is the last resort for any nasal reconstruction, so it is in the patient's best interest to save it in case of failure or recurrence.

13.2.1 Nasolabial Perforator-Based Flap

For patients with alar defects that extend beyond the lower third of the nose or those with symmetric bilateral alar defects, the midline forehead flap is a well-justified reconstructive option. This flap is often favored for its robust vascular supply and the ample tissue it can provide for substantial nasal reconstruction. Conversely, in scenarios involving unilateral alar defects or perioral alar defects that do not exceed the lower quarter of the nose, the preference shifts away from the midline forehead flap. The reluctance to employ this flap

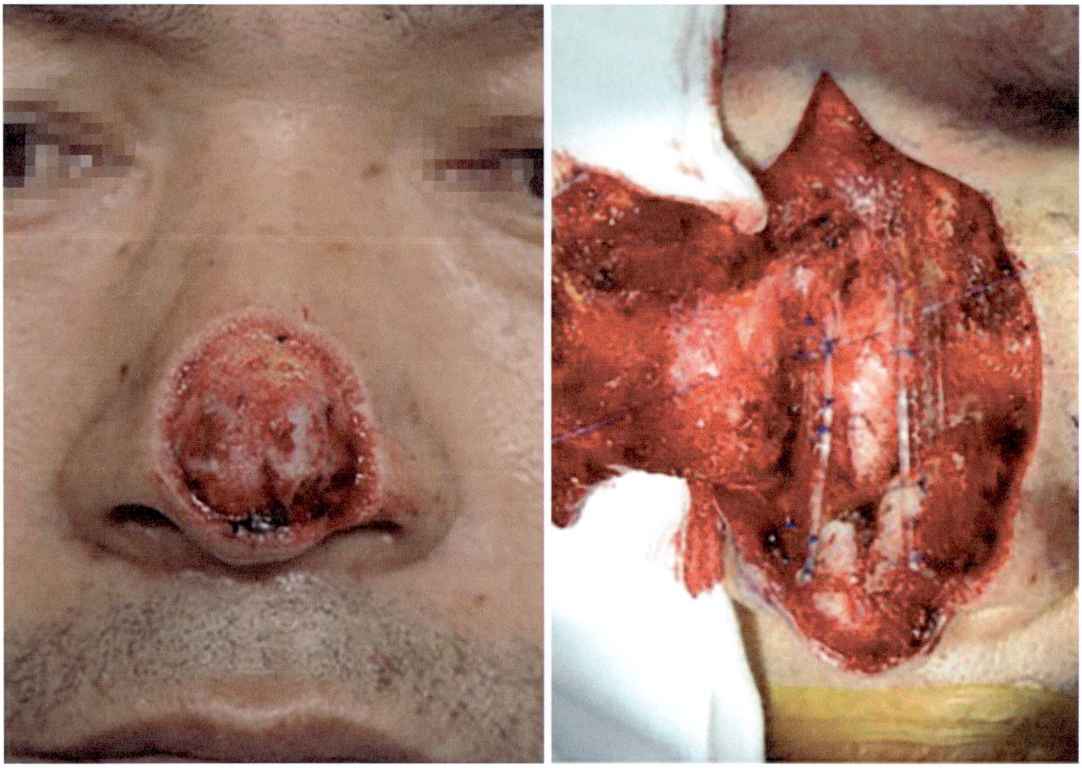

Fig. 13.10 Total nasal tip defect. (Left) Preoperative view. (Right) Dorsal nasal flap with two absorbable plates for tension relief

Fig. 13.11 Long-term postoperative view of total tip defect. (Left) AP view. (Right) Lateral view

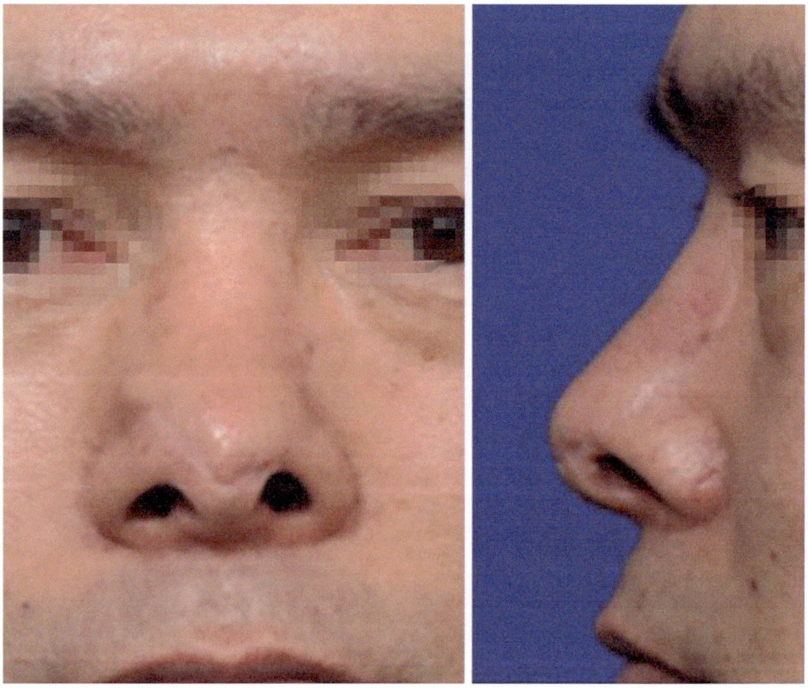

in such cases is not due to doubts about achieving satisfactory outcomes but concerns about potential aesthetic compromises. The midline forehead flap, while effective, may lead to the use of normal skin from a highly visible area, which could be deemed less desirable from a cosmetic standpoint.

In cases where the unilateral defect encompasses the entire alar region, the nasolabial perforator flap emerges as the author's preferred choice. This flap, sourced from the nasolabial fold area, is valued for its color and texture match, which can lead to more discreet and aesthetically pleasing reconstructive results. Its use underscores carefully considering functional restoration and aesthetic integrity in nasal reconstruction.

The recent introduction of a laser Doppler in the operating room helps to secure a more secure perforator, which allows the larger flap to be sent farther.

Depending on the patient, the perforator is sometimes in different places; hence, the Doppler is used. There is no way to ensure safety by surgical design other than using magnification to check circulation during the procedure. The only way is to rely on the pulsation heard on the Doppler and leave adequate soft tissue. Along with preserving the zygomaticus muscles, preserving the essential perforator, which comes from the gap between the minor and major, and the perforator present in the upper part of the minor will be the key to the operation (Fig. 13.12). The nasolabial perforator flap can be suitable for older patients with a more pronounced nasolabial fold, providing a less conspicuous donor site. However, younger patients, who often seek cosmetic rhinoplasty, may have a significantly adverse reaction to the resultant scar. Given their typically less pronounced nasolabial folds, scarring can be more apparent and aesthetically displeasing, making this flap a less desirable option for nasal reconstruction in this demographic. Age must be considered, as many patients disagree with the nasolabial scar (Fig. 13.13).

When reconstructing the columella, for example, it's essential to recognize that using a buried pedicle flap might not yield the most suitable results due to the inherent differences in skin thickness and texture compared to the native columellar skin. The cheek's larger fat compartment contributes to this discrepancy, lacking the cartilaginous support in the nasal structure.

Furthermore, issues like color mismatch, flap heterogeneity, and dissatisfaction with the donor site scar present additional challenges separate from flap survival. These factors underscore the need for a meticulous approach in selecting the most appropriate reconstructive technique, considering both functional and aesthetic outcomes.

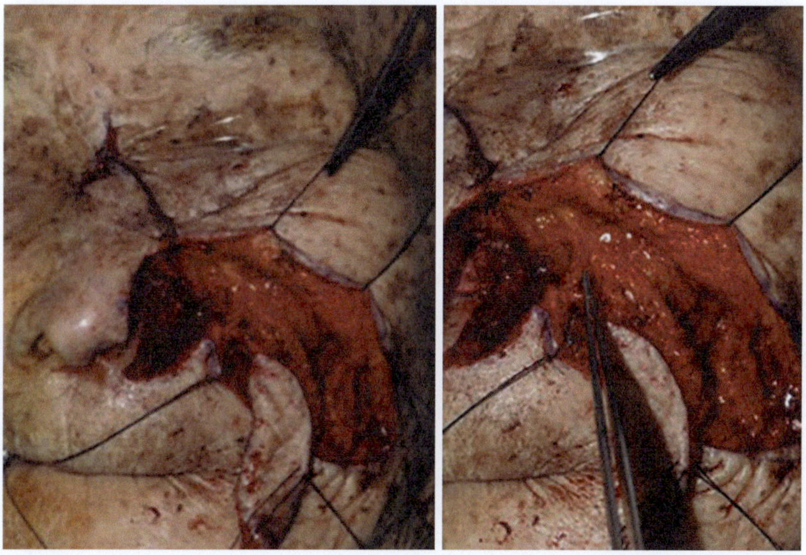

Fig. 13.12 Nasolabial perforator flap. (Left) Nasolabial flap with dorsal nasal flap. (Right) Perforator from facial artery medial branch

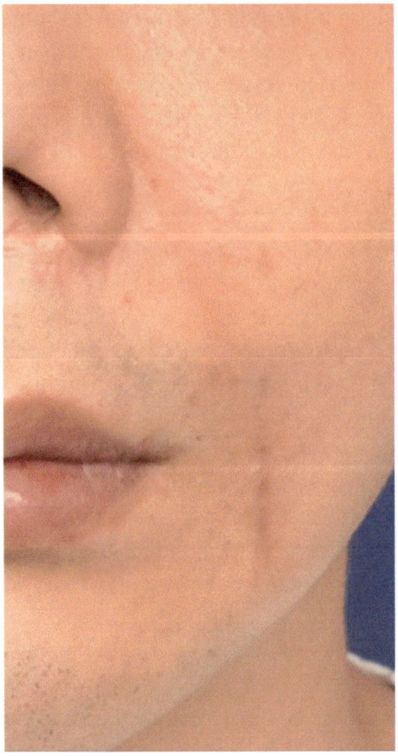

Fig. 13.13 Unfavorable scar of nasolabial flap: transferred due to columellar defect

13.3 Did I Adequately Explain the Composite Graft to the Patient?

Notably, the literature has predominantly documented using the ear's anterior surface for graft harvesting. However, for cosmetic considerations, some practitioners, including the author, prefer harvesting from the posterior aspect of the ear, utilizing both the skin and deeper cartilage layers.

Yet, their success rates are notably varied, with reports ranging from as low as 10% to as high as 70%. This wide range underscores the unpredictability and complexity associated with the survival of these grafts.

The context of composite graft success is further complicated when comparing the field of rhinoplasty to that of reconstructive surgery for fingertip reattachment. The latter often boasts lower success rates, but the clinical scenarios are markedly different. Fingertip composite grafts are more complex, encompassing bone, fatty tissue, skin, or nail bed, and are typically larger in volume than those used in nasal reconstruction.

Patient acceptance becomes a significant factor when considering alternatives for nasal reconstruction, such as the midline forehead flap or nasolabial perforator flap. Many patients, particularly those referred after unsatisfactory outcomes from previous cosmetic surgeries, may feel they have limited options. Despite this, there is often a low tolerance for additional scarring, which poses a challenge in selecting the most appropriate reconstructive approach. This patient sentiment highlights the importance of thorough preoperative counseling to manage expectations and ensure informed decision-making regarding reconstructive technique.

13.3.1 Vasculogenesis, Angiogenesis vs. Revascularization

Vasculogenesis is a concept that refers to the overall process of making blood vessels in the embryo. In short, it is the in situ differentiation of angioblast. Angiogenesis is endothelial regrowth that causes microvascular regrowth, which is a phenomenon that occurs in the long term of composite graft take. On the other hand, revascularization, which is achieved by vascular inosculation, is the reconnection of the severed microvasculature. This occurs within 4–5 days and is an essential requirement for the survival of the composite graft. To keep the microvasculature open, there must be little tissue edema, a clean-cut wound edge, and many vessels at the cutting edge of the appropriate tissue. The success of direct inosculation is the most essential factor in graft survival.

13.3.2 Improving the Survival Rate of Composite Graft

In the past, several agents have been tried in animal studies to increase survival rates.

Good results have been reported with heparin, or PRP, injected deep into the graft or with EGF,

FGF, or basic fibroblast growth factor (b FGF). Cooling as a local therapy has also been reported to be helpful.

Pharmacological agents such as corticosteroids, dimethyl sulfoxide, and heparin have been tested. Cooling and hyperbaric oxygen therapy have also been investigated. Angiogenesis was promoted by directly injecting growth factors such as basic fibroblast and platelet-derived growth factors (PDGF) [1–3].

Hyperbaric oxygen (HBO) requires specific equipment, which may not be available in private clinics. However, the author considers HBO to be the best modality.

The advantages of HBO include direct wound vasoconstriction, which reduces tissue edema, activates the immune system, increases relative tissue oxygen tension, reduces toxins involved in inflammation and reperfusion, and reduces obstacles to revascularization that can occur during periods of tissue ischemia, which also has an antibiotic effect.

In the author's case, HBO was performed two times daily for less than an hour.

13.4 Pre-conditions to Be Taken

As introduced in the literature, the composite recipient's condition has been considered the most important. It is accepted that graft take is good when the bed is clean without granulation tissue, bleeding is good, the repair margin is clear, and sharp debridement is performed to the area where the dermal-epidermal junction is well preserved. Revascularization is more likely to occur at the skin margin than at the undersurface, so securing a sharp skin edge is considered a prerequisite for taking.

There is no disagreement that the first revascularization in composite tissue is from a clean skin margin. Still, the environment differs depending on the composition of the composite tissue.

If the fat layer under the skin is thick, the cut surface's sharpness at the skin's edge is the most essential factor for take. However, when cartilage is included, it is a different matter. Cartilage has the advantage of being able to be taken and supported more widely than skin.

There is a report of composite grafts using pig skin in the literature that perpendicular angiogenesis originating from the fat bed was beneficial for taking [4].

13.4.1 The Importance of the Perichondrium in Technique and Survival

Incorporating a larger area of cartilage than the required skin surface area allows for the utilization of cartilage support to facilitate repair to the surrounding lower lateral cartilages (LLC), thereby reducing the amount of skin suturing needed. Moreover, preserving the perichondrium that covers the cartilage while simultaneously including it on one or both surfaces of the cartilage can enhance revascularization through the perichondrium of the cartilage and the undersurface of the skin flap encompassing the wound margin (Fig. 13.14).

Over the past 10 years, the author has been employing composite grafts that incorporate more cartilage than the skin defect to cover defects in the columella, which necessitates cartilage, and also for defects in the alar, lobule, and soft triangle areas.

13.4.2 Nasal Lining Composite Graft

In numerous Asian individuals, a congenital underdevelopment of the lower lateral cartilage is observed. This, coupled with the underdevelopment of the soft triangle facet, can precipitate alar retraction. Additionally, a loss of the appropriate lateral genu divergence angle, attributable to the excessive cephalic rotation of the lateral crus or over-rotation of the lateral genu following rhinoplasty, may exacerbate the appearance of alar retraction post-enhancement of tip projection.

For correction, an initial step involves lowering the rim margin through a comprehensive sleeve-down technique. This is subsequently complemented by grafting to address deficiencies in the internal nasal lining [5, 6].

Creating a soft triangle in rhinoplasty involves the precise placement of a composite graft, partic-

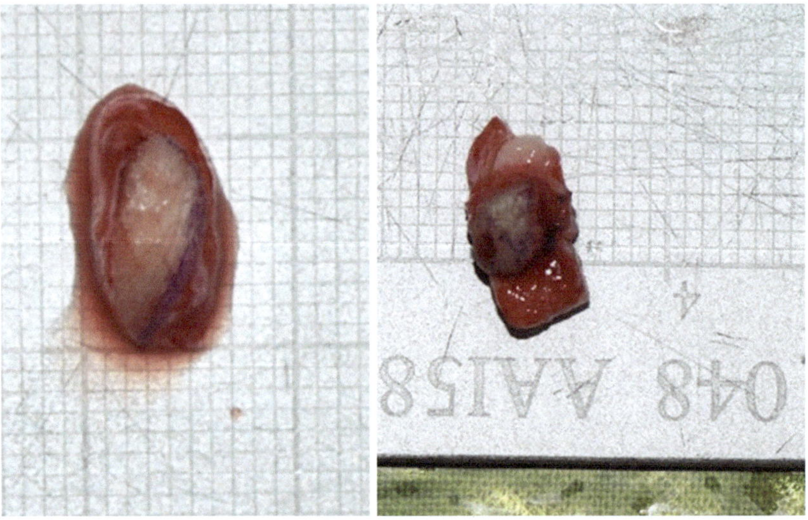

Fig. 13.14 More cartilage with perichondrium than skin. (Left) For alar extension. (Right) For columellar defect

ularly effective when positioned in the caudal portion of the dome-defining point. This area's convexity adds technical complexity, but pre-anchoring the cartilage enhances support, often alongside a shield graft. The graft aims for a caudal extension for alar retraction, supporting the lower lateral cartilages (LLC). In cases of complete LLC detachment from the upper lateral cartilages (ULC), as seen in contracted noses, additional support may be required through lateral crural strut or batten-type onlay extension grafts. Correction of soft triangles and alar retraction is challenging in Asian secondary rhinoplasty, with the risk of increased contracture following composite graft failure. Often, repositioning the rim flap or using a composite graft for new internal nasal lining defects becomes a last-resort solution, especially in secondary surgeries where nasal lining defects persist post-contracture release.

13.5 Creating a De Novo Soft Triangle

Correcting soft triangle deformities presents a significant challenge among the post-surgical deformities encountered in secondary rhinoplasty. The soft triangle lacks cartilaginous support at its base, meaning repeated surgical interventions can exacerbate the deformity. Soft triangle contracture may arise from multiple factors, mainly when surgeons have made multiple incisions in this area (Fig. 13.15).

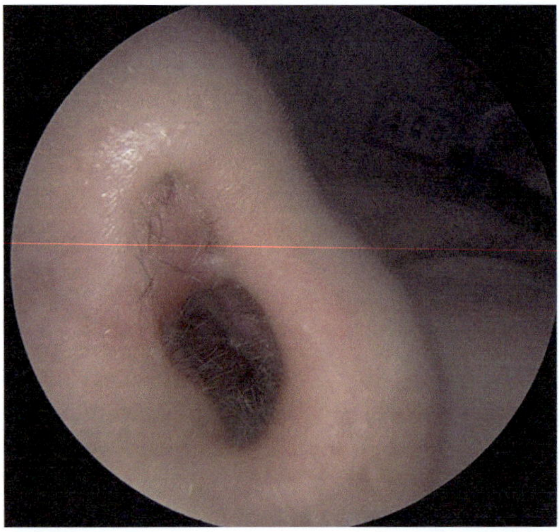

Fig. 13.15 Contracture below the soft triangle: incorrect repetitive incisions and lack of understanding of the middle crura

13.6 Causes of Soft Triangle Disappearance

13.6.1 Incision Applied to the Rim

This caution is warranted because the lower lateral cartilages (LLC) are the primary structural elements capable of withstanding the longitudinal or transverse tensions that arise at the incision margins during the healing process. Repetitive incisions near the rim can progressively diminish the size of the soft triangle if multiple incisions are made in different parts of the soft tissue. Naturally, contracture of the nasal internal lining will occur along with hardness due to scarring of the incision site. Eventually, changes in the length and thickness of the soft triangle will occur. Therefore, incisions close to the rim should never be made unless it is a secondary cleft lip and nose deformity.

13.6.2 Incision Without Considering Middle Crus

Incorrect incisions in the lower part of the lateral crus are common, especially during the transition to the middle crus, due to the complex anatomy. A thorough understanding of the anatomical transition from the lateral to the middle genu is essential to avoid such errors. The key to crafting a natural soft triangle at the nasal tip is preserving the natural divergence and angle between the medial and middle crura. Disruption of this relationship can prevent the formation of an aesthetically pleasing soft triangle, highlighting the importance of the substantial soft tissue located caudally to the middle crus in nasal tip aesthetics.

13.6.3 Invalid Tip Suture

Augmenting the caudal aspect of the medial crura enhances the divergence of the lateral genu while simultaneously reducing the caudal prominence of the soft triangle. In East Asian tip rhinoplasty, a non-physiological suture technique, often termed "lateral crural medialization," involves repositioning the lateral crus toward the medial side. This approach, once favored by many surgeons, is now recognized as detrimental to the integrity of the soft triangle.

Moreover, excessive transdomal and tip extension sutures can compromise the natural angulation of the middle crus at the nasal tip. Any suture technique that interferes with the middle crus's double break undermines the tip lobule's harmonious proportions, which is crucial for a natural appearance.

13.6.4 Contracture

Scar tissue tightening can lead to distortion of the nasal tip's shape and position, often resulting in a contracted, shortened nasal tip with an unnatural appearance. The soft triangle, devoid of cartilage support, is especially susceptible to scarring, rendering it more rigid, altering its natural contour and possibly leading to a pinched look. Consequently, the natural roundness is compromised, typically resulting in a triangular shape.

Among the techniques to augment the volume of the lower portion of the middle crus following contracture release, a large midcrural batten graft stands out as an effective method that requires minimal cartilage.

13.7 Technique for Reconstructing Soft Triangles

13.7.1 Prerequisites

Assuming an imbalance in the integrity of the lower lateral cartilages (LLC), prioritizing scar management is paramount. Various techniques, such as Z-plasty, have been proposed to address this issue, with the understanding that different patients may necessitate distinct approaches [7]. Addressing and minimizing scar tissue within the soft triangle area is critical, as excessive scarring can contribute to rigidity and distortion. Effective strategies involve careful placement of incisions and, potentially, utilizing a marginal vestibular skin flap turned down (sleeve-down) to reconstruct a soft triangle. This modified skin flap should be bolstered by sufficient volume and structural support to ensure optimal outcomes.

13.7.2 Techniques for Restoring the Support from LLC

Achieving adequate structural support for the nasal tip and soft triangle is crucial, often necessitating cartilage grafting techniques such as alar rim grafts, strut grafts, or shield grafts. In the Asian demographic, alar rim grafts tend to be less effective due to the thicker skin at the alar margin and the well-developed alar muscles. The author has explored combining wing grafts with shield grafts for robust support, as well as the use of alar extension grafts [8]. However, successful outcomes are only partially dependent on support strength. The management of relaxed skin pockets in conjunction with substantial support is pivotal. These grafts are instrumental in redefining the nasal tip and averting retraction or collapse of the soft triangle. The role of the suture technique cannot be overstated, with precise suture methods being essential for refining tip definition and the soft triangle's appearance without inducing undue tension or distortion. Techniques may include dome-binding, interdomal, or transdomal sutures tailored to the reconstruction's specific requirements. Yet, in many secondary cases where the LLC is compromised, grafting often proves more beneficial than suturing alone.

Restoring volume is crucial, particularly when addressing volume loss or thinning in the soft triangle area. Soft tissue fillers or grafts can be essential for reinstating a natural contour and averting concavity. This step ensures the soft triangle maintains its natural fullness and contributes to the overall harmony of the nasal aesthetics.

13.7.3 Where Will the LLC Get Its Staying Power?

The sesamoid complex plays a significant role in the stability of the LLCs. However, this complex alone may not provide sufficient support. A lateral crural extension graft extending to the sesamoid complex and possibly sourced from a rib graft can be particularly beneficial.

The lateral crura's attachment to the pyriform aperture and surrounding soft tissues also contributes to lateral stability. Additionally, the area of overlap between the LLCs and ULCs, known as the scroll region, aids in LLC stability through intercartilaginous connections. Nonetheless, providing support in the scroll region can be challenging in secondary cases. While it is feasible to bolster the LLC by applying pressure from the ULC, this approach typically requires a substantial amount of cartilage grafting. Moreover, scar tissue and other complicating factors may hinder achieving adequate support. A lateral crural strut graft that reaches the sesamoid complex is helpful if a rib graft is available.

References

1. Aden KK, Biel MA. The evaluation of pharmacologic agents on composite graft survival. Arch Otolaryngol Head Neck Surg. 1992;118:175–8.
2. Li EN, Menon NG, Rodriguez ED, Norkunas M, Rosenthal RE, Goldberg NH, et al. The effect of hyperbaric oxygen therapy on composite graft survival. Ann Plast Surg. 2004;53:141–5.
3. Hom DB, Winters M. Effects of angiogenic growth factors and a penetrance enhancer on composite grafts. Ann Otol Rhinol Laryngol. 1998;107:769–74.
4. Son D, Jeong H, Choi T, Kim J, Han K. A new mechanism associated with compositae graft success. J Plast Reconstr Aesthet Surg. 2010;63:1900–9.
5. Dhong E-S, Na M-W. Correction to: controlling Asian tip: facet and supra-alar groove. In: Dhong E-S, Na M-W, editors. Asian septorhinoplasty: conundrums and solutions. Singapore: Springer Nature Singapore; 2021. p. C1–3.
6. Dhong E-S, Na M-W. Controlling Asian tip: facet and supra-alar groove. In: Dhong E-S, Na M-W, editors. Asian septorhinoplasty: conundrums and solutions. Singapore: Springer Nature Singapore; 2021. p. 103–19.
7. Nguyen DQA, Motley R, Cooper MA. Repair of nasal soft triangle notching. J Plast Reconstr Aesthet Surg. 2008;61:966–8.
8. Kim HS, Roh S-G. The alar extension graft for retracted ala. J Korean Soc Plast Reconstr Surg. 2009;36:66–74.

14 Unusual Complications in Asian Rhinoplasty: Chronic Post-rhinoplasty Neuropathic Pain (CPRNP) and Others

Pitfalls

- Chronic post-rhinoplasty neuropathic pain (CPRNP) is a persistent pain condition that outlasts the expected healing period after rhinoplasty.
- While acute pain diminishes shortly after surgery, a small percentage of patients experience long-term pain, with characteristics varying by individual and region, notably in Asian patients undergoing multiple surgeries.
- Management of CPRNP is complex, requiring careful evaluation and a multidisciplinary approach.
- Osteotomy-related neuropathic pain in nasal surgery involves damage to facial nerves, such as the ophthalmic and maxillary branches of the trigeminal nerve.
- Treatment for CPRNP includes a comprehensive approach with anticonvulsants like gabapentin and pregabalin to modulate pain signals, antidepressants to enhance neurotransmitter activity, interventional nerve blocks for localized relief, and psychological support through cognitive-behavioral therapy to manage pain perception.
- The multidisciplinary strategy addresses the complex nature of CPRNP, considering both physical nerve damage and the psychological impact of chronic pain.
- Paraffin injections in Asian patients for nasal enhancements have led to severe complications like paraffinomas, necessitating complex treatments to manage inflammation, migration, and cosmetic deformities.
- Irradiated homologous costal cartilage in rhinoplasty can lead to complications like fibrous encapsulation, reduced integration, and the potential for increased resorption, which can impact aesthetic and structural outcomes.

14.1 Overview of Chronic Post-rhinoplasty Neuropathic Pain (CPRNP)

Chronic post-rhinoplasty neuropathic pain (CPRNP) is described as a persistent pain that lasts longer than the typical healing period of 3–6 months despite the absence of any ongoing healing defects. This type of pain is most often unexplained but strongly related to continuing processes involved in pain development, including nerve damage or other alterations in the pain sense. CPRNP is the most challenging condition to manage in the outpatient clinic.

Neuropathic pain is a broad term encompassing various conditions, including trigeminal neuralgia, a specific, highly localized form of neuropathic pain affecting the facial region [1]. Trigeminal neuralgia is characterized by sudden, severe, electric shock-like or stabbing pain. This pain can be triggered by everyday activities such as eating, talking, or touching the face.

There have been few studies regarding chronic post-rhinoplasty neuropathic pain that investigate

E. S. Dhong, *Asian Septorhinoplasty*, https://doi.org/10.1007/978-981-96-6127-5_14

the duration and intensity following open septorhinoplasty.

One study included 77 patients using a Visual Analog Scale (VAS) for pain assessment over 6 months. The findings indicate that acute pain significantly decreased from the first to the tenth postoperative day and was minimal by the sixth month, with chronic pain reported in only 4% of patients. The study concludes that pain typically resolves within the first month and does not significantly impact the resumption of daily activities, suggesting that concerns over pain in septorhinoplasty may be overstated. Postoperative pain after septorhinoplasty was mainly aching (40.3%) and localized to the nasal dorsum (34.3%). Pain disappeared mainly by the end of the first month, and daily activities resumed by the second week. Chronic pain was observed in 4% of patients, usually aching (36.8%) and localized to the nasal tip (39%). The incidence of chronic pain after septorhinoplasty is low, but understanding its characteristics is essential for patient counseling [2].

However, the Asian group of CPRNP patients the author has encountered has not yet been defined as the same disease group as the above. Still, it is a much larger group of patients and a challenging condition not controlled by medication, so the author dedicates a special chapter to discussing it. These patients are different from those with rhinogenic headaches, and most of them do not have a contact point on the septum.

14.2 Nature of Persistent Neuropathic Pain

Postoperative pain is usually mild and short-lived, with rare cases of chronic pain or delayed-onset neuropathic pain. Only one report presents a unique case of delayed-onset neuropathic pain after septoplasty in an asthmatic patient, successfully managed with intranasal local anesthesia [3].

Persistent neuropathic pain occurs when nerve fibers are damaged, dysfunctional, or injured. These damaged nerve fibers send incorrect signals to other pain centers. The impact of nerve fiber injury includes a change in nerve function both at the injury site and in areas around the injury. Initially, damaged nerves may send signals to the brain even without an actual harmful stimulus. There can also be a reduction in the effectiveness of the body's natural pain-control mechanisms. Emotional and cognitive factors can influence the perception of pain. Stress, depression, and anxiety can exacerbate neuropathic pain through various pathways, including increased sensitivity to pain and reduced pain inhibition.

Asian patients with CPRNP who have had multiple surgeries may not experience chronic pain after the first surgery and then begin to experience pain in a single episode. They may find that the surgery is often unsuccessful again, and the pain persists afterward. The severity of the pain can vary from an intense knife or pinprick pain to intermittent dull aches and pains with a heavy feeling and strange sensations. Some people report numbness and tingling, while others report hypersensitivity. The nature of this pain is very similar to that of a peripheral neuroma. However, in long-standing CPRNPs with suspected CNS changes, some may complain of pain that is not relieved even by injection of local anesthetics.

The specific nature of the pain, its occurrence in patients who are satisfied post-surgery, and the fact that the pain can be more controlled with medication suggest that CPRNP should be differentiated from conversion disorder within the DSM-5 category.

14.2.1 Asian-Specific CPRNP

There are several types of chronic post-rhinoplasty neuropathic pain (CPRNP) following Asian septorhinoplasty. Most patients seek consultation after undergoing surgeries, often experiencing pain following a specific incident during one of these procedures. The patient's surgical history and complaints typically include detailed accounts of such episodes. The list describes potential causes of pain following Asian septorhinoplasty.

1. Trauma from osteotomy to the nasal bones (Fig. 14.1)
2. Complications from implant removal: wide capsule excision
3. Specific surgical techniques like grafting and suturing for nasal tip extension and projection
4. Post-surgical inflammation, infection
5. Particular issues such as a pinched tip and nasal obstruction associated with internal nasal valve collapse
6. Post-preservation rhinoplasty-related pain (Fig. 14.2)

The issues mentioned could result from a single postoperative event or a mix of various factors. As noted in prior studies, chronic neuropathic pain following septoplasty is a possible underlying cause of these complications [3]. The cause of chronic neuropathic pain after septoplasty, especially with a delayed onset, is not fully understood but may involve trauma to the trigeminal nerve during surgery. This can lead to neuropathic pain syndromes like allodynia, where non-painful stimuli cause pain.

Asian septorhinoplasty, involving complex grafts or implants, often requires multiple surgeries, necessitating further research. The treatment approach for chronic post-rhinoplasty neuropathic pain (CPRNP) should be cautious, with surgical intervention considered only after thorough consultation with a neurologist and exhaustive medical management.

14.2.2 Clinical Case of CPRNP After Capsular Contracture Release

14.2.2.1 Past History

A 38-year-old female patient had undergone surgery three times before the visit. Two surgeries had been performed 15 years ago, and a third surgery was in 6 months before her visit.

- The first surgery, conducted 15 years ago, involved hump removal and lateral osteotomy, followed by the implantation of Gore-Tex and tip plasty using cartilage from the right ear.
- A few months after the first surgery, the Gore-Tex was replaced with silicone due to cosmetic dissatisfaction.
- The third surgery, conducted 6 years later, involved the removal of the implant due to capsular contracture around the silicone implant, a septal extension graft using septal cartilage, and a tip graft using cartilage from the left ear. Tip derotation graft and tip extension suture were performed with a double-layer strut graft.
- Postoperative pain continued 5 months after the surgery and visited the author's clinic.

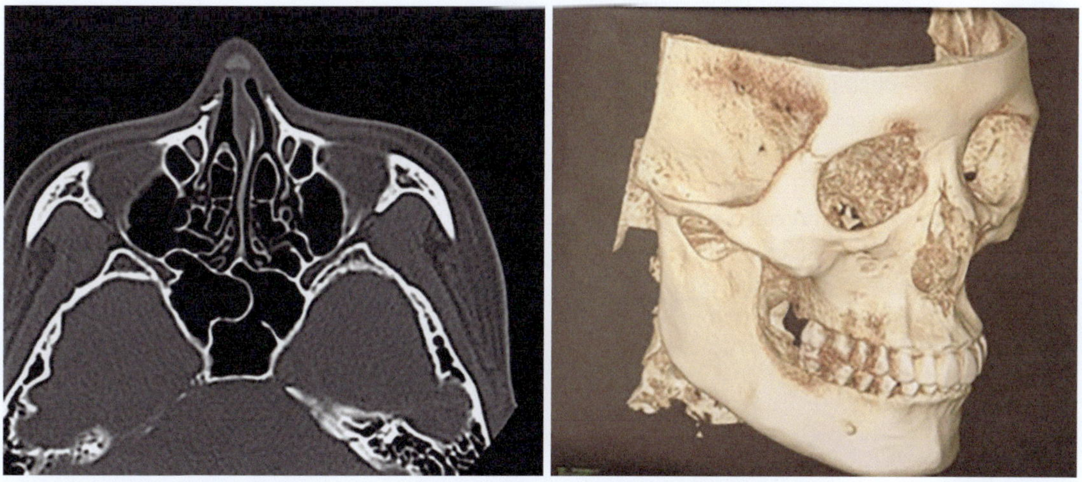

Fig. 14.1 CPRNP after osteotomy to the nasal bone. (Left) Axial CT scan. (Right) 3D view

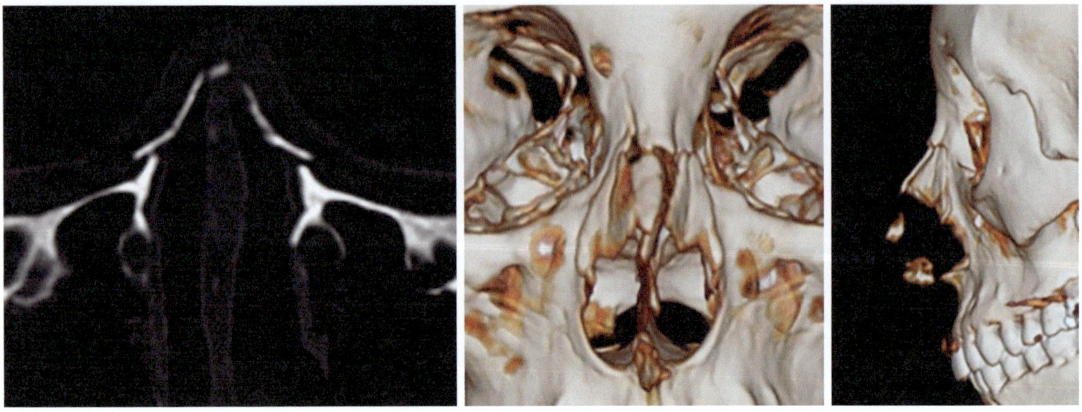

Fig. 14.2 CPRNP after preservation rhinoplasty. (Left) Axial CT scan. (Middle) 3D view. (Right) 3D lateral view

- She had been taking tramadol and gabapentin for 2 weeks before her visit, but they did not affect her pain.

14.2.2.2 Subjective Symptoms

1. The hardness of the nasal tip and pain on the touch lasted for hours after each touch.
2. Pain that interferes with sleep does not go away with medication.
3. Pins and needles throughout the day.

14.2.2.3 Preoperative Assessment

- On palpation, a hard scar was palpable at the supratip and tip. Tip cartilage graft was visible in the lobule and infralobule.
- Gabapentin dose was titrated up and down over months by a neurologist, but overall pain decreased to a non-significant level on the VAS score.
- Douleur Neuropathique 4 Questions (DN4) and Leeds Assessment of Neuropathic Symptoms and Signs (LANSS) were positive as a neuropathic pain.
- Acoustic rhinometry revealed no evidence of obstruction. Endoscopic examination revealed a right-sided convexity but no significant findings other than extensive secretions and crusts.

14.2.2.4 Surgery by the Author

- Excising supratip and tip scar, including tip graft.
- Caudal reposition of lateral genu of lower lateral cartilage after removing tip extension suture: widening the pinched tip.

The author removed the tip graft and replaced the dorsum of the nose and all the scars from the supratip and tip area, leaving lower lateral cartilage (Fig. 14.3).

14.2.3 The Outcome of Long-Term Follow-Up

The patient's level of pain decreased, but for the following year, medication adjustments were continuously made in collaboration with a neurologist. During the last visit, the patient complained that the pain had not completely disappeared. Continuous follow-up is being conducted to date (Fig. 14.4).

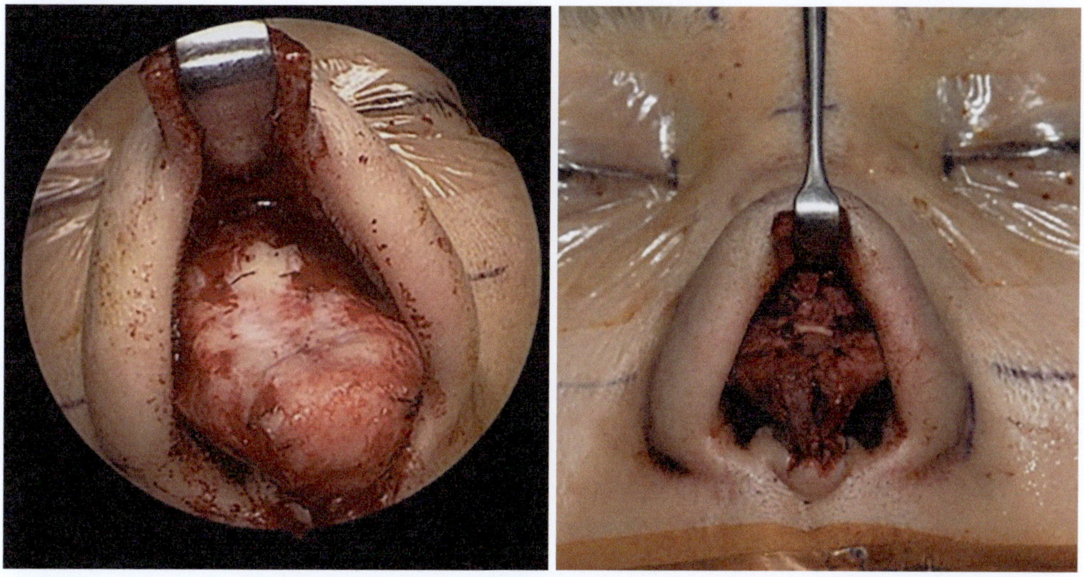

Fig. 14.3 CPRNP after multiple septorhinoplasty. (Left) Intraoperative findings of tip. (Right) After removing the scars and restoring the angles of the LLCs

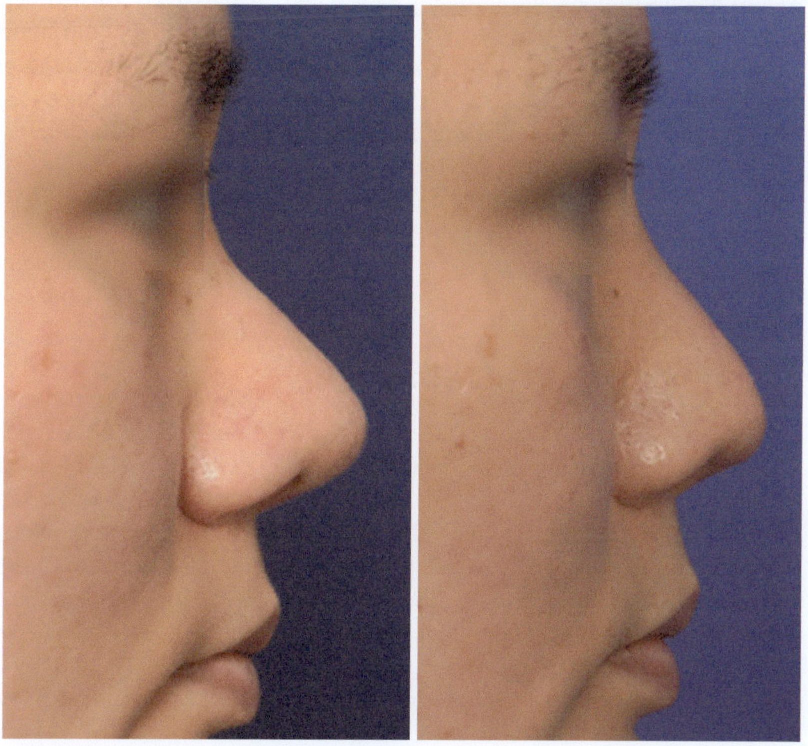

Fig. 14.4 Lateral tip position change. (Left) Preoperative lateral view. (Right) Postoperative 1 year

14.3 Osteotomy-Related Neuropathic Pain

The nerves affected by nasal osteotomy are primarily the ophthalmic nerve (V1), which supplies the upper parts of the face. The related branch of the ophthalmic branch to the nose is the nasociliary nerve. This nerve gives off several branches, including the infratrochlear nerve, which provides sensation to the medial skin of the eyelids and the sides of the nose. Above all, the main branches are governed by the external nasal nerve, a terminal branch of the anterior ethmoid nerve, which is a branch of the nasociliary nerve. It supplies the skin of the ala and dorsum of the nose. Another possibility is damage to the maxillary nerve (V2), the second branch of the trigeminal nerve, which provides sensory innervation to the center of the face. Relevant branches to the nose area include the infraorbital nerve, which emerges from the infraorbital foramen and provides sensation to parts of the nose area, including the lower eyelids, upper lip, and around the nasal bone.

Trigeminal neuralgia following orthognathic surgery has been reported previously, but its prevalence is very low and is thought to be caused by axonal injury to the infraorbital alveolar nerve [4].

14.4 Inhaling Pain: Obstruction Versus Foul Odor

Chronic nasal dysfunction is a clinical concept in managing sinonasal diseases. It considers the nose composed of three organs: the olfactory nose, the respiratory nose, and the paranasal sinuses. Etiological diagnosis accounts for the possible pathophysiological independence of nasal symptoms based on these three nasal organs' different origins and physiology [5].

The sensation of nasal obstruction or pressure often accompanies the co-occurrence of CPRNP or headaches. The Asian-specific excessive tip projection and extension commonly result in internal valve issues. The diagnosis of CPRNP becomes complex in patients who also experience nasal obstruction. Persistent perception of foul odors may result from alterations in the nasal airway or septal perforations and often do not improve with repeated nasal cleansing. Instead of being caused by vortices in the nasal airflow, the most likely explanation is the direct encountering of the lateral and medial crura of the lower lateral cartilage, combined with the increased resistance due to the significantly reduced height in the upper lateral cartilage with relatively projected lower lateral complex. Asian septorhinoplasty often presents unique challenges related to internal nasal valve dysfunction. In specific techniques for tip projection, both lateral crura are excessively rotated cephalad, and the lower lateral cartilages are sutured with a columellar strut or a septal extension graft. Although such techniques can enhance projection, they may result in an abrupt reduction of minimal cross-sectional area at the INV area. This is because the caudal portion of the ULCs may not be adequately aligned with the LLC complex, leading to a relatively lower area than the external nasal valve. Postoperative images often paradoxically show a depressed INV (Fig. 14.5).

A stable tip tripod with robust LLCs is rarely adopted in Asian patients. Tip projecting techniques need to be reconsidered, as they may not be effective due to changes in the shape of the internal nasal valve. Furthermore, heavy supratip grafting and additional dorsal implantation using alloplastic materials provoke complex uncertainties. The compression from the heavy graft and the tension from the soft tissue envelope being tightly held by gravity can lead to adverse effects such as INV depression [6, 7].

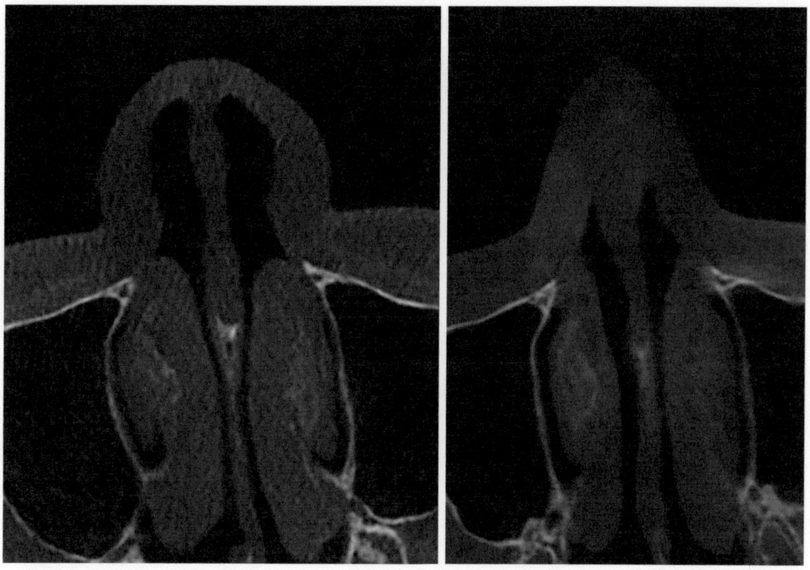

Fig. 14.5 Internal nasal valve problem. (Left) Preoperative axial view. (Right) Patient's current state when transferred

14.5 Medical Treatment of Chronic Post-rhinoplasty Neuropathic Pain (CPRNP)

The medical treatment of CPRNP involves a multifaceted approach, as this type of pain is complex and arises from nerve damage or dysfunction. Here are the primary medical treatments used for chronic neuropathic pain. Based on the author's experience, anticonvulsants were initially prescribed with the diagnosis that the pain was neuropathic. The effectiveness of anticonvulsants mainly surpasses that of traditional painkillers, and it is advisable to monitor patients for over 6 months. Referring a patient to a neurologist solely because CPRNP is perceived as an intractable or psychological issue would be a poor decision. Given that the condition stems from surgery, it is incumbent upon the surgeon to treat the patient with the highest degree of compassion.

14.5.1 Anticonvulsants (Gabapentinoids)

Gabapentin and pregabalin are commonly prescribed medications. They work by modulating calcium channels on neurons to reduce the release of neurotransmitters and dampen pain signals.

- **Gabapentin (Neurontin)**
  Gabapentin is relatively safe to use in first-time patients. They are generally well tolerated and have a relatively safe side-effect profile compared to opioids and non-steroidal anti-inflammatory drugs (NSAIDs). However, they require titration from a low dose to reach an effective dose and often need to be taken three times a day, which can affect adherence. Common side effects include dizziness, fatigue, weight gain, and peripheral edema. Cognitive impairment and sedation have also been reported, especially in older people. However, it is essential to note the delayed onset of action to achieve full effectiveness. It may take several weeks to achieve optimal pain relief. Gabapentin doesn't work for everyone. About 30–40% of people who take gabapentin can reduce their pain by half. However, up to 60% of people don't experience pain relief but do have side effects.
- **Pregabalin (Lyrica)**
  Pregabalin is absorbed more quickly than gabapentin, allowing for faster onset of pain relief.

Typically, it requires dosing only twice a day due to its longer half-life, which can improve patient compliance. Similar to gabapentin, pregabalin also has side effects, including dizziness, somnolence, dry mouth, and potential for weight gain. It is classified as a Schedule V controlled substance in the U.S. due to the potential for abuse and dependence, albeit lower than opioids.

Both medications interact with the alpha2-delta subunit of voltage-gated calcium channels in the central nervous system to reduce the release of several neurotransmitters, thereby diminishing pain signals. The choice between gabapentin and pregabalin will depend on the individual patient's medical history, the specific neuropathic pain condition, potential side effects, and cost considerations. It's essential to determine the most appropriate option.

14.5.2 Antidepressants

Tricyclic Antidepressants (TCAs), Such as amitriptyline, nortriptyline, and desipramine, are effective in treating neuropathic pain by inhibiting the reuptake of serotonin and norepinephrine, increasing their levels in the synaptic cleft, and modulating pain pathways.

14.5.3 Interventional Treatments

Nerve block: Injections of local anesthetics, sometimes combined with corticosteroids, near the affected nerves can provide temporary relief. However, injections into the nasal dorsum or sidewall should be cautiously administered, as they can lead to skin thinning.

14.5.4 Psychological Support

Cognitive-Behavioral Therapy (CBT): Helps patients cope with chronic pain by changing pain perception and developing strategies to manage pain.

14.6 Paraffinoma in Asian Patients

Paranasal paraffin injections were historically used for cosmetic enhancements, such as augmenting the nasal dorsum or filling facial defects. However, the use of paraffin injections has largely been abandoned due to serious long-term complications, known collectively as paraffinomas or sclerosing lipogranulomas. These complications arise as the body reacts to the non-biodegradable paraffin, leading to various clinical sequelae.

14.6.1 Clinical Sequelae of Paranasal Paraffin Injection

The body recognizes paraffin as a foreign substance, leading to a chronic inflammatory response. This can result in the formation of granulomas, which are small nodules of inflammatory cells. The injection sites can become infected, leading to abscess formation and skin necrosis, which may exacerbate the inflammatory response.

Paraffin can migrate from the original injection site to adjacent tissues. Over time, the ongoing inflammation can lead to fibrosis and deformities in the affected areas.

14.6.2 Nasal Skin Changes

The skin overlying the injection sites can become thin, discolored, and ulcerated, leading to problems (Fig. 14.6).

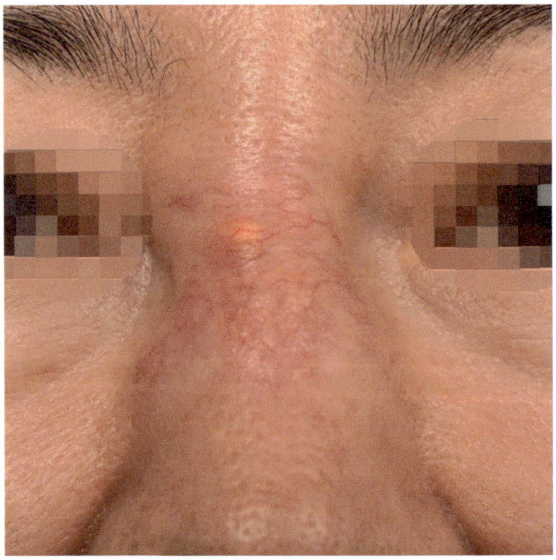

Fig. 14.6 Skin change in long-standing paraffinoma

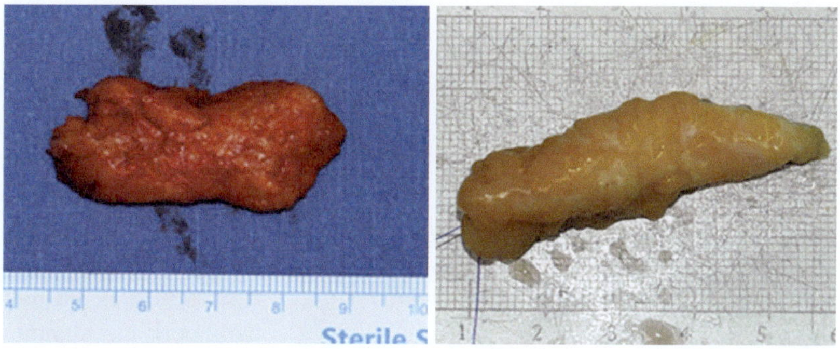

Fig. 14.7 Volume replacement of paraffinoma. (Left) Specimen of paraffinoma. (Right) Dermis-in rolling of sacral dermis graft for large-volume filling

14.6.3 Skin Incision of Paraffinoma

Treating paraffinomas, particularly mainly in the dorsal area, is challenging. The surgical approach is usually limited to the open rhinoplasty incision. Nasion and more cephalic parts may need to merge open sky incisions or sub-brow incisions.

14.6.4 Skin Flap Salvaging

If a midline forehead flap is not considered available, or if the patient objects to a forehead scar, the flap should be elevated to preserve the skin and subdermal circulation. Paraffinomas that are not entirely excised are at risk of regrowth; however, based on the author's experience, the extent of paraffinoma infiltrating deep into the subdermis. Consequently, a compromise may be necessary to maintain skin circulation when subcutaneous paraffinomas cannot be entirely removed.

14.6.5 Managing Loss of Volume and Irregularity

Due to the complex nature of these lesions and the potential for significant cosmetic impacts, volume replacement should be managed by an autologous tissue, including a dermis-fat graft. The goal is to remove as much of the paraffinoma as possible while minimizing damage to the skin flap and addressing cosmetic concerns. If concerns arise regarding irregularities in the dorsal skin, or if only a very thin skin flap is available, a dermis-fat graft in the form of a fat outlay is utilized. When a large volume is needed, tissue harvested from the sacral midline proves beneficial [8] (Fig. 14.7).

14.7 Consequences of Irradiated Homologous Costal Cartilage Use

Even in patients without septal deviation, septal harvesting for tip projection was often accompanied by the simultaneous insertion of alloplastic materials into the dorsum or septum. More recently, the use of synthetic materials like absorbable mesh and Medpor has become common, rendering the application of alloplastic materials in the septum more complex and aggressive [9, 10]. However, it is losing popularity in Korea due to multiple complications reports, except for a few reckless doctors [11].

However, in recent years, a new complex complication has been trending with the introduction of donated costal cartilage allografts.

A popular approach in East Asia, particularly in Korea, involves using donated rib allografts for tip projection and silicone for the dorsum. This combination offers convenience for secondary operations when autografts are insufficient or even for primary rhinoplasty. While this technique avoids the labor-intensive process of rib harvesting, surgeons should be mindful of the potential issues outlined below.

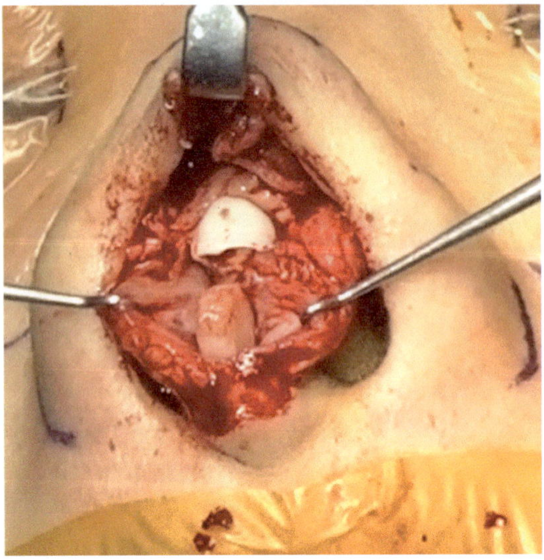

Fig. 14.8 Dorsal silicone with columella IHCC strut: Capsule formation around the IHCC

14.7.1 Capsule Forms Around the IHCC

Intraoperatively, a fibrous capsule usually forms around the IHCC. At least the IHCC is not integrated with the septal cartilage in the long term, so this is just a form of dead graft. The capsule formed around the IHCC is thin, but all the complications in alloplastic material are eventually found (Fig. 14.8).

14.7.2 Potential Problems

- Constriction and contracture: The fibrous capsule may contract over time, exerting pressure on the allograft. This may affect the aesthetic outcome of the graft.
- Reduced integration: The presence of a fibrous capsule can impede the integration of the allograft with the surrounding native tissues. Poor integration can compromise the graft's stability and longevity, potentially leading to displacement or migration.
- Impaired vascularization: Reduced vascularization can affect the health and viability of the overlying skin and surrounding tissues.
- Increased risk of late-onset inflammation.
- Resorption: The encapsulation process and the potential for reduced integration and vascularization can lead to increased allograft resorption over time. This can result in volume loss and fracture, necessitating additional corrective procedures.

It should be noted that in secondary rhinoplasty with poor circulation, IHCCs used for lack of autologous tissue may cause more problems.

References

1. Zakrzewska JM, Linskey ME. Trigeminal neuralgia. BMJ. 2015;350:h1238.
2. Aydemir L, Celik M, Sen C, Cayonu M, Comoglu S, et al. Assessment of acute and chronic pain after open technique septorhinoplasty: should we really be concerned about this topic? Eur J Rhinol Allergy. 2020;3:55–8.
3. Koumpa F-S, Ferguson M, Saleh H. Delayed-onset neuropathic pain after septoplasty. Case Rep Otolaryngol. 2021;2021:9966318.
4. Politis C, Lambrichts I, Agbaje JO. Neuropathic pain after orthognathic surgery. Oral Surg Oral Med Oral Pathol Oral Radiol. 2014;117:e102–7.
5. Jankowski R, Nguyen DT, Russel A, Toussaint B, Gallet P, Rumeau C. Chronic nasal dysfunction. Eur Ann Otorhinolaryngol Head Neck Dis. 2018;135:41–9.
6. Dhong E-S. Functional surgery 2: consideration of internal valve problems in Asian rhinoplasty, and turbinate reduction. In: Suh MK, editor. State of the art rhinoplasty techniques: perspectives from Korean masters. Singapore: Springer Singapore; 2022. p. 275–84.
7. Dhong E-S, Na M-W. Nasal obstruction in Asian rhinoplasty. In: Dhong E-S, Na M-W, editors. Asian septorhinoplasty: conundrums and solutions. Singapore: Springer Nature Singapore; 2021. p. 51–65.
8. Dhong E-S, Na M-W. Asian Septorhinoplasty: conundrums and solutions. Springer Nature; 2021.
9. Hyun S, Cho SW, Baek R-M. Polycaprolactone mesh for Asian rhinoplasty: outcomes and complications of composite septal extension graft compared to mesh-only graft. Facial Plast Surg. 2022;38:207–13.
10. Park YJ, Cha JH, Bang SI, Kim SY. Clinical application of three-dimensionally printed biomaterial Polycaprolactone (PCL) in augmentation rhinoplasty. Aesth Plast Surg. 2019;43:437–46.
11. Vila PM, Jeanpierre LM, Rizzi CJ, Yaeger LH, Chi JJ. Comparison of autologous vs homologous costal cartilage grafts in dorsal augmentation rhinoplasty: a systematic review and meta-analysis. JAMA Otolaryngol Head Neck Surg. 2020;146:347–54.

capsule [6, 7]. In other words, any material exposed to macrophages beyond the normal wound healing period will react to the fibrous capsule reaction and form a capsule.

Therefore, the late-onset inflammation described in this chapter can occur around capsules from irradiated homologous cartilage (IHCC), a type of silicone, Gore-Tex®, and any allograft with silicone.

15.1.2 Is Late-Onset Inflammation Found in Western Operations?

While late-onset inflammation in Western rhinoplasty, where alloplastic implants are not utilized, is unexpected, there have been instances of mucus cysts forming post-septal surgery, albeit rarely. Such occurrences may stem from the entrapment of respiratory epithelium. Although these cases bear similarities to long-term outcomes of septoplasty, the situation diverges in Asian patients, where the presence of a capsule is more common. The genesis of these conditions is thought to be related to the invagination of septal mucosa resulting from nasal trauma, osteotomy, and septal surgeries. Recent findings have identified the presence of pseudostratified columnar epithelium in such cases [8–10].

15.2 Differential Diagnosis of Late-Onset Inflammation

15.2.1 Subclinical Infection

The author remembers that not long ago, post-rhinoplasty swelling, which used to be controlled with empirical antibiotics, was misnomered as subclinical infection by Asian doctors.

A subclinical infection is characterized by an absence of noticeable symptoms in the host, with any minor symptoms often resolving spontaneously. During this phase, the individual may feel well and show no or minimal signs of illness despite being infected with a pathogen. This contrasts with late-onset inflammation following nasal surgery, which this chapter discusses. Late-onset inflammation typically presents with nasal symptoms, predominantly swelling or firmness, often leading to morphological deformities.

Examples of subclinical infections include Hepatitis B and C, asymptomatic Herpes infections, and poliomyelitis. A notable case is the SARS-CoV-2 virus caused a global pandemic; many infected individuals were asymptomatic or had very mild symptoms. Despite appearing healthy, they could transmit the virus to others, making them contagious. The challenge in identifying subclinical infections post-rhinoplasty is that tissue cultures from many patients do not yield the causative microorganism.Late-onset inflammation and subclinical infection should be distinguished, as they represent separate clinical entities. Healthcare professionals must avoid using these terms interchangeably during conferences and in medical discourse.

15.2.2 Latent Infection

A latent infection is characterized by a pathogen within a host without manifesting any active disease. The pathogen is not active. During this phase, the pathogen remains dormant and asymptomatic. Typically, individuals harboring a latent infection do not transmit the disease. Individuals with a latent infection generally are not contagious during the dormant phase. However, the infection may become active and potentially infectious under certain circumstances, such as immunosuppression.

An illustrative example of these concepts is the herpes simplex virus (HSV). An individual may carry a subclinical HSV infection, capable of shedding the virus without exhibiting any symptoms, thus posing a risk of transmission to others. Concurrently, HSV can enter a latent state within nerve cells, remaining inactive until specific triggers lead to its reactivation, resulting in symptomatic episodes, such as cold sores. This clinical presentation is distinct from late-onset inflammation post-nasal surgery.

15.2.3 Acute Surgical Site Infection (SSI)

Acute surgical site infection (SSI) is an infection that manifests following a rhinoplasty procedure at the healing stage. Per the clinical guidelines set by the Centers for Disease Control and Prevention (CDC), an acute SSI typically presents within 30 days post-operation or a year if an implant remains post-surgery. However, this chapter focuses on late-onset inflammation, distinct from acute SSI, which emerges 7–10 days post-rhinoplasty during the critical wound healing phase. This condition is characterized by a different clinical profile, including purulent discharge, painful swelling, and systemic symptoms such as fever or headache, often accompanied by systemic leukocytosis. Blood cultures can be instrumental in diagnosis, and appropriate antibiotics are recommended.

While SSIs are relatively rare in reduction rhinoplasty, their occurrence in Asian rhinoplasty, which often involves extensive grafting and alloplastic materials, can have severe consequences proportional to the surgical dissection involved.

15.2.4 Late-Onset Inflammation (LOI)

Late-onset inflammation after rhinoplasty, especially when alloplastic implants are used, is a rare but significant complication. It can occur months to years following a complicated septorhinoplasty. A study on this issue found that in cases of late-onset inflammation, there was an increase in edematous granulation tissues, inflammatory cellular content, and a disorganized collagen layer compared to healthy cases with or without pus-draining infection. The presence of mucin deposition and the synovial membrane was also noted in multiple cases, suggesting these factors might play a crucial role in developing late-onset inflammation, especially in the fibrous capsules around the implant [11].

In this chapter, we will discuss the different clinical manifestations of LOI.

15.3 Clinical Manifestations of Late-Onset Inflammation

15.3.1 Swelling: Waxing and Waning

Late-onset swelling following Asian rhinoplasty starts with edema in the nasal area that manifests well after the initial postoperative phase. This inflammation can vary in intensity, waxing and waning naturally or with over-the-counter drugs (Fig. 15.2). Several factors contribute to this phenomenon.

Here are some possibilities to consider

1. Physical trauma: Even though the initial surgical site may have healed, the capsule continues to undergo remodeling and repair. This ongoing healing process can cause intermittent inflammation as the body adjusts to the implants or grafts. Many people experience swelling after sustained nasal trauma, sports accidents, or trauma in daily life. It can also be caused among young women by bumping into a baby's head.
2. Foreign body reaction: Implants or grafts used during rhinoplasty, such as silicone implants or donated cartilage grafts, can trigger a foreign body reaction in some individuals. This reaction may manifest as late-onset swelling as the body attempts to integrate these foreign materials.
3. Allergic reactions: Some patients may experience late-onset inflammation due to allergic reactions to materials used during surgery, such as sutures or implants.
4. Contamination: While relatively rare, late-onset inflammation can also be a sign of low-grade infection or inflammation related to bacterial colonization around biofilm around the implant.
5. Delayed healing: Individual differences in healing capacity, underlying medical conditions, and lifestyle factors can contribute to delayed healing and persistent inflammation.

Clinically, some patients respond to empirical antibiotics, and the swelling decreases with no problems found, while others progress to the

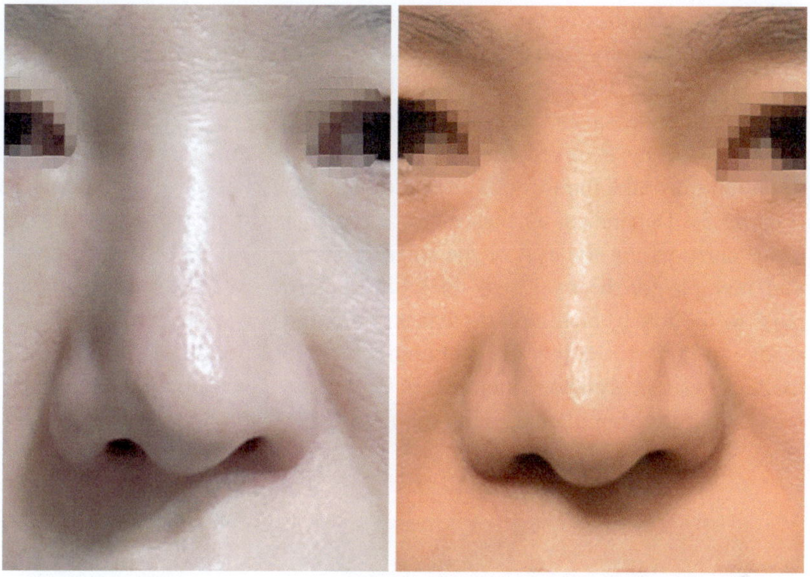

Fig. 15.2 Waxing and waning of swelling: selfies. (Left) When swollen due to poor condition. (Right) After taking antibiotics, the swelling subsided

stage described below and require secondary surgery. Therefore, this is a stage that requires close follow-up.

15.3.2 Persistent Hardness with Pain, Capsular Contracture

Capsule maturation results from fibroblast proliferation and collagen deposition. Over time, the collagen matrix becomes more organized and dense, forming a peri-implant capsule. The thickness and density of the capsule can vary depending on several factors. However, the hard tissue found in Asians is due to excessive alloplastic material or in combination with other grafts. Combining artificial dermis or cartilage and alloplastic materials in rhinoplasty can form dense, hard tissue around the implants due to several interconnected processes. There are reports of ADM solving the capsular problem [12], but ADM seems more of a problem than a solution regarding rhinoplasty. The expected effect of a single layer of ADM in direct-to-implant procedures appears to differ from the role ADM plays when used in the nose.

1. Avascular scar formation: An avascular ADM has limited access to these essential healing components, which can slow down or impair the healing process. This can result in impaired scar tissue that is different in composition and structure compared to scar tissue formed in well-vascularized areas.
2. Dense scar: In avascular areas, the balance between collagen production and degradation may be disrupted, leading to excessive collagen deposition and a hard, dense scar, later scar contracture: the silicone implant applied to the dorsum, in combination with the use of multiple layers of ADM onlay creates a scar of unimaginable hardness.

The results of one layer of ADM and multiple layers of ADM will be different. The authors are confident that vascularization does not occur with multiple layers of ADM and that this will be the same for thicker ADM applied over or under silicone.

15.3.3 Skin: Cystic(Mucoid) Lesion

These lesions are characterized by their mucoid content, a thick, viscous, gel-like substance. Depending on their size and location, these cysts may be asymptomatic or cause symptoms such as swelling and discomfort. If the cyst interferes with nasal structures or passages, it might lead to breathing difficulties or nasal obstruction. These lesions are typically smooth, round, or oval and can vary in size. They may be palpable beneath the skin or mucosa and could be mistaken for other types of cysts or growths. The clinical presentation may take the form of an epidermal cyst (Fig. 15.3). Depending on the extent of the scar tissue surrounding the cyst or the stage of synovial metaplasia, the cyst may feel like a hard mass to the touch, or it may be soft and red and ready to burst. Pathologic findings include mucoid cysts or synovial metaplasia, and more recent findings of epithelial lining require further study.

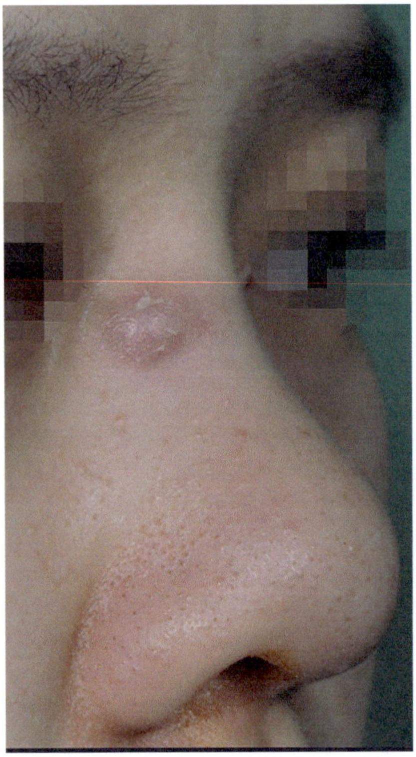

Fig. 15.3 Late-onset inflammation with skin cystic lesion: Epidermal cyst-like feature

15.3.4 Puncture with Cystic Lesion: With or Without the Pus Drainage

Puncture with the cystic lesion is the last stage of late-onset inflammation and is an urgent stage of implant exposure or pus drainage from the patient's perspective.

Material strands are not always found in the draining pus because most patients are taking over-the-counter medications, but in many cases, potentially infectious normal flora (PINF) is found [13, 14].

It is expected to find mucoid tissue at the tip of a ruptured cyst, and even if it is squeezed out several times, it will continue to drain the next day (Fig. 15.4).

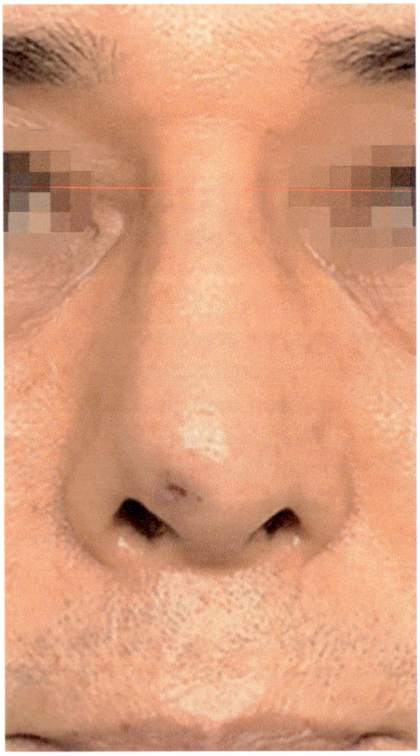

Fig. 15.4 Late-onset inflammation with a puncture with skin cystic lesion

15.4 Pathological Features of Late-Onset Inflammation

Pathologic classification of late-onset inflammation is challenging because the whole specimen is significant. Without close communication with the pathologist, it is easy to fail to get the pathology of the desired area. Obtaining accurate pathology by excising the implant and removing the capsule is impossible. It is more accurate to send the capsule with the implant in situ to the pathologist.

15.4.1 Capsule with Synovial Metaplasia

Synovial metaplasia is a condition in which the lining of the synovial membrane is found in a non-articular area. This transformation can occur in response to trauma, inflammation, or foreign materials. Synovial metaplasia is often associated with a reaction to foreign bodies, such as implants (Fig. 15.5). Histologically, synovial metaplasia is characterized by synoviocyte-like cells and vascularized connective tissue resembling the synovial lining of joints. You may also find some fluid inside the bare synovium at this stage. This is distinctly different from a mucocele and is often asymptomatic due to the thin layer of the cyst.

This has sometimes been referred to as a healthy capsule, and many doctors are known to use it [15]. Clinically, even capsules without mucus drainage cannot be excluded from the possibility of synovial cysts, even if they do not have a cellular lining. Therefore, if fluid is draining around the implant from the incision, it is recommended that the capsule be removed by total resection. However, this can be a difficult decision as it can be confused with infiltration of local anesthetics.

15.4.2 Capsule with Thick Avascular Scar Layer

The avascular layer plays a crucial role in capsular contracture. A reduced blood supply in the avascular layer can lead to a less effective healing response. It might contribute to an increased risk of fibrosis, where excessive fibrous tissue forms, leading to peri-implant capsular contracture. At the same time, the avascular nature of the peri-implant layer may modulate the inflammatory response, either by reducing the delivery of inflammatory cells, leading to a milder fibrotic response, or by contributing to a chronic, low-

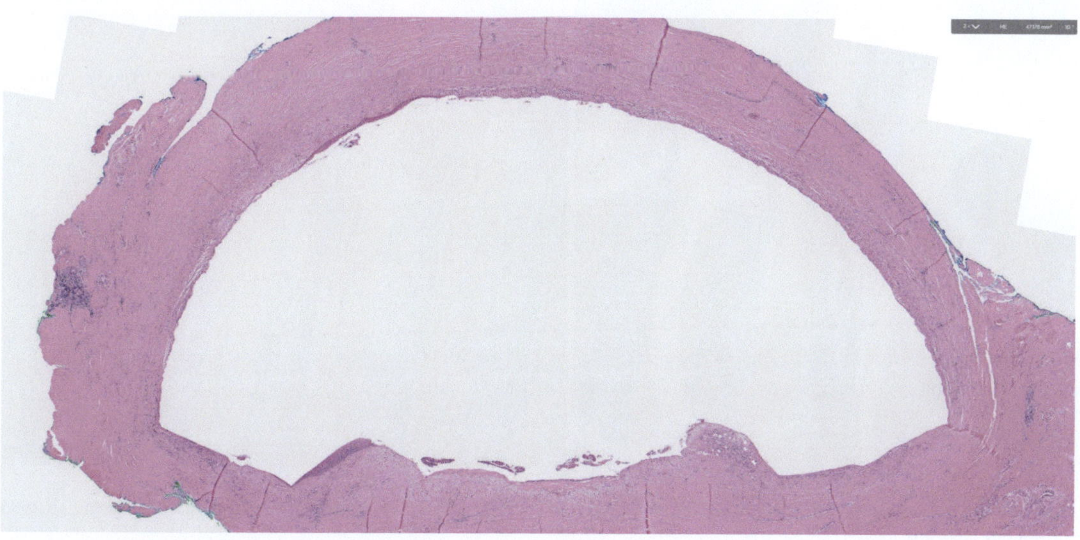

Fig. 15.5 Synovial metaplasia of capsule: whole capsule trans-section view (H&E)

grade inflammation that could stimulate fibrosis and contribute to contracture. Hypoxic conditions can stimulate fibroblasts to produce more collagen, potentially leading to a thicker and more fibrous capsule, which could increase the risk of contracture [16]. The avascular layer might inhibit the formation of new blood vessels (angiogenesis) around the implant. Reduced angiogenesis can contribute to a chronic hypoxic environment, further promoting fibrosis and the risk of capsular contracture. Clinically, there is a difference between reports that indicate a single layer of ADM reduces breast implant contracture and multiple layers of ADM applied to the nasal dorsum or tip, which form a dense scar mass and can cause contracture from the perspective of peri-capsular avascular condition.

15.4.3 Unhealthy Capsule with Mucocele Formation

A mucocele is a mucus-filled cystic lesion commonly occurring in the oral cavity, but an implant-specific nasal mucus cyst refers to an intracapsular mucocele formation.

A nasal mucus cyst in the context of a silicone implant could arise from the trapping of mucus-producing glandular tissue within or adjacent to the fibrous capsule surrounding the implant (Figs. 15.6 and 15.7). This could be due to surgical trauma, implant migration, or chronic irritation caused by the implant. Mucocele formation is an exceedingly rare complication in previous reports. Despite the large number of rhinoplasty procedures performed, only 26 documented cases of postoperative mucoceles have been reported [9]. Most cases involve the nasal dorsum, but other locations (such as the inner canthus, glabella, alar cartilages, nasal tip, and paranasal region) have also been affected. It was suggested that mucoceles develop when nasal mucosa grows postoperatively through osteotomy lines into subcutaneous pockets [9, 17]. The authors believe that the manipulation of incomplete septal mucosa—for example, the use of implants with wide dissection between upper lateral cartilages and septum, such as alloplastic implants placed on an open roof after septal harvest or hump removal—is one of the most likely causes.

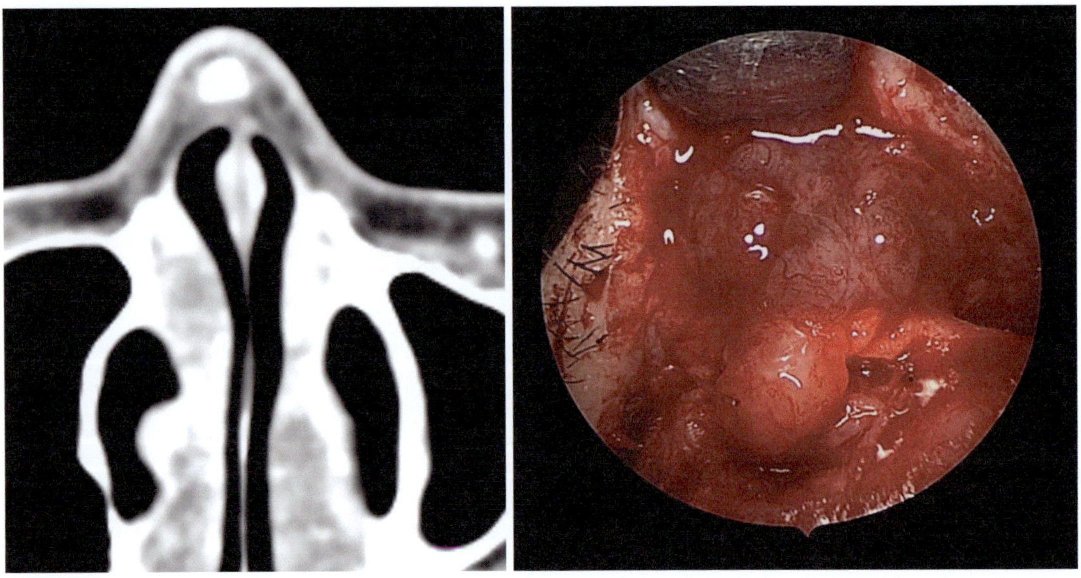

Fig. 15.6 Mucus-producing cyst over the silicone implant. (Left) Cyst around the implant: CT scan. (Right) Intraoperative view

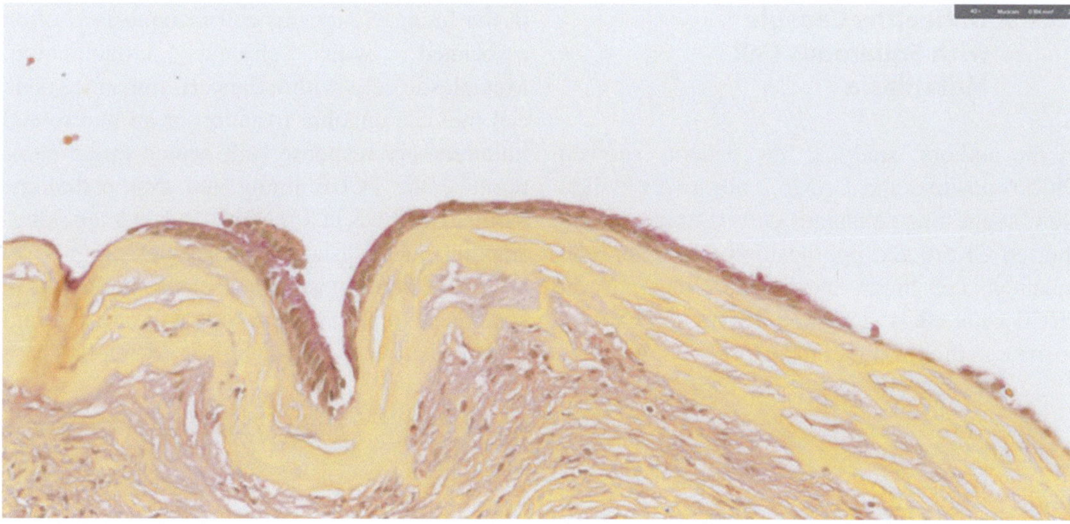

Fig. 15.7 Mucicarmine positive surface: Mucin-producing retention cyst

15.4.4 Unhealthy Capsule with PCCE Lining

The pseudostratified ciliated columnar epithelium (PCCE) is not found in every patient's mucocele. There are technical difficulties with biopsy, and it is unlikely that PCCE will be present in all areas. However, in addition to previous reports, the authors observed PCCE growth in intracapsular mucoceles in many patients. Hematoxylin and eosin (H&E) staining, performed for histological examination, revealed a cell lining on the inner side of the capsule with the upper respiratory epithelium consisting of pseudostratified ciliated columnar epithelium (PCCE) and goblet cells (Fig. 15.8). Additionally, D-PAS, Alcian blue at pH 2.5, and mucicarmine were positive around the PCCE and goblet cells inside the capsule, confirming the presence of a mucinous lining. This indicates an intracapsular mucin-producing retention cyst. Contrary to previous reports, we found a population of upper respiratory cells growing within the capsule formed by the silicone implant.

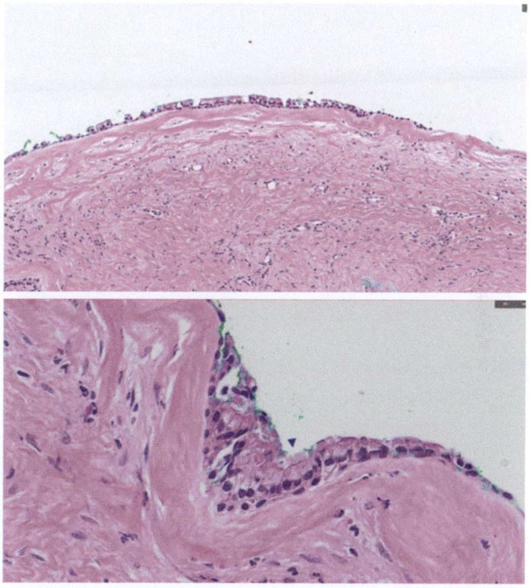

Fig. 15.8 Unhealthy capsule. (Above) Cell lining. (Below) Pseudostratified ciliated columnar epithelium (PCCE) and goblet cells with cilia (H&E)

15.4.5 Unhealthy Capsule with Squamous Cell Metaplasia

In the authors' study, a few patients showed CK/5/6 positive and CAM5.2 negative on slide view, suggesting squamous cells. Some staining showed CK5/6 and p40 positivity in areas with squamous cell lining and CAM5.2 positivity in PCCE cells (Figs. 15.9 and 15.10). CD31 was positive in the stroma of the capsule but negative in the lining. Squamous cell metaplasia is often associated with chronic inflammation. Metaplastic cells within the peri-implant capsule can indicate ongoing irritation or an unresolved inflammatory response [18], which might compromise the PCCE lining and cyst pathology. While squamous cell metaplasia is benign, longstanding metaplasia can sometimes progress to dysplasia or even squamous cell carcinoma in specific contexts. However, the risk of malignant transformation in the setting of peri-implant cap-

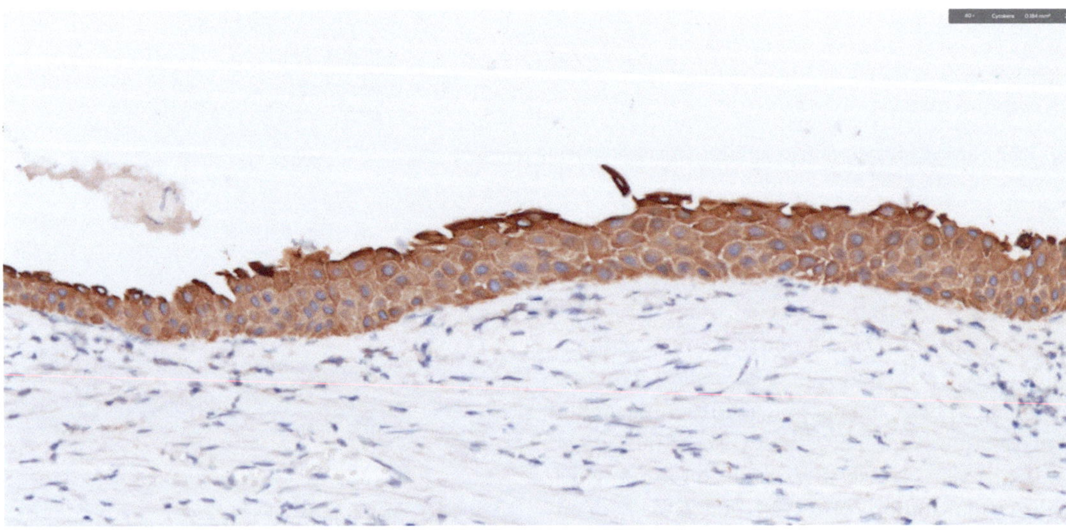

Fig. 15.9 Cytokeratin 5/6 positive cell lining: squamous cell metaplasia

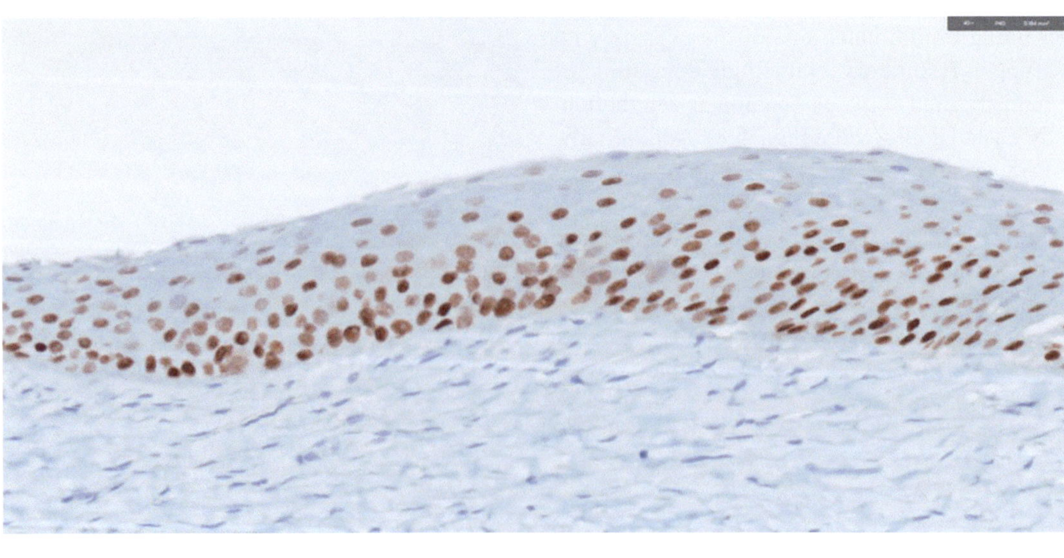

Fig. 15.10 P40 positive cell lining: squamous cell metaplasia

sules is not well-defined and likely varies depending on the implant's location and other patient-specific factors found in implants used for breast augmentation: Breast implant-associated squamous cell carcinoma (BIA-SCC) [19]. However, to date, no cases of SCC involving the nasal implant capsule have been reported.

15.5 Timing of Surgical Intervention

15.5.1 LOI Without Skin Puncture

For patients with swelling or heavy scar contracture without skin puncture, immediate surgery is not urgent. The use of empirical antibiotics is based on the patient's symptoms. Redness or tenderness of the flap around the swelling should be monitored and followed up. Delaying surgery in the presence of ongoing inflammation can lead to further complications, such as tissue damage, spread of mucocele, or even framework destruction. The risk of such complications must be balanced against the risks associated with surgery.

15.5.2 LOI with Skin Puncture

Late-onset inflammation with skin puncture is sometimes an urgent situation.

1. Flap viability: The condition of the skin flap and soft tissues around the LOI area is crucial. Poor skin flap condition with thinning can increase the risk of non-healing wounds or further exposure to the nasal graft. Early surgical intervention might address these issues and prevent further complications.
2. Infection assessment: It is essential to distinguish between a pus-draining status and a mucus-draining appearance. Prompt evaluation and systemic antibiotics are crucial. Culturing the area to identify any infectious agents can guide appropriate antibiotic therapy. An immediate response is essential to prevent the spread of infection and more severe complications.
3. Implant status: If the implant is exposed or there's evidence of cellulitis around it, immediate surgical intervention may be necessary to remove it. Even though the pus is not draining with the skin puncture, the implant should be removed as it is a contaminated wound.
4. Response to initial antibiotics: The response to antibiotics should be closely monitored after initiating them. Lack of improvement or worsening symptoms may indicate that the strain is not susceptible to the antibiotics, necessitating a change in antibiotics and prompt implant removal.

15.5.3 Which Strains Are Currently Being Drained?

In cases where patients present with purulent drainage, it is expected to find them on oral medications or receiving treatment from external healthcare facilities. However, conducting a culture to ascertain the specific strain of pseudomonas, MRSA, or other relevant pathogens is imperative. Persistent purulent discharge despite ongoing treatment may indicate resistance to the administered antimicrobial agent. Consequently, for pathogens such as *Pseudomonas aeruginosa*, methicillin-resistant Staphylococcus aureus (MRSA), methicillin-resistant Staphylococcus epidermidis (MRSE), or enterobacter species, precise identification and susceptibility testing are crucial to ensure the selection of an effective antibiotic regimen.

In cases where patients have been on oral second-generation or lower cephalosporins for over 3 days without improvement, or if symptoms are exacerbating, it is advisable to transition promptly to a broad-spectrum, second- to third-generation fluoroquinolone antibiotics, accompanied by wound culture acquisition. Crucially, the septum should be closely inspected for pus pockets, and vigilance for systemic symptoms is essential.

Above all, prompt drainage and irrigation are critical in this emergency.

There should be evidence of septal pus pockets, particularly if accompanied by systemic manifestations. Initiating systemic antibiotic therapy is warranted. Alternatively, in cases where sepsis is a concern, intensive care and hospitalization may be necessary.

Although the following symptoms are rarely seen, there are cases of death after septorhinoplasty, so they should be taken seriously. The septum should also be observed.

- Fever or hypothermia
- Tachycardia
- Tachypnea
- Chills or shivering
- Confusion or disorientation
- Edema or swelling
- Increased white blood cell count

15.5.4 Is the Pus Pocket Relatively Confined to a Single Pocket?

Late-onset inflammation confined to the dorsal pocket is generally easier to manage. Intraseptal inflammation tends to remain localized and does not spread extensively, which can be attributed to the fact that 4–5 days post-surgery, the mucosal membrane undergoes coaptation. This process reduces the available dead space, thereby limiting the spread of inflammation even if it occurs later. However, using absorbable PCL (polycaprolactone) mesh disrupts this natural defense mechanism.

In contrast to Medpor implants, where post-coaptation septal flap pain is primarily due to physical force, PCL mesh (polycaprolactone mesh: TnR Mesh ®, Korea) presents challenges mainly due to deformities caused by resorption rather than pain. The severity of inflammation with PCL mesh can lead to various deformities, including septal perforation, depending on its extent.

Due to hydrolysis during the resorption process, the PCL mesh is particularly prone to severe inflammation. Coupled with its rough physical properties, inflammation can manifest after a period, making the PCL mesh a persistent foreign body until it is entirely removed.

15.6 Types of Surgical Intervention

15.6.1 Total Extirpation of Implant Capsule and Refill

Except in some cases of synovial metaplasia, total capsulectomy is the treatment of choice in LOI. However, flap loss should be a concern if the anterior capsule is extremely thin. If complete excision is not possible, the best that can be done is meticulous curettage to prevent flap loss.

15.6.2 Partial Extirpation of Implant Capsule

The capsular flap provides additional tissue that can be used to cover or augment areas, enhancing the nasal contour or correcting deformities without the need for external donor sites. The technique allows for the effective management and utilization of scar tissue that has formed around the implant, potentially reducing the need for autogenous tissue [15]. However, synovial metaplasia can also result in fluid collection. If a membrane within the capsule is suspected in the surgical field, the author would advise against reusing the capsule as soft tissue.

15.6.3 Re-insertion of Another Alloplastic Implant

The condition of the skin-soft tissue envelope and vascular supply is critical. Healthy tissue is essential for the successful integration of the new implant. If the anterior skin flap is thin, the autogenous soft tissue mentioned below can be used with an alloplastic implant. However, the authors disagree that an alloplastic implant should be placed again in this situation. How can issues caused by alloplastic material be resolved using alloplastic material again?

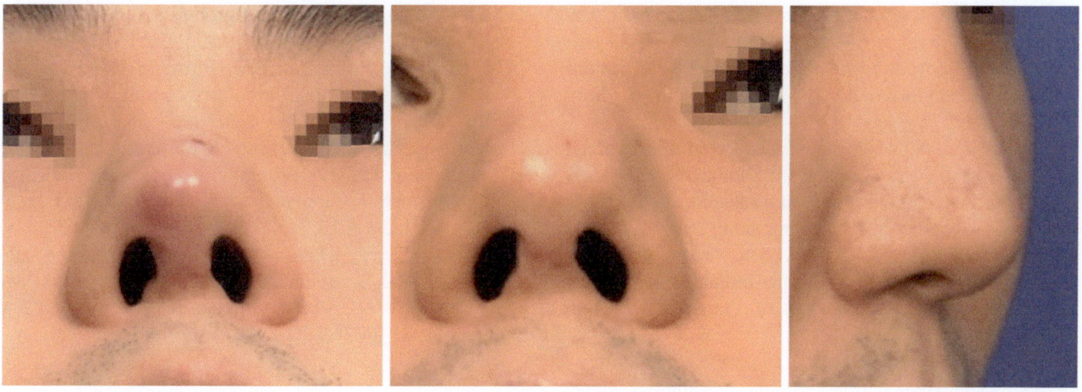

Fig. 15.11 Correction of L.O.I. with mucocele. (Left) Preoperative basal view. (Middle) Long-term postoperative basal view. (Right) Long-term quarter view

15.6.4 Autogenous Soft Tissue Graft

The supply of autogenous soft tissue is essential for resolving LOI, where intraoperative thinning of the dermal soft tissue envelope is expected. Even if the reconstruction of the framework is successful, a good outcome can only be predicted with a successful covering. The two most useful and frequently used donors are as follows:

1. Sacral dermis fat graft: If the anterior skin envelope is very thin, the anterior contour of the sacral dermis graft itself may be demarcated under the skin flap. In this case, harvesting the sacral dermis with a fatty layer and inserting the fatty portion in direct contact with the skin flap is a way to reduce contour deformity (Fig. 15.11, Video 15.1). However, if the skin has a puncture, you must apply the reverse to solve the skin problem.
2. Superficial mastoid fascia: Superficial mastoid fascia can be an excellent alternative if a small amount of volume or contour filling is needed in the tip area.

References

1. Byrd HS, Andochick S, Copit S, Walton KG. Septal extension grafts: a method of controlling tip projection shape. Plast Reconstr Surg. 1997;100:999–1010.
2. Hyun S, Cho SW, Baek R-M. Polycaprolactone mesh for Asian rhinoplasty: outcomes and complications of composite septal extension graft compared to mesh-only graft. Facial Plast Surg. 2022;38:207–13.
3. Park YJ, Cha JH, Bang SI, Kim SY. Clinical application of three-dimensionally printed biomaterial polycaprolactone (PCL) in augmentation rhinoplasty. Aesth Plast Surg. 2019;43:437–46.
4. Rajkumar K, Khalil H, Elloy M, Sheffield E, Baldwin D. Histopathological changes in the human larynx following expanded polytetrafluroethylene (Gore-Tex(R)) implantation. BMC Ear Nose Throat Disord. 2005;5:1.
5. Ustundag E, Boyaci Z, Keskin G, Kaur A, Ozkarakas H. Soft tissue response of the larynx to silicone, Gore-Tex, and irradiated cartilage implants. Laryngoscope. 2005;115:1009–14.
6. Hernandez JL, Park J, Yao S, Blakney AK, Nguyen HV, Katz BH, et al. Effect of tissue microenvironment on fibrous capsule formation to biomaterial-coated implants. Biomaterials. 2021;273:120806.
7. Bank RA. Limiting biomaterial fibrosis. Nat Mater. 2019;18:781.
8. Romo T 3rd, Rizk SS, Suh GD. Mucous cyst formation after rhinoplasty. Arch Facial Plast Surg. 1999;1:208–11.
9. Tracy LE, Badran K, Siaghani P, Wong BJ. Dorsal nasal mucocele: a delayed complication of rhinoplasty. Aesth Plast Surg. 2014;38:100–3.
10. Pausch NC, Bertolini J, Hemprich A, Hierl T. Inclusion mucous cysts of the nose: a late complication after septorhinoplasty in two cleft lip patients. Cleft Palate Craniofac J. 2010;47:668–72.
11. Moon K-C, Lee K-I, Lee J-S, Kim A-R, Dhong E-S, Kim D-W, et al. Late-onset inflammation in Asian rhinoplasty using alloplastic implants. Aesth Plast Surg. 2021;45:670–8.
12. Kook WS, Ryu DH, Baek W, Kook HM, Jang YY, Lew DH. Prevention and resolution of silicone implant-related problems in secondary rhinoplasty using a cross-linked human acellular dermal matrix. Plast Reconstr Surg. 2023;152:45–54.

13. Moon K-C, Jung J-E, Dhong E-S, Jeong S-H, Han S-K. Preoperative nasal swab culture: is it beneficial in preventing postoperative infection in complicated septorhinoplasty? Plast Reconstr Surg. 2020;146:27e–34e.
14. Dhong E-S, Na M-W. Nasal swab culture: the preparation for the safe surgery. In: Dhong E-S, Na M-W, editors. Asian Septorhinoplasty: conundrums and solutions. Singapore: Springer Singapore; 2021. p. 29–38.
15. Jeong JY, Oh S-H, Suh MK, Kim CK, Kim KK. Effective use of a silicone-induced capsular flap in secondary Asian rhinoplasty. Plast Reconstr Surg Glob Open. 2014;2:e172.
16. Morimoto C, Takedachi M, Kawasaki K, Shimomura J, Murata M, Hirai A, et al. Hypoxia stimulates collagen hydroxylation in gingival fibroblasts and periodontal ligament cells. J Periodontol. 2021;92:1635–45.
17. Flaherty G, Pestalardo CM, Iturralde JG, Laguinge R. Mucous cyst: postrhinoplasty complication. Aesth Plast Surg. 1996;20:29–31.
18. Herfs M, Hubert P, Delvenne P. Epithelial metaplasia: adult stem cell reprogramming and (pre)neoplastic transformation mediated by inflammation? Trends Mol Med. 2009;15:245–53.
19. Goldberg MT, Llaneras J, Willson TD, Boyd JB, Venegas RJ, Dauphine C, et al. Squamous cell carcinoma arising in breast implant capsules. Ann Plast Surg. 2021;86:268–72.

Part IV

Video Cases

16 Video Case of Primary Septorhinoplasty: Reduction-Augmentation Septorhinoplasty

16.1 Background of Choosing This Case

In East Asian patient populations, the most commonly encountered cases require both reduction and augmentation. Historically and presently, most of these cases have been addressed with implant insertion. Many surgeons opt for silicone implants post-humpectomy, even for generalized hump noses, due to the patient's requirements for dorsal projection. The distinction between a mild hump nose and a mild saddle nose may hinge upon the ideal height of the rhinion.

Assuming that there is no need for using an implant, if the rhinion is higher than the ideal profile, reducing the bony dorsum would be necessary; however, if enhancement is desired in the lower two-thirds area, augmentation of the cartilaginous dorsum would be indicated.

Conversely, if the rhinion is lower than the ideal profile, surgeons who prefer convenience may opt for camouflaging by inserting an implant. Even then, some reduction at the rhinion may be performed to create a flat implant platform.

Another point to consider is that many surgeons harvest the septum not for septoplasty but to obtain graft material. Surgical techniques typically focus on tip plasty, with the dorsum managed through rasping followed by implantation and additional supratip grafting to achieve a natural contour between the implant and the tip. The author does not favor this conventional approach but performs the septal L-strut extension graft (SLEG) instead.

The prominent issues associated with implant camouflage include the following:

1. An excessively elevated dorsal profile due to implantation following inadequate bony reduction.
2. Compromised stability of the nasal bony platform resulting from reduction.
3. Numerous complications at the septum and implant site due to a weakened L-strut following submucous resection (SMR): Implants inserted following hump reduction or lateral nasal osteotomy are primarily implicated in the causation of lateral septal deviation or malunion of the nasal bones.
4. As demonstrated throughout this book, SLEG's most significant advantage is depicting the lower two-thirds of the nose using an enlarged septum. This technique particularly benefits patients requiring rhinion reduction and simultaneous augmentation of the lower two-thirds of the nose.

Supplementary Information The online version contains supplementary material available at https://doi.org/10.1007/978-981-96-6127-5_16.

E. S. Dhong, *Asian Septorhinoplasty*, https://doi.org/10.1007/978-981-96-6127-5_16

16.2 Case Study

16.2.1 History

A 27-year-old female patient presented with a deviated nose accompanied by a localized hump. She reported a history of nasal trauma from a ball impact 20 years before, which had not been treated specifically at the time.

16.2.2 Physical Exam and Diagnostic Findings

The skin was in a very thin state, possessing an extremely thin dermis, commonly found in Western patients, alongside a hump nose and underprojection of the lower two-thirds. When pressure was applied to the cartilaginous dorsum, the septum did not feel particularly strong.

The ears were not overly large relative to the facial structure, but the toughness of the auricular cartilage was not weak. From a frontal view, a C-shaped deviation was present (Fig. 16.1). The patient strongly desired enhanced tip projection and a straight nasal profile.

The NOSE score was 30 out of 100, and similar degrees of blockage were on both the left and right sides.

16.2.2.1 Endoscopic Findings and CT Scan

The left side septum was convex. A contact point was between the maxillary crest and the inferior turbinate, necessitating septal cartilage and maxillary crest resection and left inferior turbinoplasty (Fig. 16.2).

16.2.2.2 Acoustic Rhinometry

Both sides were within the normal range, but the left minimum cross-sectional area (MCA) was narrower than the right. Although these are just reference values, the goal was to correct the convexity on the left side (Fig. 16.3).

16.2.2.3 Culture-Study and Antibiotics

First culture: Enterobacter aerogenes, heavily
Second culture (2 weeks after the first visit): no bacteria cultured
Third culture (operation day): no bacterial: no bacteria cultured

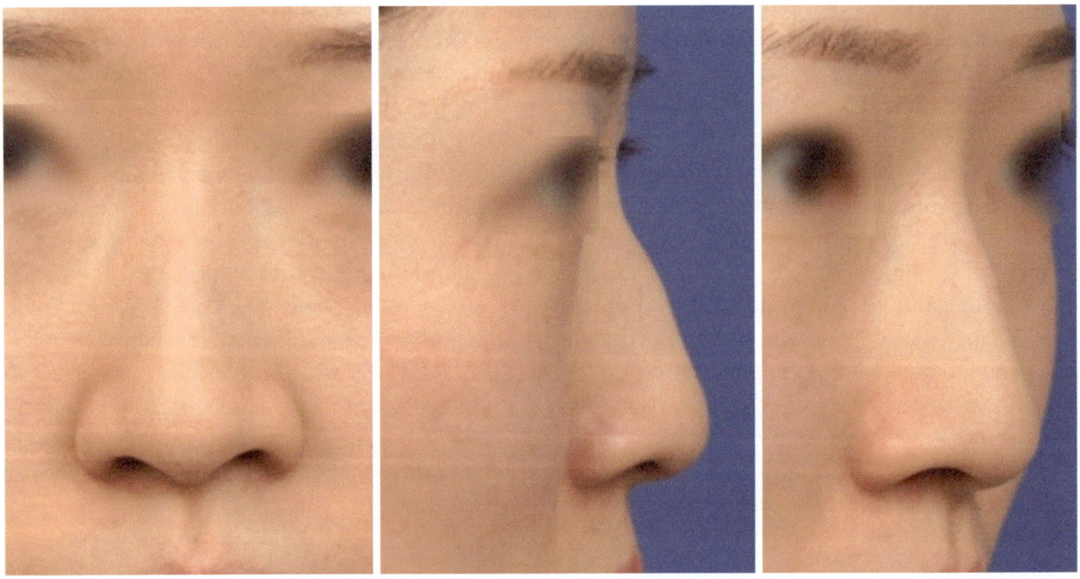

Fig. 16.1 Preoperative photo. (Left) AP view. (Middle) Modified lateral view. (Right) Quarter view

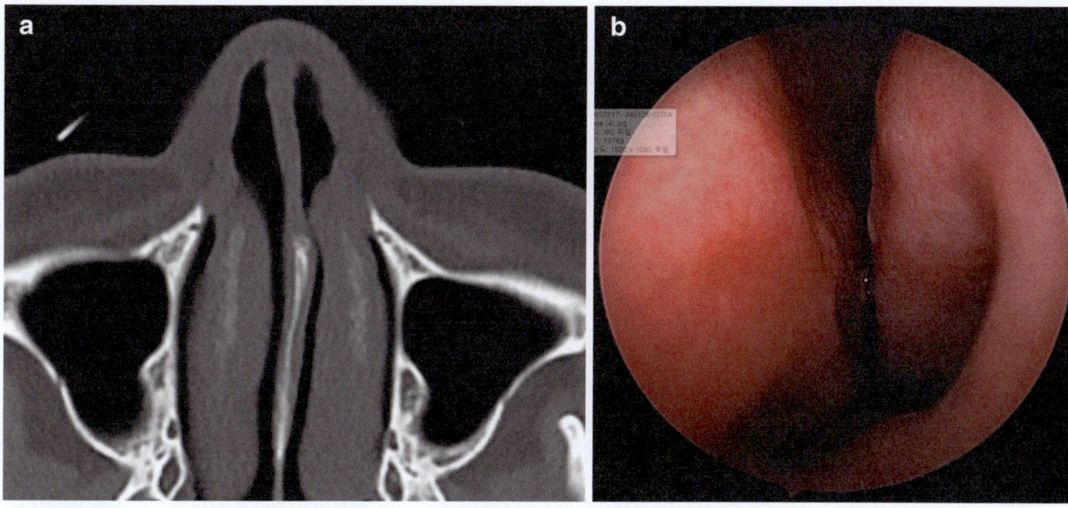

Fig. 16.2 Preoperative CT scan and endoscopic evaluation. (**a**) CT axial view shows left nasal obstruction and protrusion of the maxillary crest. (**b**) The endoscopic view shows the same point of obstruction

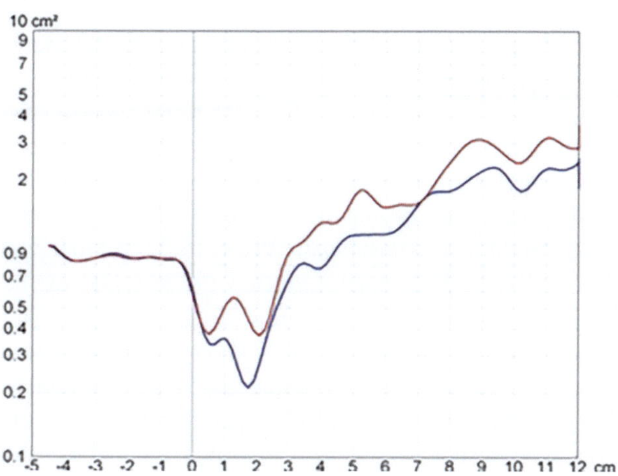

Side	Vol 0-5	Vol 2-5	Vol 0-3	MCA
#1 LEFT	2.86	2.20	1.12	0.21
#2 RIGHT	3.95	3.01	1.51	0.37
L+R	6.81	5.21	2.63	0.58
Change %	+38	+37	+34	+76

Fig. 16.3 Acoustic rhinometry shows left-side obstruction

Two weeks before surgery, a nasal swab culture heavily cultured enterobacter, which was sensitive to ciprofloxacin but resistant to amoxicillin and second-generation cephalosporins such as cefoxitin. A nose bidet with saline solution was introduced for her for 1 week, followed by a 5-day premedication regimen of ciprofloxacin ointment in the nostrils before proceeding with the surgery.

Choice of antibiotics: Tarivid ointment for 5 days preoperatively. IV ciprofloxacin for 2 days peri and postoperatively during admission after general anesthesia.

16.3 Preoperative Surgical Planning

- The bony dorsum was slightly reduced, extending from the nasion to the rhinion. A mild hump at the rhinion area was reduced.
- The hump and right side lateral nasal wall will be shaved.
- It was decided to augment the tip, including the cartilaginous dorsum (lower 2/3 of the nose).
- Due to the insufficiency of septal cartilage alone in constructing the framework, it was

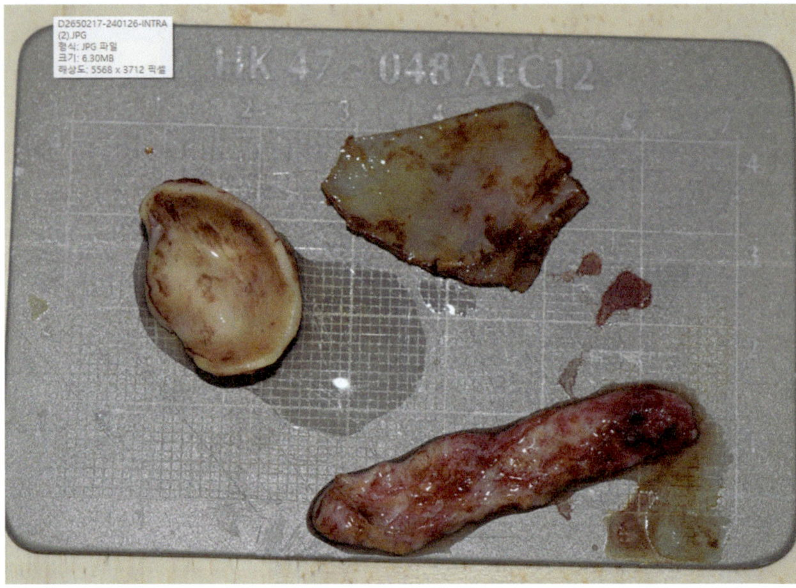

Fig. 16.4 Intraoperative preparation of septum, cymba concha cartilage, and superficial mastoid fascia

decided to harvest cymba concha. Additionally, superficial mastoid fascia was chosen for harvest to achieve minimal dorsal augmentation (Fig. 16.4).

16.4 Intraoperative Findings

From the operator's perspective, the right nasal lateral wall protrusion is observed, and the overall nose displays a C-shaped deviation. First, the inter-canthal distance is measured, followed by the inter-brow distance to delineate the midline. Care must be taken to accurately calculate the inter-brow distance in groomed eyebrows, as incorrect measurements can lead to significant discrepancies. The right lateral nasal wall is planned to be shaved only. This decision is based on the patient's lack of awareness of the protrusion of the nasal lateral wall and the presence of canting in the occlusal plane, which suggests a larger left facial aspect. To minimize maladaptation from performing an osteotomy on the right nasal wall, it is considered better to undercorrect than to risk complications of overcorrection. For the nasal tip, the tip-defining points are compared bilaterally and marked in relation to the cheeks. During this process, it is crucial for the operator to repeatedly stand and sit to ensure accurate marking from both the lateral and frontal views of the patient (Video 16.1). After elevating the soft tissue envelope, the periosteum covering the nasal bone is identified. Dissection of the subperiosteal layer is then performed, followed by electrical rasping to reduce the hump and the right lateral nasal wall (Video 16.2). Submucosal dissection is carried out on the left side of the patient to perform a caudal septal swing door and SMR. On the right side, submucosal dissection is performed while maintaining minimal attachment (Video 16.3). After performing SMR, the balance between the left and right sides was assessed, focusing on the stability above the maxillary crest of the caudal septum. Any extra bony spurs were corrected, and the posterior septal angle was secured at the anterior nasal spine (Video 16.4). The cymba concha has been prepared for CSEG. As previously described, the perichondrium is always harvested to include the cartilage on the back of the cymba (Video 16.5). The CSEG is first performed using folded cymba cartilage for the spreader graft (Video 16.6). Subsequently, bilateral spreader grafts are performed to complete the de novo anterior septal angle for the anterior extension of the cartilaginous dorsum.

The extended spreader graft on the left is first applied, followed by the right to secure sta-

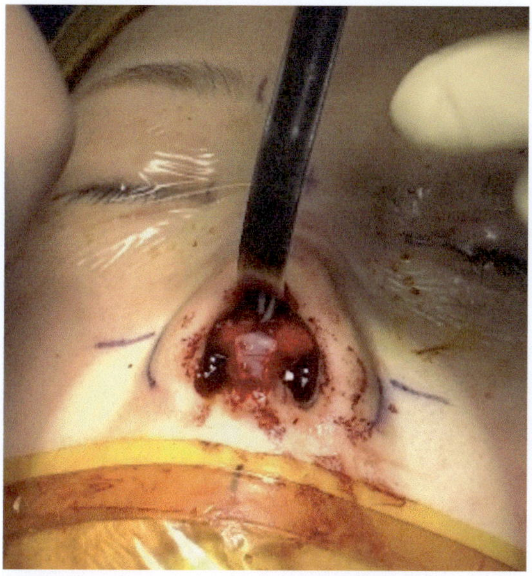

Fig. 16.5 Application of shield graft: the height of cartilaginous septum enhanced by bilateral anterior extended spreader grafts

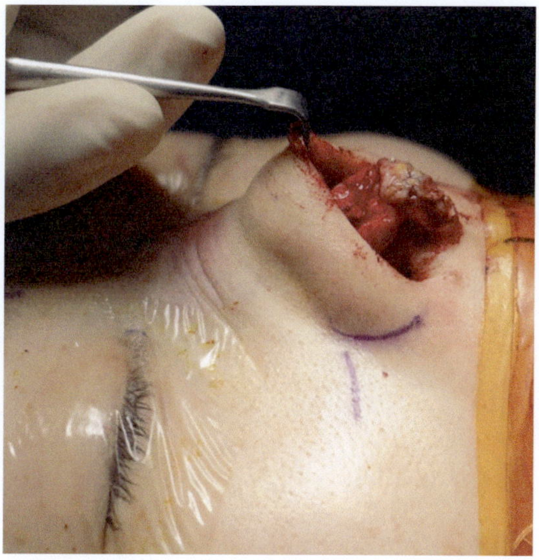

Fig. 16.6 Final tip and application of lobule graft with the remnant of superficial mastoid fascia

bility. In the preoperative design, AESG was initially planned to be applied in one or two layers only on the patient's left side. However, during the swing door procedure and septal dissection from ULCs, it was found that the tension of the quadrangular cartilage was released, significantly alleviating the C-shape deformity of the high septum. Therefore, it was determined that placing a thinner AESG on the patient's right side would be more advantageous for stability. Afterward, the de novo anterior septal angle is created, and the tip-defining point of the LLC is connected to form the desired tip position (Video 16.7). Finally, the relationship with the high septum of the LLC is established using a lateral spanning suture, completing the nasal framework. After the tip shield graft, a superficial mastoid fascia graft was performed to achieve minimal augmentation from the nasion to the supratip (Fig. 16.5, Video 16.8). The final grafts for the tip and supratip were completed using a lobule graft made from the remaining superficial mastoid fascia (SMF) (Fig. 16.6).

16.5 Operative Strategies

- Folded cymba cartilage was applied to the caudal septum for the caudal septal extension graft (CSEG).
- The missing dorsal volume was filled with superficial mastoid fascia.

16.6 Postoperative Results

- The patient's tip projection and cartilaginous dorsum have been improved to achieve the straight line desired by the patient.
- The patient's slightly deviated nose has also been corrected (Fig. 16.7).

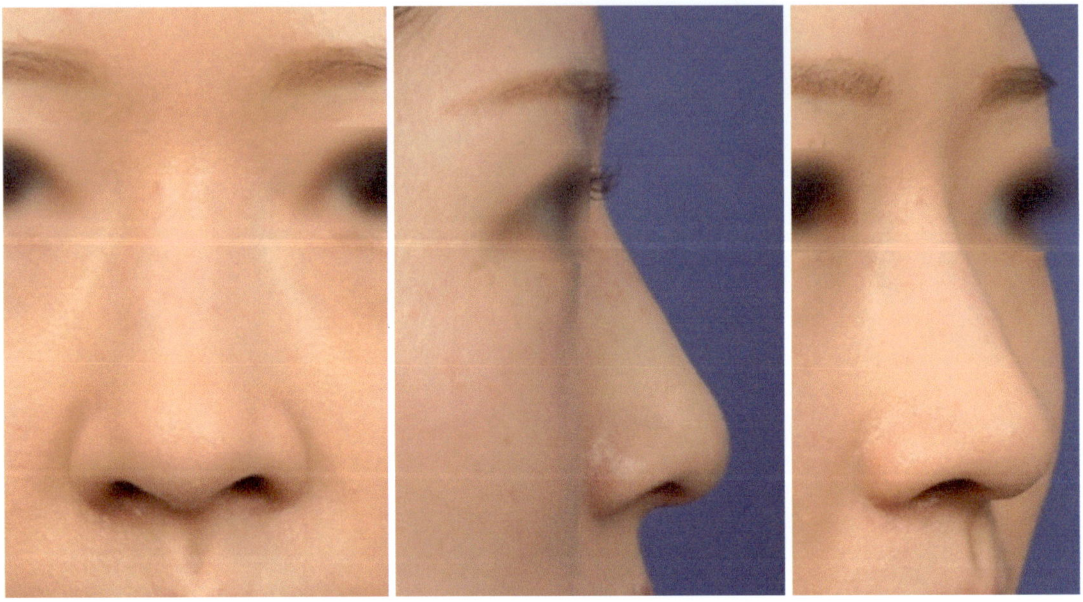

Fig. 16.7 Postoperative photos. (Left) AP view. (Middle) Modified lateral view. (Right) Quarter view

17 Video Case of Primary Septorhinoplasty: Deviated Nose with Hypoplastic Lower 2/3 of Nose

17.1 Background of Choosing This Case

A deviated nose invariably necessitates septal surgery. Among the methods to achieve functional improvement of the nose and alteration of its profile, the septal L-strut extension graft (SLEG) technique stands out as a unique approach. However, employing the caudal swing door technique often weakens the L-strut in most patients. If dorsal implantation is performed as part of camouflage under these circumstances, it may exacerbate the deviation.

Perfect repositioning of the septum to the midline is rare. The objective is to reduce the convex septum. The majority of Asian patients desire tip projection in addition to correction of the deviation. Without a stable septal foundation, all dorsal grafts risk recurrent deviation.

It is advisable to distinguish between the bony and septal axes during surgery. The author prefers to correct the septal axis first, followed by the bony correction. The support for SLEG comes from only two points: the keystone area and the anterior nasal spine (ANS) support. The support from the upper lateral cartilages (ULC) at the keystone area and the bilateral mucoperichondrium at the ANS are beneficial. Therefore, deciding whether a complete dissection is necessary in these areas or if only a minimal space should be left through tunneling is crucial.

17.2 Case Study

17.2.1 History

A 20-year-old female patient visited the clinic with complaints of nasal obstruction and a deviated nose, which occurred after colliding with a friend 8 years ago. She had no history of previous surgeries.

17.2.2 Physical Exam and Diagnostic Findings

The patient exhibited a severe C-shaped deviation. The underprojection of the lower two-thirds of the nose and hump was observed. The nasal obstruction was not as severe as it appeared, with a NOSE score of 25 out of 100 (Fig. 17.1).

17.2.2.1 Endoscopic Findings

The patient's left nasal cavity was narrow, with a contact point between the lower septum and the inferior turbinate. Although a submucosal resection was initially planned, the primary objective shifted to removing the bony spur at the contact point. Along with widening this area, an inferior turbinoplasty was also planned (Fig. 17.2).

Supplementary Information The online version contains supplementary material available at https://doi.org/10.1007/978-981-96-6127-5_17.

E. S. Dhong, *Asian Septorhinoplasty*, https://doi.org/10.1007/978-981-96-6127-5_17

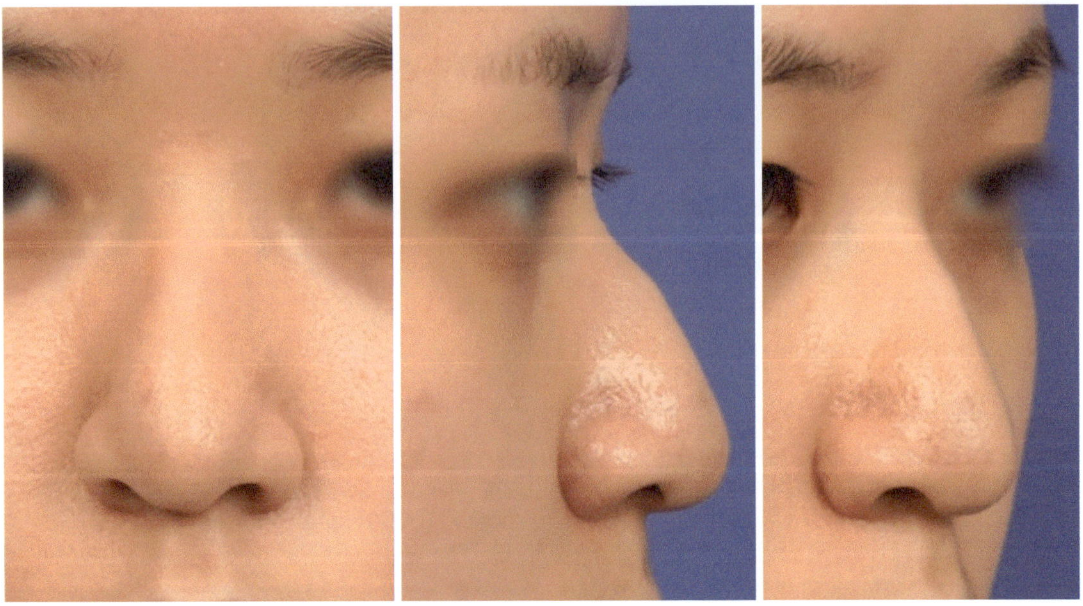

Fig. 17.1 Preoperative photo. (Left) AP view. (Middle) Modified lateral view. (Right) Quarter view

Fig. 17.2 Endoscopic evaluation and CT scan. (Left) Endoscopic examination of left nasal cavity. (Middle and Right) CT scans

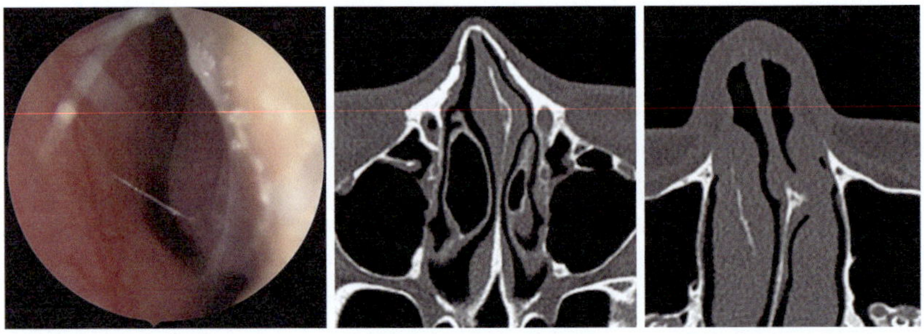

17.2.2.2 CT Scan

The entire nasal bony axis was deviated, necessitating a bilateral nasal osteotomy. Along with a deviation of the entire septum, bilateral concha bullosa of the middle turbinate was observed, with the right side being more severe. This suggests that the long-standing nasal deviation likely originated congenitally (Fig. 17.2).

17.2.2.3 Acoustic Rhinometry

The nasal obstruction on the left side was more severe, consistent with the endoscopic examination and CT scan findings (Fig. 17.3).

17.2.2.4 Culture-Study and Antibiotics

First culture: no bacterial growth
Second culture(operation day): no bacterial growth

Choice of antibiotics: Mupirocin ointment for 5 days preoperatively and postoperatively IV first-generation cephalosporin for 3 days peri- and postoperatively.

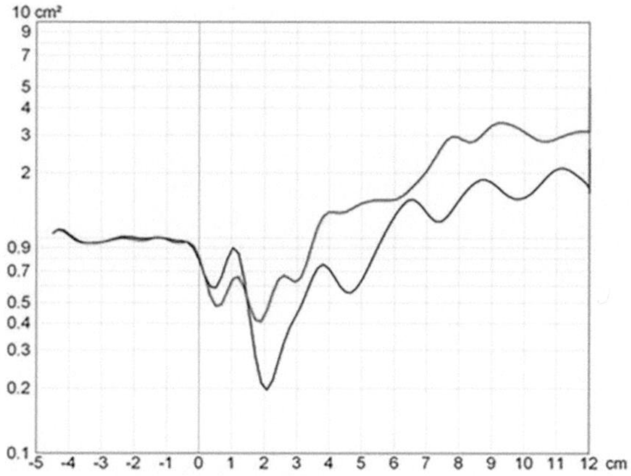

Fig. 17.3 Acoustic rhinometry

Side	Vol 0-5	Vol 2-5	Vol 0-3	MCA	Dist.
#2 LEFT	2.76	1.54	1.52	0.20	2.07
#3 RIGHT	4.02	2.92	1.71	0.41	1.90
L+R	6.78	4.46	3.22	0.60	-
Change %	+46	+89	+12	+108	-

17.3 Preoperative Surgical Planning

- The septal cartilage is anticipated to be reasonably available, so ear cartilage will not be used.
- Depending on the situation, the in-fracture of the right nasal sidewall was primarily considered, possibly performing an out-fracture on the left sidewall.
- The possibility of placing a double layer of anterior extended spreader grafts on the left side of the septum was explained. However, it was explained that the decision would be made after observing the changes in the high septum following the septal swing door procedure.
- If the septal cartilage is weak, cymba concha cartilage may be necessary.
- It was also explained to the patient that if a slight augmentation is needed at the nasion area, removed septal cartilage or an incidentally obtained bony spur, mixed with diced or crushed bone and fibrin, can be used.

17.4 Intraoperative Findings

The midportion of the inter-canthal and inter-brow distances was established, and the ideal position of the sellion, as determined in the preoperative analysis, was defined. The midpoint Si was chosen accordingly because slight augmentation of the nasion area was considered in the analysis.

The current position of the tip-defining point was determined, and it was decided to enhance its projection while maintaining the same position, avoiding any clockwise or counter-clockwise movement. A plan was made for a low-to-high curved lateral osteotomy on the right side, and the medial osteotomy was curved from high to low medial to the component reduction point of the hump (Video 17.1).

For the submucous resection, the mucoperichondrium on the patient's left side was dissected completely from the maxillary crest. After the submucosal resection, the dorsal hump was addressed through a component resection (Fig. 17.4, Video 17.2). After rasping for hump removal, a 3 mm osteotome and Jansen-Middleton forceps were used to excise the bony spur of the left maxillary crest and remove any protruding contact points. Subsequently, the posterior septum was removed to facilitate a caudal swing door, and for stability, the posterior septal angle and anterior nasal spine were fixated (Video 17.3).

On the right side of the caudal septum, with the anterior nasal spine (ANS) in between, a caudal septal extension graft was performed for reinforcement. Then, anterior extended spreader grafts were applied to both sides of the septum. During this process, multiple sutures were used to enhance the strength of the L-strut (Video 17.4). After positioning the nasal tip, interdomal

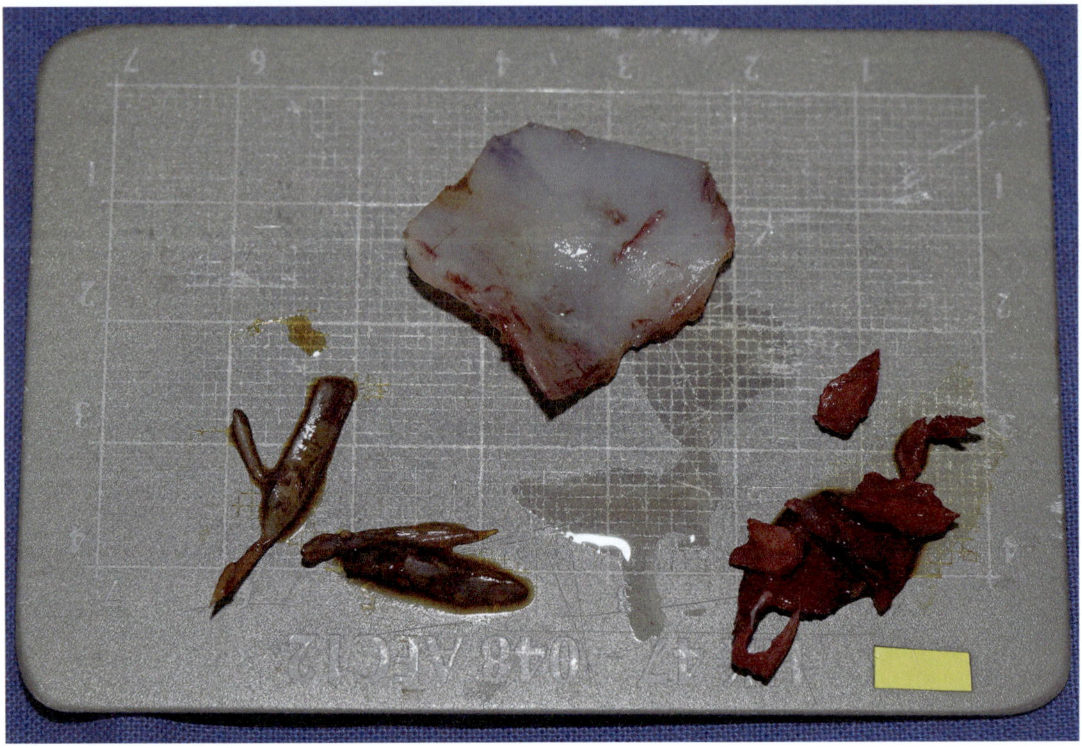

Fig. 17.4 Intraoperative preparation of septum, reduction of the hump and maxillary bony spurs

sutures and lateral crural spanning sutures were applied to secure the tip-defining point. This allowed direct fixation to the elevated high septum provided by the anterior extended spreader grafts (AESG). Subperiosteal tunnels were created for the osteotomy. Following this, the tip projection was enhanced using subdomal grafts, a columellar strut, and a shield graft (Fig. 17.5, Video 17.5).

For the corrective osteotomy on the right side, a medial oblique osteotomy was performed, followed by a lateral low-to-high osteotomy to complete the in-fracture. After coaptation of the upper lateral cartilage and the anterior septum, the nasion and supratip area were grafted with a mixture of diced bone and diced cartilage in fibrin glue. This mixture was then grafted into place (Video 17.6). Usually, tip grafting is done after osteotomy to ensure stability, but in this case, an attempt was made to avoid nasal osteotomy as much as possible. However, a noticeable bony axis deviation was still apparent even after rasping and the anterior extended spreader graft (AESG), necessitating performing right osteotomy later.

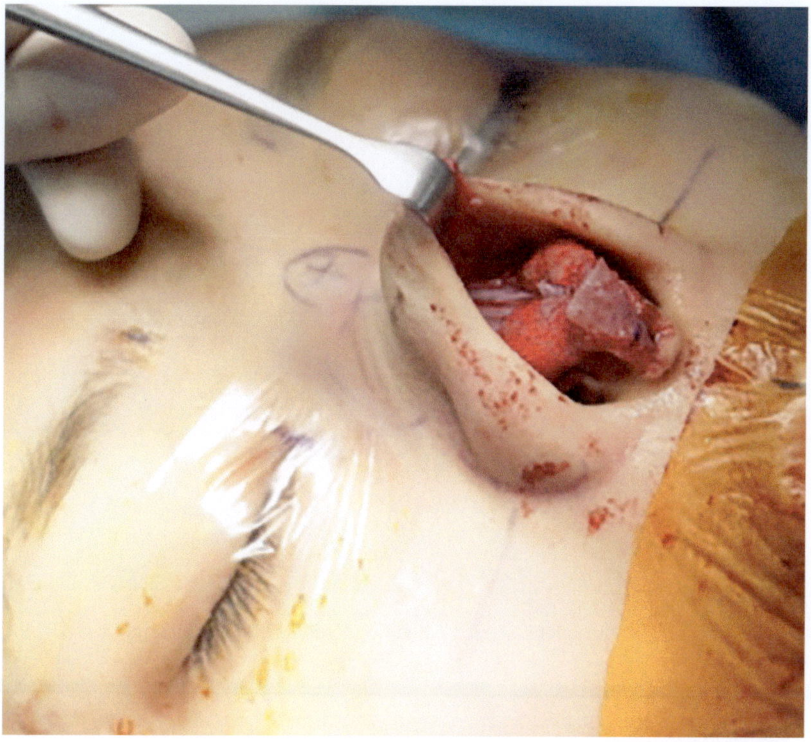

Fig. 17.5 Application of shield graft after bilateral anterior extended spreader grafts

17.5 Operative Strategies

- A single septal strut was applied to the caudal septum for caudal septal support.
- Initially, a double-layered anterior spreader graft on the left side was anticipated. However, after the septal dissection, the tension in the high septum was relieved, and the tension in the septum forming the hump was released. This led to applying bilateral anterior extended spreader grafts (AESG).
- The missing dorsal volume was filled with diced bone and cartilage with fibrin glue.
- The right side convexity of the nasal bone was corrected with an in-fracture, while the left side out-fracture was not performed.

17.6 Postoperative Results

- The patient's tip projection, along with the correction of the dorsal deviation, has been improved to achieve the straight line desired by the patient.
- Along with the correction of the patient's hump nose, the lower two-thirds of the nose were augmented using the patient's septum.
- This improved the overall nasal profile to a more straight-line appearance (Fig. 17.6).

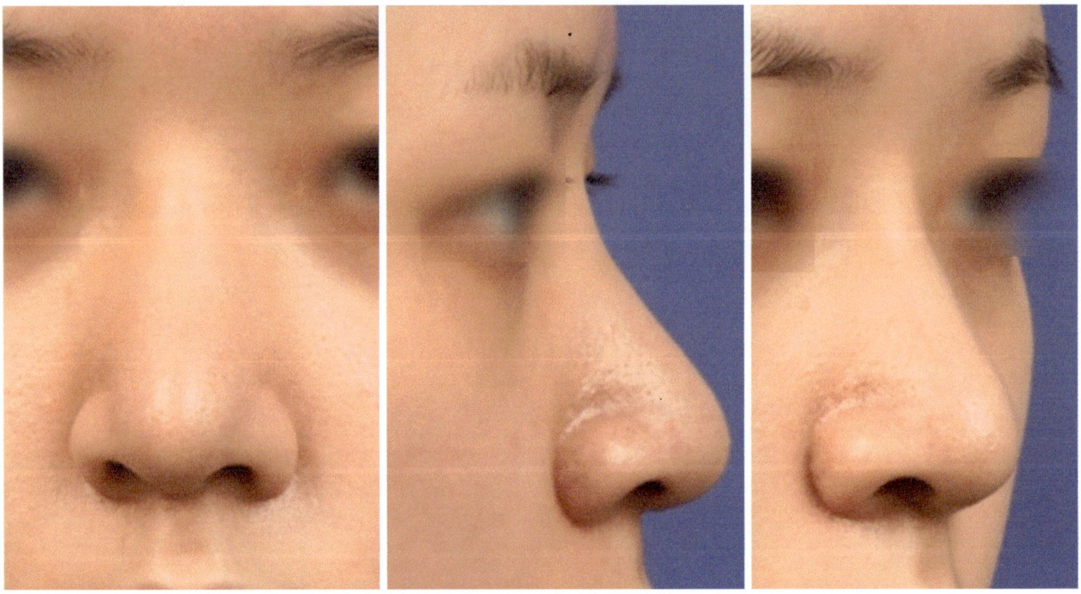

Fig. 17.6 Postoperative photos. (Left) AP view. (Middle) Modified lateral view. (Right) Quarter view

18 Video Case of Secondary Septorhinoplasty: Contracted Nose

18.1 Background of Choosing This Case

In a contracted nose, the septal L-strut is a critical structure. The apparent reason for the severe constriction, rarely seen in Western rhinoplasty but common in Asian secondary cases, lies in the loss of septal support leading to central mucosal contracture. Inflammation in the soft tissue envelope does not result in significant contracture if the septum remains intact. Even in patients with severe implant intracapsular pus drainage, severe contracture leading to the adhesion of the tip and rhinion is unlikely following explantation and irrigation, despite some contraction of the soft tissue envelope.

The nose can appear shortened even without severe inflammation in the soft tissue envelope in patients lacking septal support. But, continued intraseptal inflammation can lead to a surprisingly significant reduction in nose length.

The decision between septal reconstruction and camouflage using a cantilever graft hinges on the feasibility of dissecting the septum. When septal dissection is not possible, camouflage becomes the only option. Overzealous septal dissection can lead to weakened L-strut, potentially starting another tragic cycle.

Forcing the extension of the skin's soft tissue envelope when the septal mucoperichondrium does not stretch well will inevitably encounter limits in lengthening. The most significant challenges in secondary septorhinoplasty for Asian patients are the uncertainty regarding nasal extension and the strange, unexpected implants from past surgeries that can only be discovered during the surgical procedure.

A donor can be prepared if such grafts are identified on preoperative CT scans. However, if unexpected materials such as donated ribs or Medpor are discovered, the surgery enters a new phase.

This chapter addresses a typical secondary septorhinoplasty case that the author commonly encounters. Nevertheless, the reasons for choosing this patient for a septal L-strut extension graft include discovering unexpected materials during surgery and the need for septum reconstruction.

18.2 Case Study

18.2.1 History

The patient underwent her seventh surgical procedure. Her surgical history is as follows:

- Five years before her current visit, she underwent an open rhinoplasty using a silicone implant and ear cartilage at a local clinic.
- Two months later, dissatisfied with the height of the silicone and its deviation, she had the silicone implant changed at another local facility.

Supplementary Information The online version contains supplementary material available at https://doi.org/10.1007/978-981-96-6127-5_18.

E. S. Dhong, *Asian Septorhinoplasty*, https://doi.org/10.1007/978-981-96-6127-5_18

- One year after that, she visited an ENT hospital where the silicone implant was removed. A capsulectomy was performed, and grafts using her seventh rib cartilage were implemented for spreader and caudal extension purposes.
- Three months later, she complained about a low nasion. At the same hospital, she underwent radix augmentation using an 8 mm silicone and Gore-Tex, during which some donated rib was also utilized.
- One month following this procedure, a surgical site infection occurred, leading to the removal of all implants and the donated rib, although the previously inserted autogenous rib was retained.
- Two months following this event, she continued to experience pus drainage, necessitating ongoing irrigation until her current presentation.
- There is currently no alloplastic material, and she stated that pus drainage had stopped 6 months before the visit.

18.2.2 Physical Exam and Diagnostic Findings

Due to the inability to insert a finger into the nasal cavity, the caudal septum could not be palpated. However, nasoscopic examination revealed no palpable septum, and the nostrils were severely upturned. The nose tip was very hard, and a midline scar from the nasion to what appeared to be a pus drainage site was visible on the front. According to the patient, pus had been draining from this area and the right nostril for over a month (Fig. 18.1).

18.2.2.1 Endoscopic Findings

No signs of septal perforation were observed, but fluttering was detected when a cotton swab was inserted and pushed against the center portion. The caudal septum seemed not palpable; only a rigid framework serving as an L-strut was expected in the high septum and columella. The STCA image shows the surgical plan, but the endoscopic findings did not allow for that release level (Fig. 18.2).

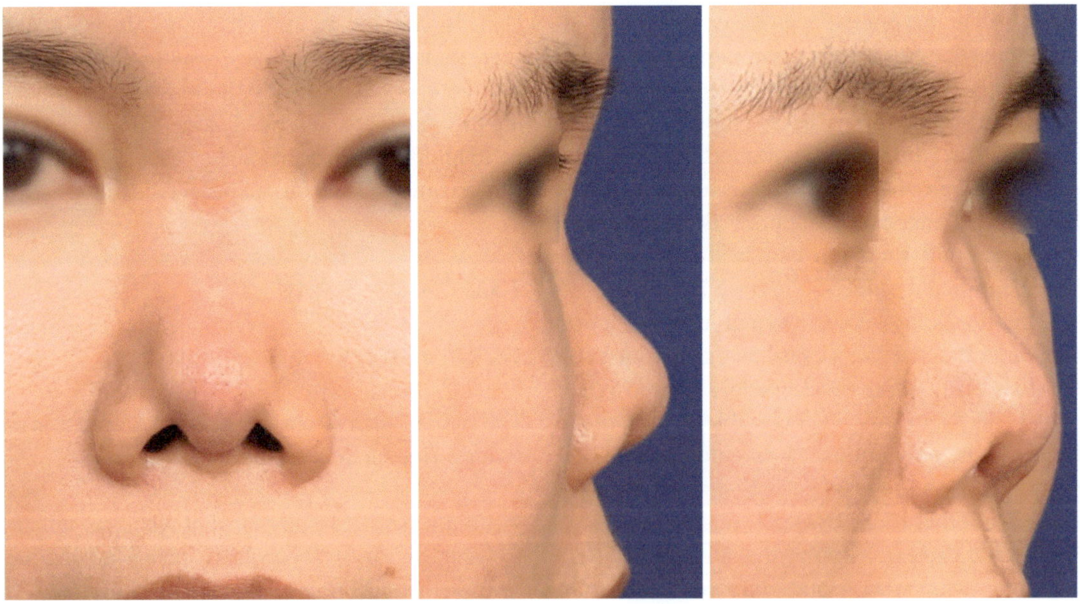

Fig. 18.1 Preoperative photo. (Left) AP view. (Middle) Modified lateral view. (Right) Quarter view

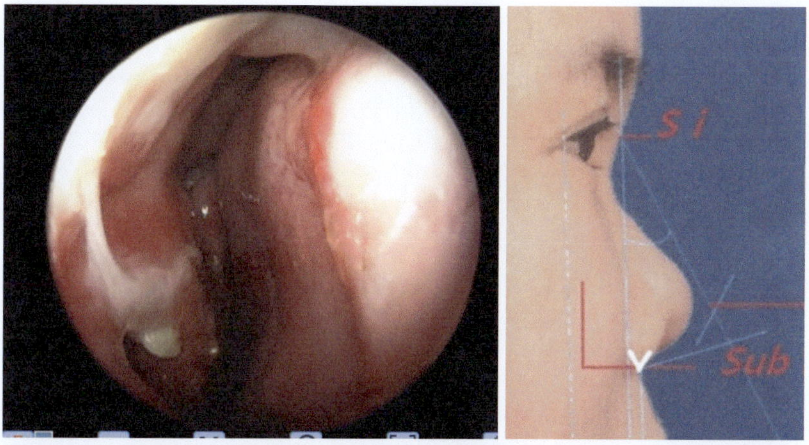

Fig. 18.2 Endoscopic evaluation and preoperative analysis using STCA

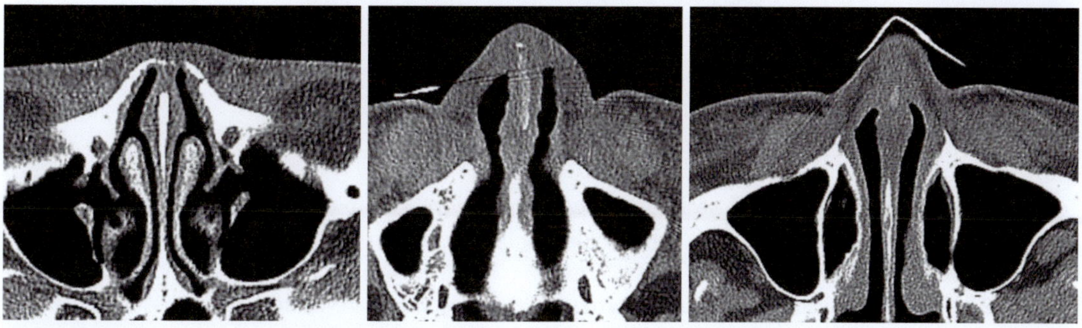

Fig. 18.3 CT scan, preoperative (mediastinum shadow). (Left) The lateral nasal wall is thicker than the midline, distal resorption of the nasal bone. (Middle) Lowered nasal roof and heavy scar

18.2.2.2 CT Scan

A very low nasion was observed, and the lateral sides where the capsules had been placed were thicker than the midline dorsum. This appearance suggested that the thickening was not due to silicone or Gore-Tex resorbing the nasal bone but because a previous capsule had not been removed.

A high-density cartilage-like shadow was visible in the columella and the septal area of the nose, which the author suspected to be previously inserted rib cartilage. Slight bony resorption was observed in the caudal portion of the nasal bone, and a very thick soft tissue appeared to be pressing down on the entire roof above the upper lateral cartilage, resulting in a markedly low nasal roof. Compared to the very hard features, this was determined to be a capsule or a pericapsular scar mass (Fig. 18.3).

18.2.2.3 Acoustic Rhinometry

Despite the lowered roof of the nose, the patient did not complain of severe nasal obstruction. The NOSE score was 20/100, which differed from the apparent physical findings. In AR, the right's minimal cross-sectional area (MCA) was reduced compared to the left, but the patient did not report any clinical symptoms (Fig. 18.4).

18.2.2.4 Culture-Study and Antibiotics

First culture (first visit): MRSE lightly

Second culture (2 weeks before surgery): *Pseudomonas aeruginosa*, moderately

Third culture (operation day): *Pseudomonas aeruginosa*, lightly

Choice of antibiotics: intraoperatively and postoperative 3 days ciprofloxacin + Teicoplanin

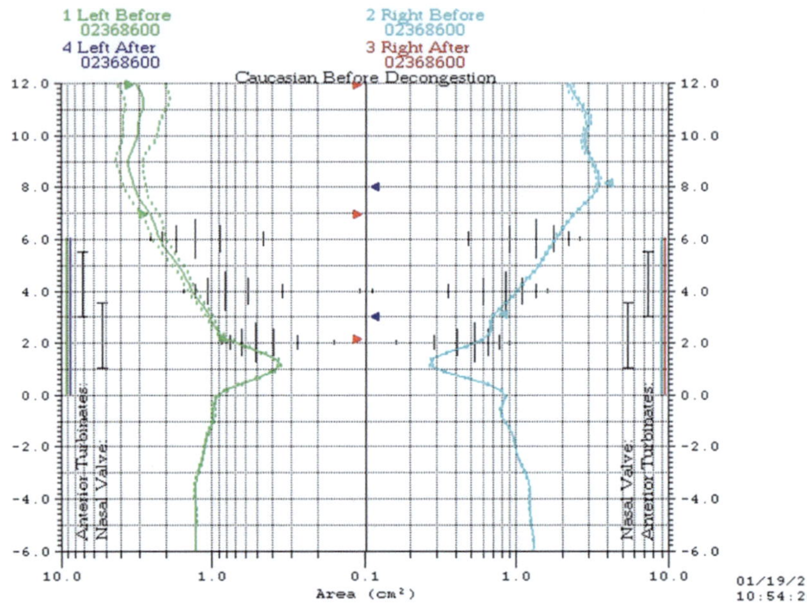

Fig. 18.4 Acoustic rhinometry, preoperative

During the initial visit, a nasal swab identified methicillin-resistant Staphylococcus epidermidis (MRSE). The patient was advised to use a nose bidet, and a subsequent nasal swab was performed 2 weeks before surgery for routine lab work identified pseudomonas. The pseudomonas was susceptible to ciprofloxacin, and the patient was recommended to apply ciprofloxacin ointment to the nostrils 5 days before surgery. On the day of surgery, vancomycin was not used due to a systemic side effect. Ciprofloxacin, which had reduced susceptibility, was used instead. The third culture performed just before surgery also identified the same pseudomonas, and ciprofloxacin, along with teicoplanin, was chosen as the antibiotic for use during surgery and the subsequent 3 days.

18.3 Preoperative Surgical Planning

- It was determined that septal dissection would be feasible to some extent. Removing the existing rib graft that maintained the framework was expected to create sufficient space.
- A laminated rib will be used for septal L-strut extension based on the extent to which septal dissection is possible.
- A dorsal rib block and a soft tissue graft will be necessary to fill the extensive defects in the area below the nasion and the scar tissue occupying the to-be-removed soft tissue envelope.
- After dissecting the septum and the mucoperichondrium, the extent of its expansion will be assessed to determine the amount of graft needed.
- Thus, the plan includes using a septal L-strut extension graft (SLEG) supplementing with a soft tissue graft to support the weakened framework and the volume deficiency.

18.4 Intraoperative Findings

The current positions of the patient's nasion and tip were marked. Due to a history of infection, care was taken to repeatedly apply and dry betadine, a skin disinfectant, before draping (Video 18.1). Since the previous incision was close to an almost rim incision, special attention was made to recreate the middle crus during the nostril incision by securing as much intranasal lining as possible near the cephalic side to form a soft triangle. Efforts were made to maintain a consistent thickness of the skin flap while removing the underlying scar. A hard scar mass, presumed to be a capsule and allograft, was encountered along with the columella's previously applied rib, which was bloodless. Wrapped in a thin capsule, the bloodless yellowish rib was brisker than an autologous rib. While showing some integration with the existing septal cartilage by a few millimeters, it is presumed to cause erosion of the existing septal cartilage. The patient stated that all donated rib material had been removed, but materials resembling columellar strut, caudal septal extension, and spreader grafts made of rib cartilage were discovered (Fig. 18.5). As the cartilage was found to lack circulation, it was strongly suspected to be residual donated rib cartilage. The main issue was that the hard framework was not resilient. Additionally, severe scar tissue was present around both the upper and lower lateral cartilages, and its removal was difficult even with a scalpel, suggesting the possible use of alloderm (Video 18.2).

Using the patient's previous incision, the eighth rib was harvested. Several laminated ribs and a rib block for dorsal onlay were prepared. For the soft tissue, rectus fascia was prepared, and perichondrium was layered and sutured beneath the rib block (Fig. 18.6, Video 18.3).

Only some existing septal cartilage remained around the ANS and parts of the cephalo-posterior EPP. In contrast, the cartilage around the rest of the previously donated rib L-strut showed signs of resorption. The CSEG was first positioned in the subperiosteal pockets on both sides of the ANS, and then the surrounding tissue was repaired to begin building the framework (Video 18.4). To aid in the stability and extension of the CSEG, a small strut graft was implemented to connect it with the remaining septal cartilage. Subsequently, anterior extended spreader grafts were applied to both sides. However, attempts to secure these grafts with transcutaneous transosseous cerclage sutures faced issues due to the lateral nasal walls being too low for adequate stability. A small wedge was added to the proximal laminated rib to assist in fixing the distal nasal bone (Video 18.5) [1]. Scar tissue above the ULC was removed, and the scar tissue in the hinge and scroll areas was eliminated. Subsequently, an interdomal suture was placed at the high septum for tip positioning and coapted with the high septum (Video 18.6). A shield graft was performed after the lateral crural spanning suture for tip positioning. Subsequently, a rib

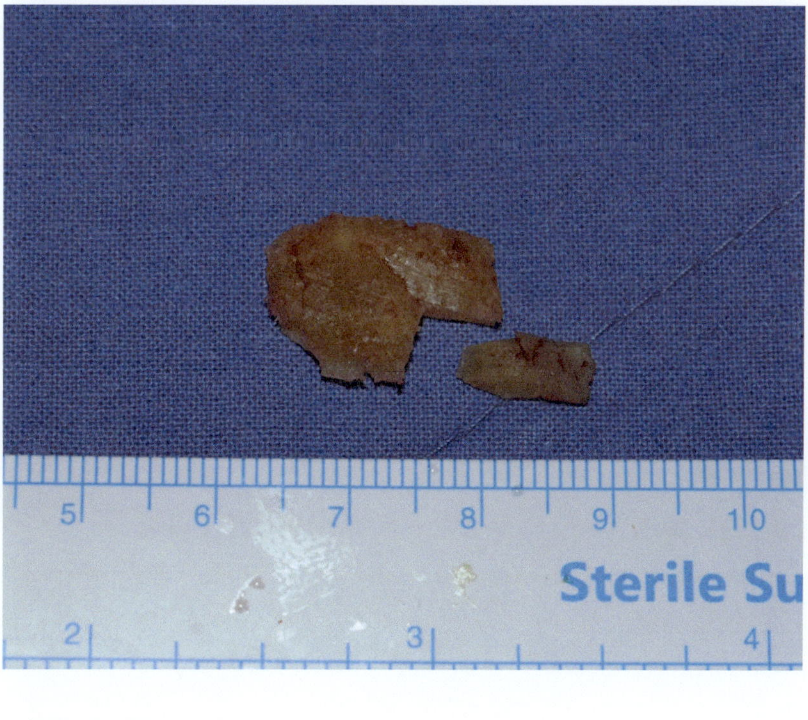

Fig. 18.5 Thin encapsulation presumed to be a donated rib found in the septum

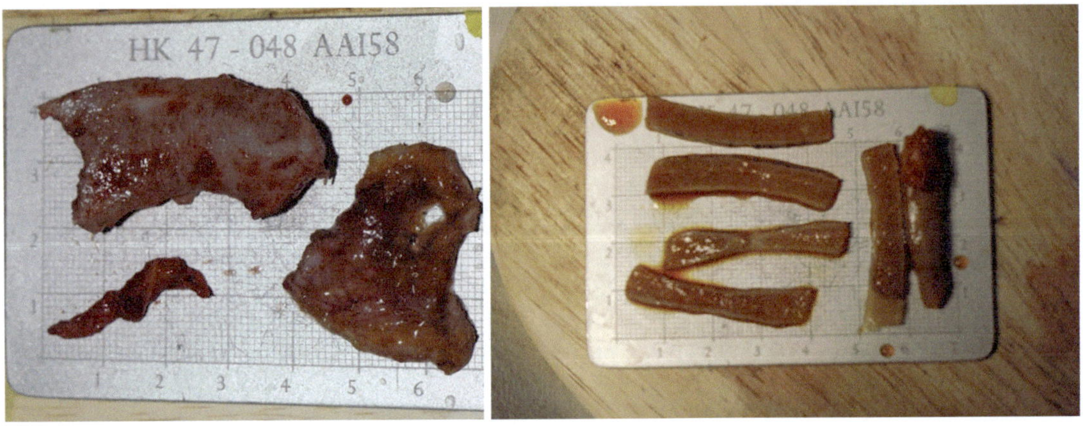

Fig. 18.6 Intraoperative preparation of rib. (Left) Eighth rib, periosteum, and rectus fascia. (Right) Laminated rib and block

Fig. 18.7 Final tip after grafts

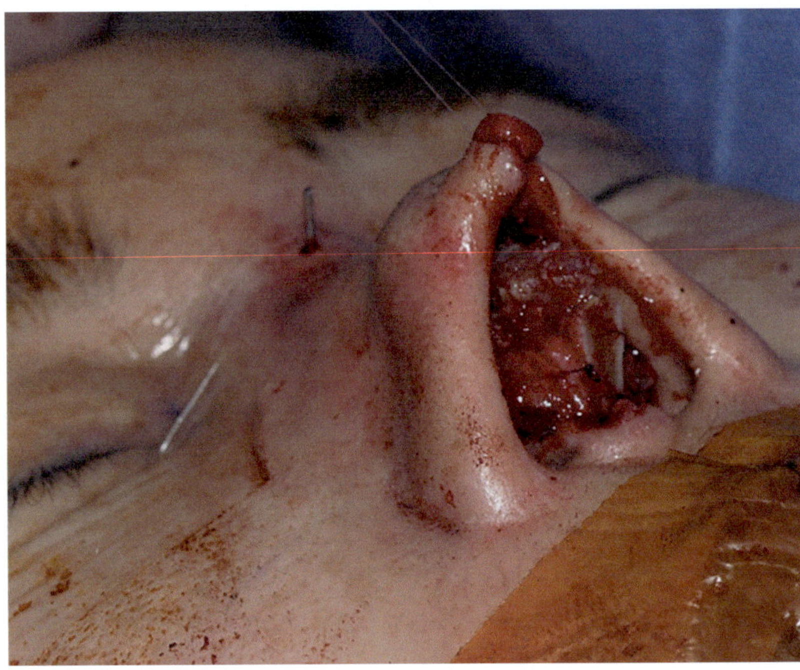

block was grafted at the nasion, and its fixation was achieved using a medium K-wire for vertical transcutaneous fixation (Fig. 18.7, Video 18.7). Afterward, diced cartilage with fibrin and the remaining rectus fascia were grafted onto the supratip (Fig. 18.8). The sub-dermis was injected with diluted triamcinolone solution. The remaining perichondrium was grafted onto the lobule and the LLC to prepare for potential spreading at the incision site (Video 18.8).

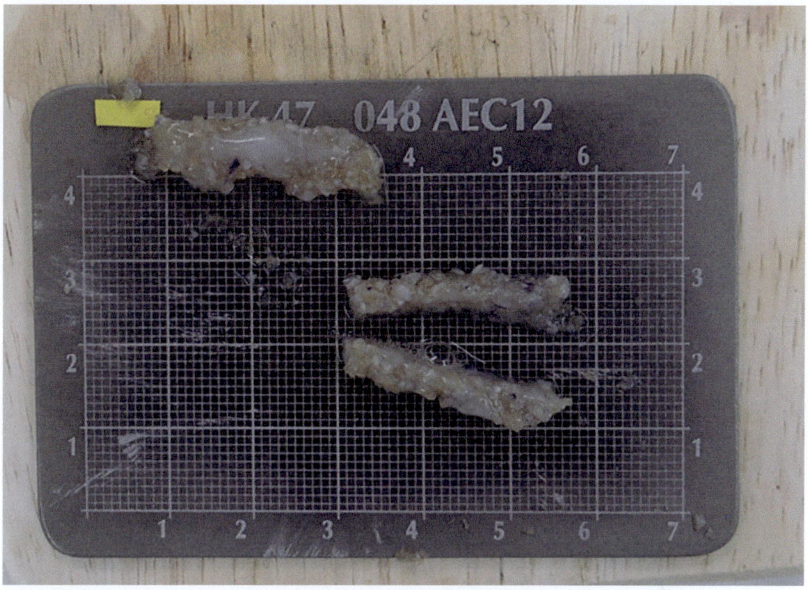

Fig. 18.8 Diced rib with fibrin glue

18.5 Operative Strategies

- The patient, who had a history of surgical site infection (SSI) that had resolved 6 months prior, decided to advance the surgery due to concerns about nasal foreshortening. However, the possibility of another SSI occurring could not be ruled out.
- Efforts were made to use the appropriate antibiotic, but due to side effects from Vancomycin, a second-choice antibiotic was used, and extra caution was taken during surgical irrigation.
- All existing allografts were removed, and an extension of the nose was planned within the limits allowed by the release of the skin-soft tissue envelope (SSTE) and the septum's mucoperichondrium.
- To rebuild the nasal framework, a septal L-strut extension graft (SLEG) and a dorsal rib block graft were planned to refill the lacking volume.
- It was determined that forming a caudal septal extension graft (CSEG) first, followed by an anterior extended spreader graft (AESG), would be advantageous.
- To ensure the stability of the dorsal rib block, it was planned to maintain the nasion K-wire for more than 4 weeks.

18.6 Postoperative Results

- During the long-term follow-up, the K-wire at the nasion became unstable on the fourth week and was removed (Fig. 18.9).
- Significant amounts of diced cartilage and the soft tissues of the supratip and lobule had resorbed. While a complete 18-month follow-up for an accurate volume check was not completed, data up to 12 months was available, and the patient's satisfaction was high (Fig. 18.10).
- A slight soft tissue bulge was observed on the right side of the nasion, but continuous compression and rehabilitation were recommended.
- Monitoring for further resorption and warping is needed, but no notable issues were reported within the first year.
- Postoperative acoustic rhinometry showed some improvement, and no signs of nasal obstruction were observed, which was better than the data observed before surgery (Figs. 18.11 and 18.12).

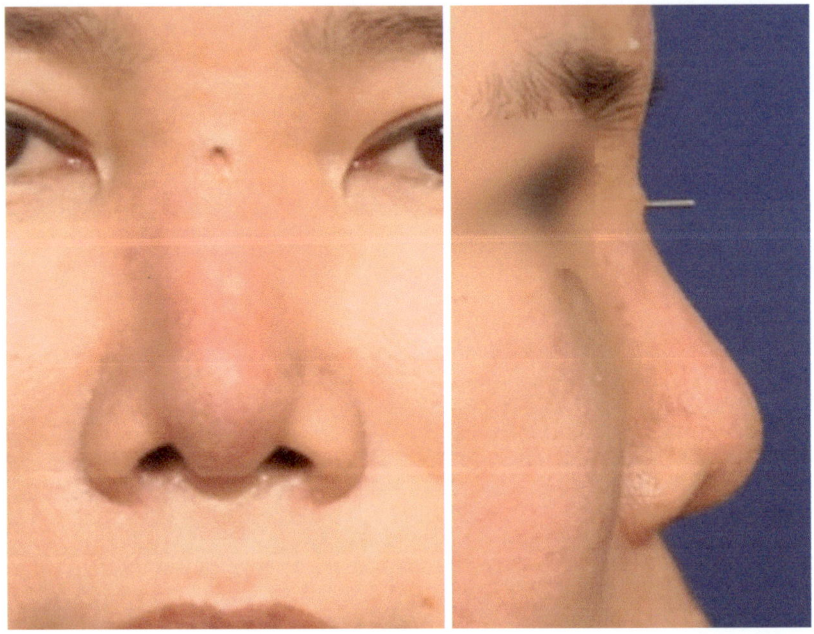

Fig. 18.9 Postoperative photos, 1 month. (Left) AP view. (Right) Modified lateral view

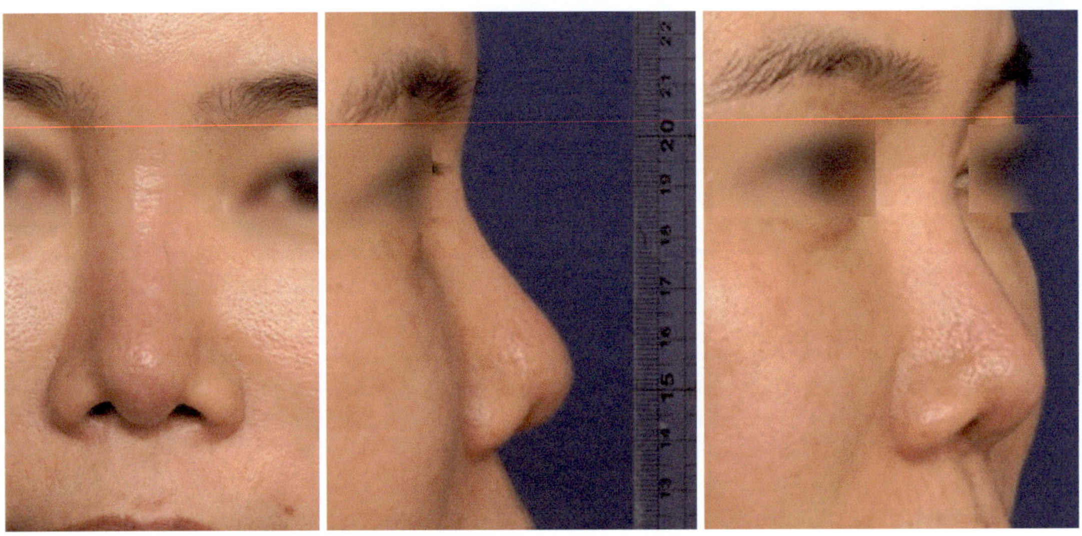

Fig. 18.10 Postoperative photos, 12 months. (Left) AP view. (Middle) Modified lateral view. (right) Quarter view

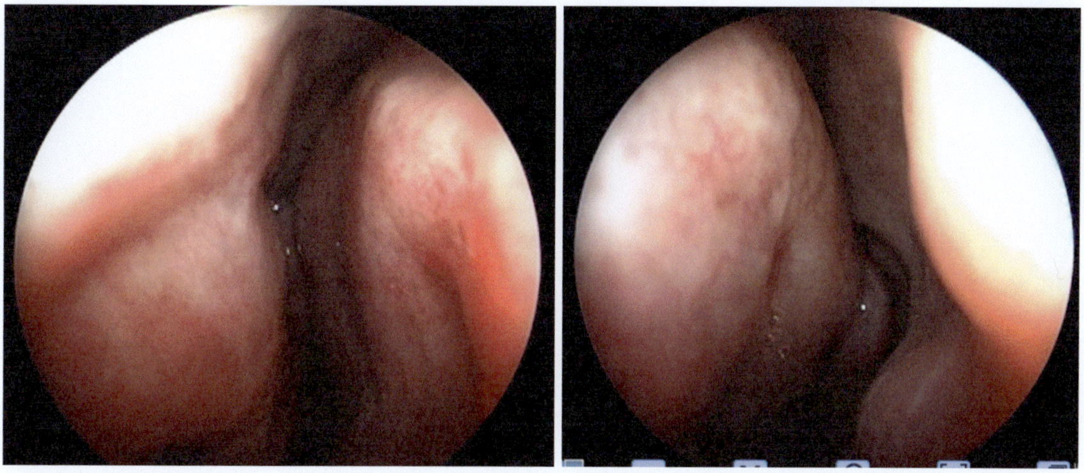

Fig. 18.11 Endoscopic evaluation postoperative 12 months. (Left) Right nasal cavity. (Right) Left nasal cavity

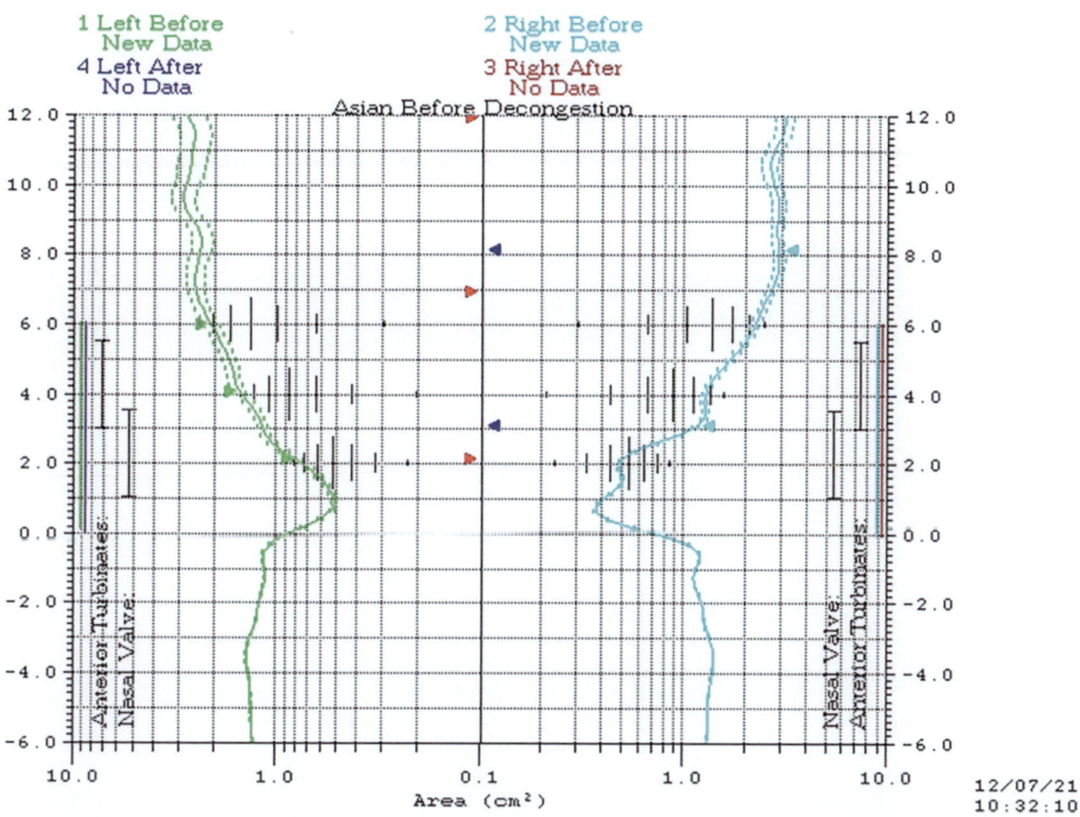

Fig. 18.12 Acoustic rhinometry, postoperative 6 months

Reference

1. Rezaeian F, Gubisch W, Janku D, Haack S. New suturing techniques to reconstruct the keystone area in extracorporeal septoplasty. Plast Reconstr Surg. 2016;138:374–82.

19 Video Case of Secondary Septorhinoplasty: High Septal Defect Repair

19.1 Background of Choosing This Case

The most challenging aspect of septal L-strut reconstruction is addressing defects in the high septum. The primary causes of mucoperichondrium loss in the high septum include iatrogenic defects due to alloplastic implant problems, severe contracture, and associated saddle deformities corrected during surgery or accidental damage incurred during the septal surgery. When L-strut reconstruction is imperative, two approaches are available: creating a local flap to cover the insufficient mucoperichondrium or allowing for natural healing using biological covering.

A mucoperichondrial flap is not advisable when a significant septal graft is required, mainly because rotating the flap inevitably creates another defect nearby. Therefore, the graft that requires healing is exposed to the nasal cavity, which can lead to infection. The most crucial and needed areas are subjected to the highest tension, often rendering the flap unable to fulfill its intended purpose.

Flaps near the ethmoidal perpendicular plate (EPP) or those encompassing the entire septum, including areas near the maxillary crest, can be feasible for recovering the high septum. However, it is challenging to create a tension-free flap. Reaching the high septum from a distant side is difficult because the highest tension mentioned above gets caught on the defect again. Consequently, the author does not employ recently reported methods due to resistance at the high septum's location. Nevertheless, there is potential for using such techniques for the membranous septum or septal perforations closer to the nostril. However, it is challenging to use for defects in the septal framework, including a high septum. The author has found that covering with perichondrium, especially when applying septal L-strut reconstruction, is an effective alternative to mucoperichondrial flaps for high septal defects. This chapter presents a case where the sequential healing of costal perichondrium, used to cover a high septal perforation arising from late-onset inflammation over septal alloplastic materials, is discussed. The larger the defect, the longer the waiting period and the higher the risk of prolonged exposure to variables such as acute surgical site infection. In most cases, no infection has occurred at the septal reconstruction site. However, there has been rapid resorption of the transplanted costal cartilage due to delayed healing compared to other patients.

It is well understood that mucoperichondrial coverage is essential for rapidly healing the transplanted cartilage, and a low burden of microorganisms in the intra-nasal environment is crucial.

Supplementary Information The online version contains supplementary material available at https://doi.org/10.1007/978-981-96-6127-5_19.

E. S. Dhong, *Asian Septorhinoplasty*, https://doi.org/10.1007/978-981-96-6127-5_19

19.2 Case Study

19.2.1 History

The 46-year-old male patient presented to our clinic, having sustained a nasal bone fracture 3 years before his visit. Dissatisfied with the shape of his nose after the injury, he underwent septorhinoplasty and enhancement of the dorsum using Gore-Tex 6 months later. During this procedure, an absorbable mesh (T&R mesh, Korea) was also used in the septum. Seven months following this, the Gore-Tex in the dorsum was replaced, and a derotation graft using the cymba and cavum concha was performed. Two years later, he frequently experienced swelling and pus drainage, leading to the removal of the Gore-Tex. Cultures identified Staphylococcus epidermidis, and after more than a month of antibiotic treatment, he sought further care.

The patient wanted to extend his shortened nose and correct irregularities on the bridge. He did not complain of nasal obstruction but did report a foul odor.

19.2.2 Physical Examination and Diagnostic Findings

The skin of the nose was very hard, and the tip did not move. Irregularities could be felt along the dorsum, which showed signs of a saddle nose deformity. The nostrils were triangular in shape, indicating the destruction of the soft triangle. The longitudinal axes of the left and right nostrils differed, and there was a noticeable tilt in the columella and a previous ugly scar. The length of the nose had significantly shortened when compared to pre-operative photos provided by the patient (Fig. 19.1).

19.2.2.1 Endoscopic Findings

The endoscopic findings revealed multiple perforations in the nasal septum. There was severe convolution on both sides, and signs suggestive of a collapse of the nasal septum were observed (Fig. 19.2).

19.2.2.2 CT Scan

In the axial CT scan, severe destruction of the nasal bone was observed, along with an open roof. There was no evidence of lateral osteotomy

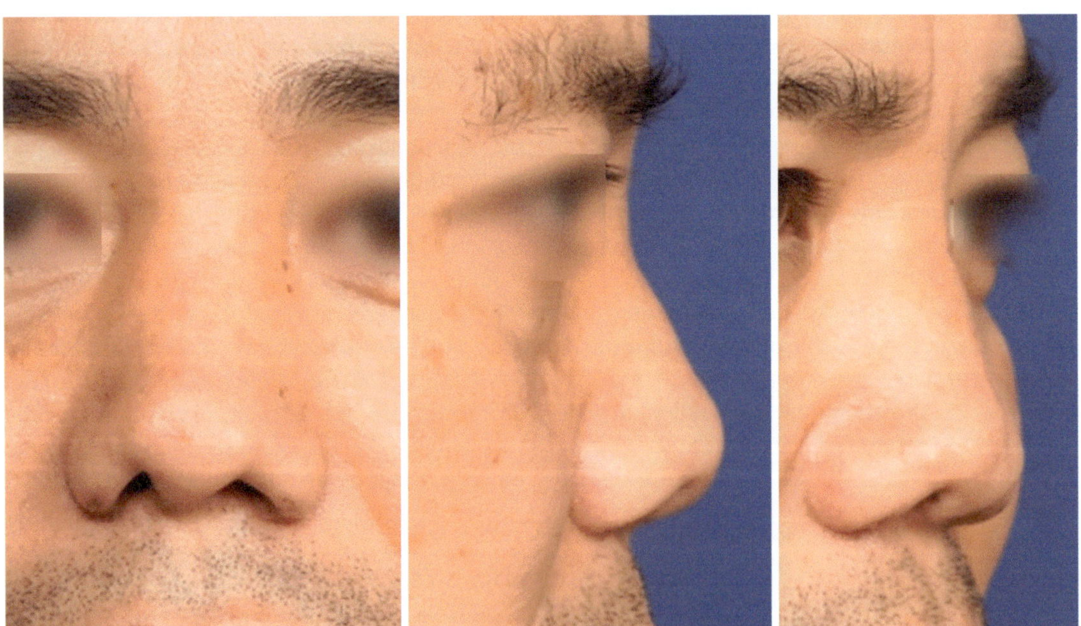

Fig. 19.1 Preoperative photo. (Left) AP view. (Middle) Modified lateral view. (Right) Quarter view

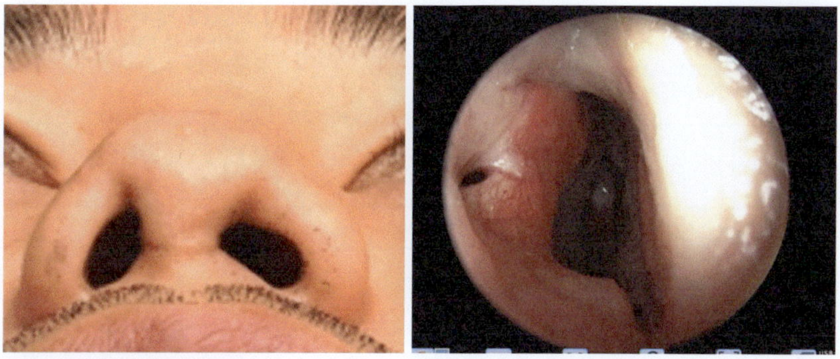

Fig. 19.2 Basal view and preoperative endoscopic evaluation. (Left) Worm's-eye view. (Right) Left nasal cavity

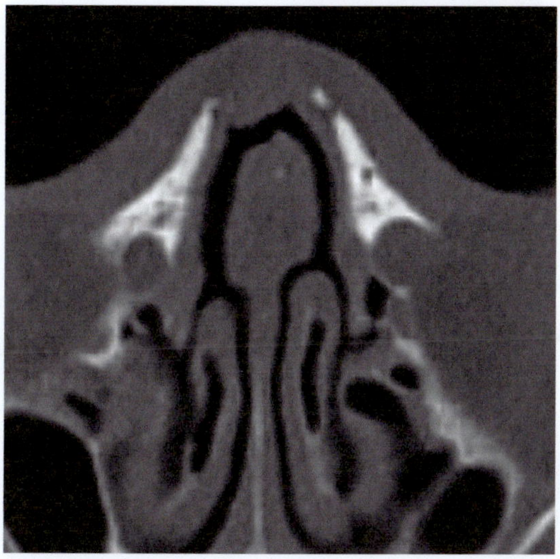

Fig. 19.3 CT scan, preoperative (mediastinum shadow): high septal perforation

(Videos 19.1 and 19.2). A large perforation in the high septum revealed a connection between the left and right nasal cavities (Fig. 19.3).

19.2.2.3 Acoustic Rhinometry

Before the surgery, the patient did not complain of nasal obstruction (Fig. 19.4).

19.2.2.4 Culture-Study and Antibiotics

First culture: Corynebacterium accolens, heavily
Second culture (2 weeks before operation): no bacterial
Third culture (operation day): Staphylococcus haemolyticus, lightly

From the initial visit, nasal swabs were taken monthly, consistently showing a heavy presence of corynebacterium, which was unresponsive to first- and second-generation cephalosporins. Continuous nasal irrigation with a nasal bidet was recommended.

For the choice of antibiotics, ciprofloxacin ointment and mupirocin were alternately applied to the nostrils 5 days before surgery. Perioperative antibiotics initially included vancomycin, but on the second day, based on culture results, the identified strain was sensitive to ciprofloxacin, which was then administered for 3 days.

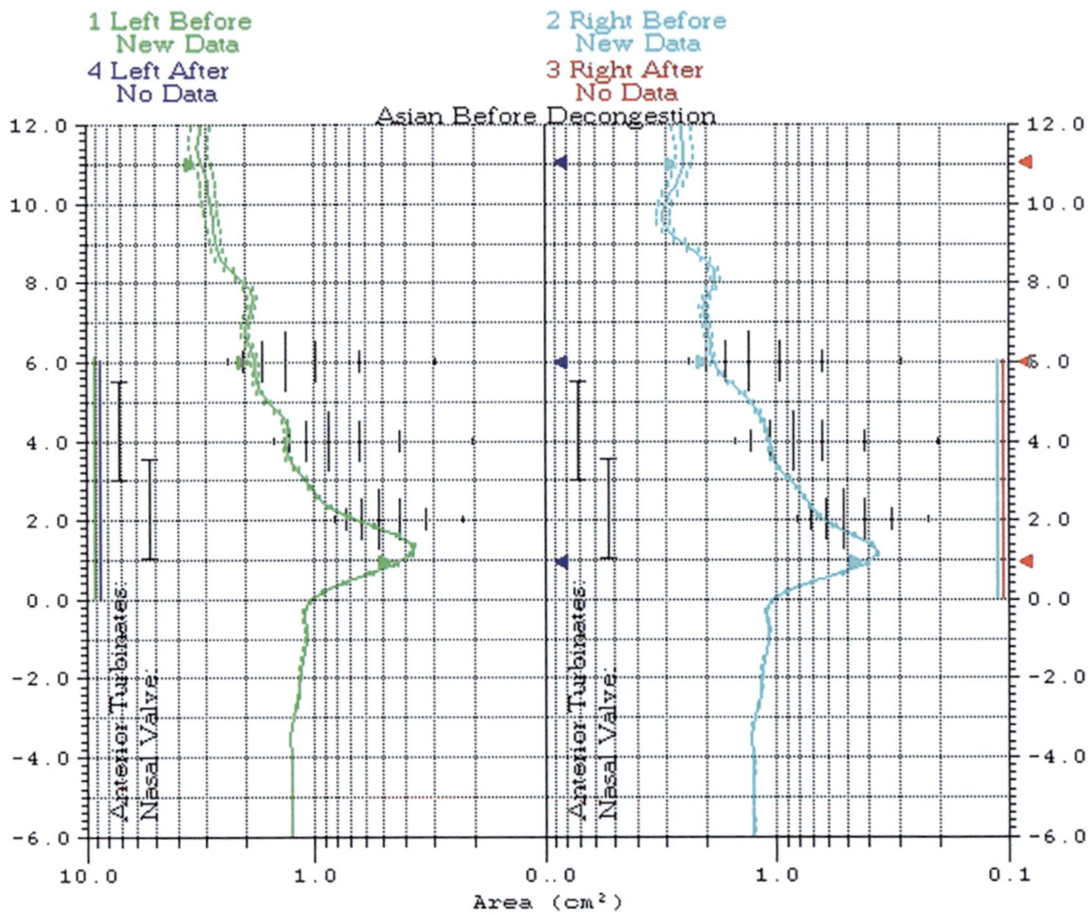

Fig. 19.4 Preoperative acoustic rhinometry

19.3 Preoperative Surgical Planning

- Given the septum's characteristics, there was a potential for a huge, high septal defect, necessitating a mucosal cover.
- After the scar tissue was removed, measures were taken to prevent the collapse of the framework by attempting to reconstruct the septum. Additionally, a strategy was needed to address the huge volume deficiency on the dorsum.
- The surgical goals were set to restore a normal, functional nose for daily activities, emphasizing preventing recurrence by meticulously removing potential inflammatory scar tissues.
- The decision on whether to rotate a mucosal flap from the ethmoid perpendicular plate (EPP) or allow for healing after covering with perichondrium was made based on the size of the defect.
- Along with extending the septal L-strut, preparations were made to replace the dorsal volume using the seventh rib and a significant amount of perichondrium and rectus fascia (Fig. 19.5).

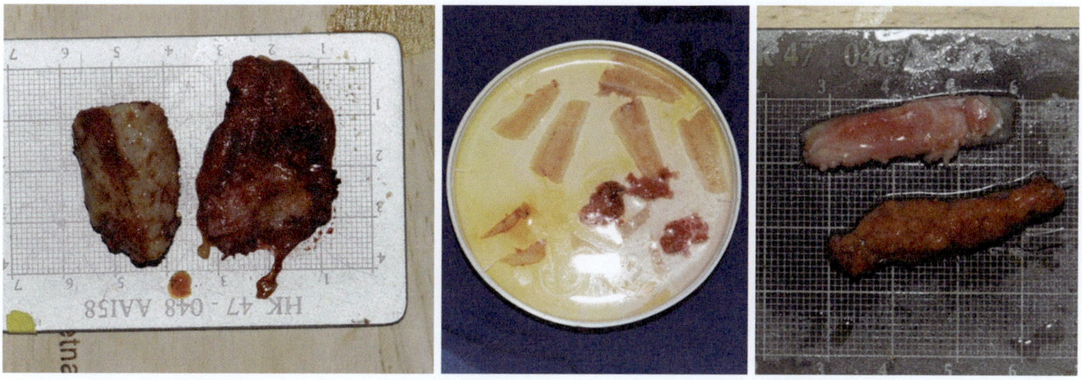

Fig. 19.5 Intraoperative preparation of rib. (Left) Seventh rib and rectus fascia. (Middle) Laminated rib and periosteum. (Right) Laminated rib sutured with periosteum and rectus fascia and rolled rectus fascia

19.4 Intraoperative Findings

A wide dissection of the skin-soft tissue envelope was performed to excise the entire scars. Dissection began at the caudal septum after dissecting through the middle of the lower lateral cartilages (LLC) to facilitate an anterior approach. Significant destruction of the lower lateral cartilages (LLC) was detected. During the procedure, challenging dissection areas were found in the midportion and caudal position of the septum. It was determined that the mucoperichondrium was absent in these areas, and preparations were made for a huge perforation (Video 19.3).

Tedious dissection of hard scar tissue had to be continued. All scars that hindered the release of the mucosal flap needed to be removed to allow the flap to stretch. While controlling bleeding, efforts were made to preserve the healthy mucosal flap and remove as much of the remaining scar tissue as possible (Video 19.4).

Beyond the perforation, residual septal cartilage was located beneath it. The remaining septum in this patient was entirely as seen in the video. The initial step involved dissecting while aiming to preserve the undersurface mucosa of the upper lateral cartilage (ULC) on the patient's left side. As the dissection proceeded internally within the nasal cavity, leaving a layer of mucosa, it was discovered that most of the ULC had been eroded and lost due to the infection. Parts of the high septum were also found to have been eroded by the scar (Video 19.5). Dissection continued by connecting to the right side of the patient, and similarly, parts of the right upper lateral cartilage (ULC) were found to be lost. Rebuilding the septal defect destroyed by the previous infection and simultaneously reconstructing the missing mucosal defect proved impossible with a mucosal flap from the EPP and posterior septal mucosa. Instead, a SLEG using the seventh rib and perichondrium was chosen, along with covering the defect. A caudal septal extension graft was applied around the anterior nasal spine (ANS) on both sides, then fixed to the surrounding soft tissue with adjustments to prevent excessive thickness. Subsequently, a transcutaneous transosseous cerclage suture was performed in preparation for an anterior extended spreader graft (Video 19.6).

Perichondrium was inserted to correct defects in the high septum. Repairing scar tissue around the upper lateral cartilage achieved additional stability.

A voluminous dorsal graft was created by layering laminated rib, rectus fascia, and perichondrium. This technique ensured a robust structural enhancement to the dorsal region of the nose. After positioning the tip dependent on the high septum, the depression from soft tissue loss at the supratip, which could not be resolved with the anterior extended spreader graft (AESG), was corrected using the remaining rectus fascia as a volume-filling graft on the undersurface of the supratip (Video 19.7). Subsequently, for tip plasty, cartilage grafts were placed, and a batten graft was applied to the lower lateral cartilages

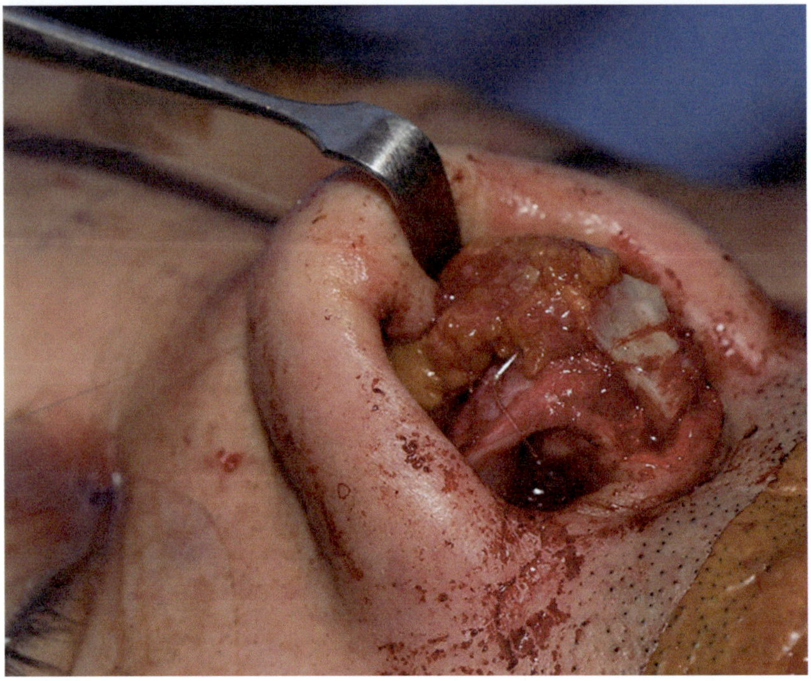

Fig. 19.6 Final tip grafts

(LLC). Any mucosal defects were covered with perichondrium to ensure adequate coverage (Fig. 19.6).

19.5 Operative Strategies

- Efforts were concentrated on releasing the mucoperichondrial flap as much as possible to construct the nose's framework.
- A perichondrial graft was performed to repair the high septal perforation.
- The missing dorsal volume was replenished using laminated rib and fascia.
- The newly rebuilt septal L-strut extension created most of the nasal volume, minimizing the amount of dorsal graft required. This approach ensures a more natural reconstruction of the nasal structure while reducing excess material on the dorsum.

19.6 Postoperative Results

The defect in the high septum was completely healed during the regular follow-up 3 months later (Fig. 19.7). Most autograft resorption appeared to have stopped two and a half years later. However, some irregularity remained in the supratip area, and there will be a minor correction under local anesthesia in the near future (Fig. 19.8). The length of the patient's nose increased, and at the 3-month post-surgery follow-up, the NOSE scale was 0/100, and it consistently showed 20/100 6 months later, with no complaints of nasal obstruction (Fig. 19.9).

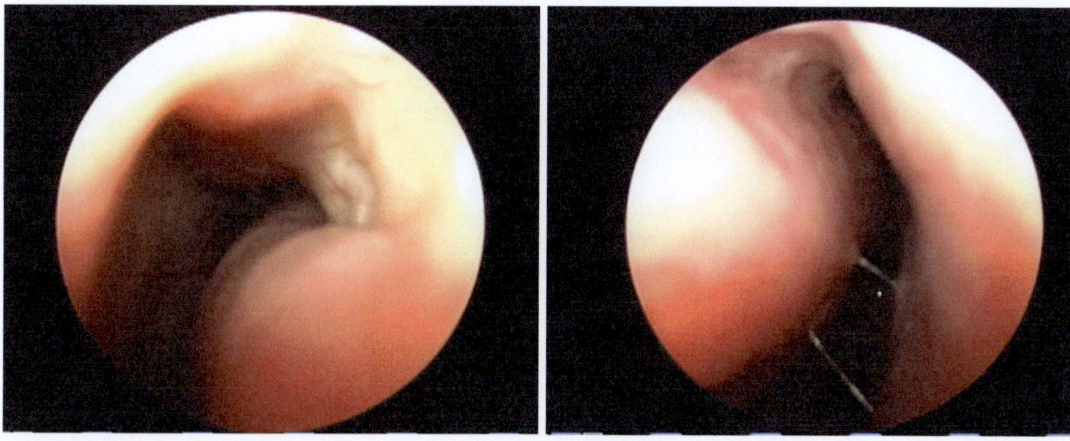

Fig. 19.7 Postoperative long-term endoscopic view. (Left) Right nasal cavity. (Right) Left nasal cavity

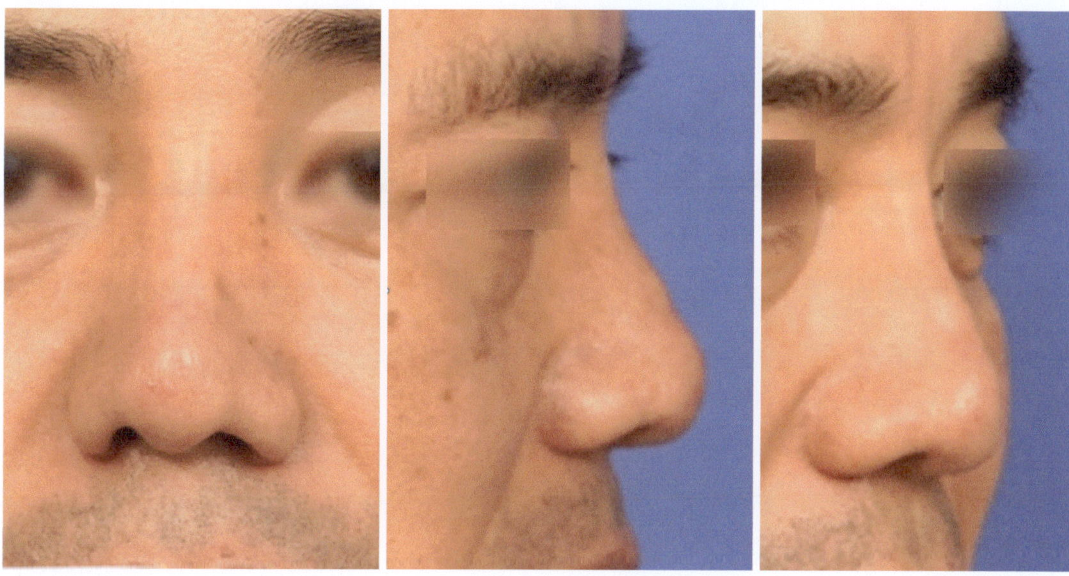

Fig. 19.8 Thirty months postoperative photos. (Left) AP view. (Middle) Modified lateral view. (Right) Quarter view

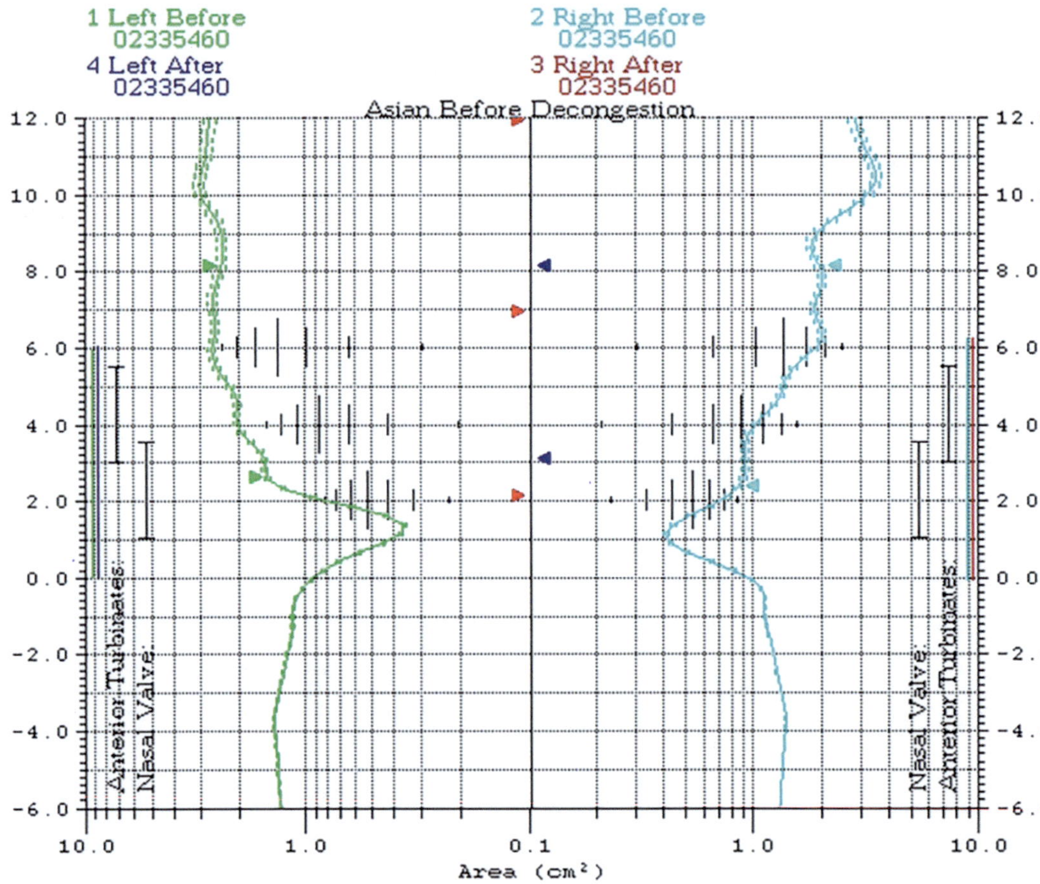

Fig. 19.9 Postoperative acoustic rhinometry

MIX
Papier aus verantwortungsvollen Quellen
Paper from responsible sources
FSC® C105338

If you have any concerns about our products,
you can contact us on
ProductSafety@springernature.com

In case Publisher is established outside the EU,
the EU authorized representative is:
Springer Nature Customer Service Center GmbH
Europaplatz 3, 69115 Heidelberg, Germany

Printed by Libri Plureos GmbH
in Hamburg, Germany